Introduction

BROKEN DOWN, BEAT UP, OR BOTTLENECKED

Broken down, beat up, or bottlenecked. Virtually everyone falls into one of these three categories. They're not separate categories, really, just different points on the same spectrum.

The *broken down* are those unlucky souls who are so riddled with pain and injuries that improving fitness and building a strong, healthy body has become all but impossible.

The *beat up* aren't quite so damaged. Yet they suffer the debilitating effects of muscle imbalances, chronic inflammation, and nagging aches and pains, all of which put a damper on exercise goals and active hobbies.

The *bottlenecked* are the healthiest of the bunch. Though joint dysfunction and pain don't sideline them completely, they continually get stuck when attempting to stretch their bodies' capabilities. Each time they progress in terms of strength, performance, or body composition, something breaks down and their bodies retrogress. Even elite athletes and professional fitness competitors suffer from this. Their limiting factor is rarely discipline or intensity or muscle-building capability or even time management. It's almost always joint problems, injuries, and connective tissue degeneration.

No matter where you fall on this spectrum, the major impediment to realizing your physical potential and moving pain-free through life is the same: *joint dysfunction*. That's the real obstacle. The central question this book seeks to answer is this:

How can we manage our exercise, lifestyle, and nutrition habits to overcome the obstacle of joint dysfunction?

HOW THIS BOOK WILL BENEFIT YOU

To walk a thorny road, we may cover its every inch with leather—or we can make sandals.

—Indian adage, from *The Art of Learning*

There's a lot in a name.

"Built from broken" doesn't just mean going from a state of *being broken* to *being built*. It signifies that the final product is made from broken pieces. All the injuries, pain, limitations, and setbacks you've experienced aren't merely obstacles preventing you from achieving your ideal body. *They are the actual pieces you build with.* In this book, I'll show you how to identify, understand, and assemble them into a unified system.

You'll learn to target the underlying issues that cause joint pain and dysfunction. If you're injury-prone, like me, you can use the principles in this book to build a strong, pain-free, injury-proof body. If you're an overtrained and beat-up athlete, you can implement the training program I recommend as a reset before conquering your next training cycle or competition. If you've been around the block a few times and your body is screaming for help, you'll learn to build muscle and strength without sacrificing joint integrity. If you're broken, in pain, and searching for relief, you can do more than just mask symptoms. You can rebuild your body's scaffolding, improve functional strength, and enjoy a body that works now and that stands the test of time.

Part 1 of this book covers the principles and strategies of rebuilding your body (and the way you think about it). It breaks down the primary causes of joint pain and dysfunction, how to resolve pain naturally, prevent injury, and build healthy connective tissue structures. In addition to laying the foundation for the training section in Part 2, it also teaches you to develop your own exercise program that fits your specific needs.

Part 2 takes the principles a step further, organizing a complete training program that folds all the concepts from Part 1 into a tactical plan with comprehensive templates and instructions.

• • •

This book doesn't claim to reveal any secrets. Instead, it focuses on illuminating a handful of principles that (when applied to resolving pain and dysfunction) allow you to achieve *your* ideal, functional body. It offers a paradigm shift in how to think about your fitness goals. *Built from Broken* is the culmination of my personal experiences, research in therapeutic sports nutrition, and face-to-face work with health clients I've helped overcome injuries, obstacles, and setbacks. Most of all, it's a product of the realization that many people don't fit into the available fitness boxes.

If you're suffering from old or new injuries—if you feel beat up, stuck, stiff, sore and falling apart at the seams, and not even close to where you want to be physically—I want you to know that all the broken pieces can be reassembled to form a stronger version of you. In this book, I'll show you exactly how.

In the coming chapters, you're going to learn the five primary causes of joint pain, how your body's pain signaling system works, and what to focus on instead of pain relief. You'll also learn about the misunderstood concept of collagen synthesis, what science really has to say about stretching, and why your connective tissue deserves as much attention as your muscles. These concepts form the backbone of the Built from Broken principles. Even if you're eager to dive into the training section, I encourage you to take your time with Part 1 of this book and internalize the concepts as best you can. You probably already know about some of the ideas we'll cover. That's OK. It doesn't matter if you've heard something already or learned about it in the past. What matters is how well you know each principle and if you understand when to apply each for maximum effect. I want you to understand these ideas on a deep, fundamental level.

PART 1

Principles and Strategy

A Case for Load Training

**When something bad happens you have three choices. You can either
let it define you, let it destroy you, or you can let it strengthen you.**

— Dr. Seuss

In 1986, cross-country skier Janine Shepherd was headed to the Olympics. Favored as one of the top contenders, she was about to realize her dream of becoming Australia's first ever medal winner at the winter games. But a freak accident would change the course of her life.

On a training bike ride through the Blue Mountains in South Wales, Janine was struck by a speeding utility truck. Her last memory before the accident was looking up and feeling the sun on her face. She woke up hours later in a body consumed by pain.

Her neck and back were broken in six places. She had five broken ribs, a broken right arm, broken collar bone, and several crushed bones in her feet. The right side of her body had been ripped open by the impact and was filled with gravel from being dragged along the road. She had a head wound so severe that parts of her skull were exposed. She had lost five liters of blood. Doctors didn't expect her to survive.

But miraculously, she did. And even though she was paralyzed from the waist down, her surgeon considered the operation to put her back together a success. The vertebrae in her low back were shattered into thousands of pieces, forcing doctors to spend hours plucking shards of bone from her spinal cord. They removed two ribs, rebuilt her back, and fused several bones together with rods and pins.

She had a little movement in one of her big toes, but that was it. The doctors explained to her that the damage to her central nervous system was permanent. She was a partial paraplegic and would have no feeling from the waist down ever again.

In a talk filmed at TEDxKC, Janine recounted her first memories after the accident, drifting in and out of consciousness in the spinal ward. She had an out-of-body experience and recalls asking herself, "Why would I want to go back to a body that's so broken?"

Strangely, a voice called back to her: "C'mon, this is our opportunity."

After 10 days, she decided to mentally return to her body. She spent the next several months lying in a room with five other spinal cord injury patients, some of them completely paralyzed.

In a moment of truly unrelatable insight, she talked about the close bonds formed among the patients in that spinal ward: "Because we were all paralyzed, we didn't know what each other looked like. How amazing is that? How often do you get to make friendships, judgment-free, purely based on spirit?"

She continued, "Lying paralyzed in the spinal ward, there were moments of incredible depth and richness and authenticity and connection that I had never experienced."

Six months later, she was released from the hospital. A nurse pushed her outside in a wheelchair, into warm sunlight she hadn't felt in months.

"How could I ever have taken this for granted?" she said to herself.

The nurse warned her that she would be depressed at home. Staying true to her nickname, "Janine the Machine," she doubted that. But depression did set in. Self-pity did rise to the surface. It wasn't until she remembered her friends in the spinal ward that the fog of depression lifted. Her friend, Maria, only 16 years old, was a quadriplegic. Though she was unable to move or even speak, Maria always smiled.

"How had she found that level of acceptance?" Janine asked the audience during her talk.

"That's when I realized it wasn't just my life, it was life itself…. I knew then, just like before, that I had a choice. I could either keep fighting this, or I could let go and accept not only my body but the circumstances of my life."

She continued, "Maybe being at rock bottom is the perfect place to start. I was free to explore life's infinite possibilities."

Janine recovered to a remarkable degree, learning to walk again with only a slight limp. Almost immediately, she began working on her next dream—to be a pilot—and became the youngest (and the only female) director of Australia's Civil Aviation Safety Authority.[1]

Throughout her recovery, Janine showed astonishing spirit, wisdom, and even gratitude. She accepted her fate and adapted, building a trail-blazing career when others might have been permanently mentally sidelined from the trauma.

• • •

How often do you play the pity game with comparably minor setbacks? How often do you say, "*Why me?*"

"*Why is my body always breaking down?*"

"*How come I can't do the things I used to do?*"

It's easier said than done, but Janine's story illustrates a higher road. One of acceptance, steadfast spirit, and adaptability.

You don't have to—and should NOT—accept pain and movement dysfunction as part of aging. Those things need to be addressed and eradicated. But if you can let go of your preconceived notions about what you are supposed to look like and what exercises you should be able to do, you'll be wiser, capable of addressing the obstacles in front of you and moving past them. The real challenge is accepting your current limitations without letting that knowledge discourage you.

Instead of asking yourself, "*Why me?*" ask, "*What is the next logical step forward?*"

Extreme examples like Janine's story show us the mind's capability to overcome adversity and the body's capacity to repair itself. It's agonizing to accept, but there is always a silver lining—always an alternative solution, a way around obstacles and setbacks.

It starts with the right mindset. It continues with the pursuit of knowledge and a plan for resolving pain, improving joint function, and rebuilding your body from the ground up.

HEALING LOADS

Load training (a.k.a. resistance training) is the most effective lever for resolving joint pain and building a resilient body. Everything else—stretching, foam rolling, manual therapy, massage, flossing, smashing, taping, cracking, and popping—is secondary. You can spend hours each week on extraneous soft tissue and recovery work, but if you don't effectively utilize load training, you won't get the relief you're looking for.

Load training has a unique benefit related to the regenerative processes in your muscles, joints, and virtually every cell in your body. It's called *mechanotransduction*—the process by which your cells sense and respond to mechanical stimuli, changing them into biochemical signals that prompt certain cellular responses.[2] Essentially, it describes how your body turns load-bearing activity into structural changes and healing mechanisms. And its impact is proportional to the load used. The more load, the greater the response.

Many people believe that weight training inevitably leads to joint breakdown and that pain and injuries are simply the cost of developing a fit body. But this is backward. Despite popular opinion, tendon breakdown and joint dysfunction can only be fixed by increasing the load tolerance of connective tissues. And how is that accomplished? Rest? Stretching? Anti-inflammatories and injections? Nope. Only through load training. But it must be well planned and well executed. Your ability to choose the correct exercises, stabilize your joints, and perform movements effectively determines how your body responds to load-bearing training. If it breaks your body down, it's because either your tissues are not prepared for the load volume or specific movements are creating unnatural stress on your musculoskeletal system.

I want you to perform a thought experiment with me. Close your eyes and imagine a gym full of weightlifters. Big, muscular, tough guys and gals moving heavy weights. Now, imagine there are no weights in the gym. No machines, pulleys, or barbells. Just the lifters in an empty room, doing the same movements. What do you see? It's a room full of people that appear to be practicing basic human movement patterns: squats, presses, rows, and lunges—sometimes performing dozens of repetitions. This is all weight training is—practicing and perfecting movement patterns under loads. It's the most functional and beneficial form of exercise there is. When you look at it this way, weightlifting morphs from a vanity-based hobby to a learned skill of absolute human necessity.

I want you to take a break from jogging, stretching, and long sessions of aerobic exercise. You are not going to run into the body you want. Nor will you stretch your way out of pain. Load training is the only logical path.

Fear of injuries and worsened joint pain fuels the common misconception that heavy weight training is only for bodybuilders, powerlifters, and athletes. And that everyone else should use light, easy weights to "tone" up and stay healthy. This couldn't be further from the truth. Though there are dozens of good reasons to focus your fitness efforts primarily on resistance training, here are two of the most relevant.

First, physical fitness (specifically, muscle mass and strength levels) is one of the strongest predictors of future health. And resistance training is the most practical and proven way to build muscle mass and strength. Having more muscle improves metabolic health markers such as insulin sensitivity, reduces all-cause mortality risk, and may reduce the risk of cardiovascular disease, heart attacks, and strokes.[3]

Second, heavy loads are required to create adaptive responses (healing responses) from connective tissue like tendons. Easy exercise and light training won't cut it. Studies show you must challenge your joints with weights around 80% of your one-repetition maximum to elicit the greatest adaptive response. This equates to a weight you can lift about eight times before reaching failure. Unsurprisingly, eight times is also in the range of recommended reps for building muscle.[4] Not only does load training build strength and muscle, it also thickens and strengthens connective tissue.[5] For building and maintaining bone mass, studies show even heavier weights initiate the greatest bone-growth response.[6] If you want muscles, joints, and bones that work well now and later, load training is a must.

STRENGTH, MUSCLE, AND MORTALITY

Say it ... what one man can do, another can do.

—from *The Edge* (movie, 1997)

Building muscle and strength isn't just a young person's game. It's even more important for older adults. A study published in *Medicine & Science in Sports & Exercise* showed that "low muscle strength was independently associated with elevated risk of all-cause mortality" among participants 50 years or older.[7] Another paper published in *Nature* showed that muscle mass is a consistent predictor of mortality in seniors.[8] Building muscle in your 20s is for fun. Building muscle in your 30s, 40s, 50s, and beyond is a smart strategy for keeping body fat down, increasing longevity, and improving well-being. It may even save your life.

A study performed at the Penn State College of Medicine tracked the habits of people age 65 or older over the course of 15 years. Researchers found that those who lifted weights had a 46% lower death rate.[9] Even after adjusting for other health variables such as body mass index and chronic disease, and lifestyle habits such as smoking and drinking, the weight-lifting group still had a 19% lower mortality rate. Resistance training has even been shown to reduce age-related cognitive decline, slowing down neurodegeneration in people at risk of developing Alzheimer's.[10] Weight training effectively boosts production of brain-derived neurotrophic factor (BDNF), a naturally occurring protein responsible for nerve cell maintenance. Researchers refer to BDNF as "Miracle Grow for the brain." Despite the dumb weight lifter stereotypes, resistance training is one of the best things you can do for your cognitive function.

If you're on the far end of the age ranges in these studies, or you haven't been able to make consistent fitness progress in recent years, you may be wondering: *Is it too late for me?* Well, let's see what the research has to say.

A study published in *Frontiers in Physiology* demonstrated that previously untrained seniors can build muscle and strength comparable to masters athletes who have been training for decades.[11] Another study from the *Canadian Journal of Applied Physiology* found that the primary driver of age-related muscle loss (sarcopenia) was not age itself but reduced neuromuscular activity. Researchers concluded that strength training could slow or even halt muscle atrophy and that sarcopenia "should not be conceptualized as a linear process" that begins in middle age.[12]

Even in advanced age, you can do more than just maintain muscle. Research from the *American Journal of Medicine* shows that aging adults can gain nearly 2.5 pounds of lean muscle and increase their overall strength by 25% to 30% with just four to five months of consistent training.[13]

With all this convincing research and these impressive case studies, most people still fall victim to the muscle-ravaging effects of age. But age alone isn't to blame. Exercise volume, training intensity, movement variability, and fitness goals all gradually change as you get older. Building muscle and strength takes a back seat to "easier" forms of exercise that don't hurt so much. Ironically, weight training (when programmed intelligently) is the most effective way to prevent joint degeneration.

It's no coincidence that the timelines of age-related muscle loss track perfectly with increased connective tissue injury accumulation in middle age. Joint degeneration (often without symptoms) reaches a tipping point in your mid-30s. In your 40s and 50s, the risk of connective tissue injuries (like Achilles tendon ruptures) peaks as decreased load tolerance combines with continued high activity levels.[14] The path of least resistance (and the one typically recommended by conventional medicine) is to stop doing the things that hurt—avoid uncomfortable movements and find easier forms of exercise. As I hope you are starting to see, that's the exact opposite of what you should do.

There is a path forward. But it doesn't involve following the typical pain management advice of rest, ice, and nonsteroidal anti-inflammatory drugs (NSAIDs), which multiple reviews have shown is not effective for treating age-related joint pain and dysfunction.[15] These methods do nothing more than treat superficial symptoms. The only viable solution is to fortify your musculoskeletal system with targeted load training.

Whether you've been training for a few years or a few decades, or haven't ever stepped foot in the weight room, it's not too late to overhaul your body, build real strength, and achieve your physical potential. The catch is, you'll have to work smarter than the 20-year-old bodybuilder or fitness model next to you. So to answer the question: No, it's not too late. It's the perfect time.

PROBLEMS WITH CONVENTIONAL APPROACHES TO RESISTANCE TRAINING

There's an obvious contradiction here. If resistance training is so great for joints, why does it break so many people down instead of building them up? If you were to walk into any commercial gym and start interviewing people, you'd find the vast majority have a nagging injury or painful joint they blame on lifting. Most fitness enthusiasts are riddled with joint dysfunction but soldier on anyway. To understand the contradiction, consider the case of "Gary," a friend of mine who keeps roughly the same workout schedule as I do. Gary is in his mid-40s. Admittedly, his strength levels and overall fitness peaked around age 30. A bum shoulder, aching low back, and shoddy knees keep him from lifting the same amount of weight he used to. But that doesn't stop him.

Week after week, he straps on his weight lifting belt and sets up under the squat bar, performing a few excruciating reps with gritted teeth and a look of horror on his face. He crawls under a heavily loaded barbell and ekes out a few bench press repetitions—arching his back and focusing on the last few inches of the movement to avoid stressing his shoulder. In between sets he shuffles around, adjusting his back and swinging his shoulders as if looking for a sudden pop that will slam everything back into place. Near the end of his grinding weight training session, he lies down on a padded bench and spends a few minutes stretching his hips and hamstrings, clearly looking for relief from the pain he just inflicted on himself. After an hour or so of this routine, Gary sighs and calls to the other exercise goers, "That's enough damage done for one day. See you all tomorrow."

Gary's story isn't unique. In fact, this struggle is the rule rather than the exception. Most people eventually get to the point where pain and mobility limitations prevent them from performing like they used to. At that point, they either keep grinding on, struggling to maintain their fitness, or they give up altogether and stop training.

How do so many well-intentioned fitness enthusiasts end up here? And is there a better way? Let's look at what got Gary into this mess in the first place.

Bodybuilding

Ask any fitness buff about the best way to build muscle and get into shape and they'll tell you to follow a bodybuilding routine. This involves training one or two body parts per day with high volume to spur muscle growth. Here's what a typical bodybuilding routine looks like:

- Monday: Chest
- Tuesday: Back
- Wednesday: Arms
- Thursday: Shoulders
- Friday: Legs

The workouts consist of set after set of mass-focused movements, usually in the form of isolation exercises and machines to target the muscle of the day. One problem with this approach is that your muscles don't work in isolation. Each primary muscle has an entire cast of stabilizing muscles that surround it. If these smaller stabilizing muscles are neglected, muscle imbalances occur that quickly create movement faults, mobility restrictions, and joint irritation. To make matters worse, a muscle-only approach often exacerbates common muscle imbalances. For example, an exercise routine that leans on heavy pressing, rows, and lat pulldowns builds the shoulder's internal rotation muscles while neglecting the posterior (rear) muscles. This front-biased training combined with slouching over a desk all day causes shoulder impingement and pain. Not to mention, most bodybuilding routines blatantly neglect all exercise that doesn't have the pure purpose of building muscle mass. Mobility work, core stabilization training, endurance exercise, and joint-building movements all get left by the wayside. As time goes on and more loads are added to compromised joints, pain and injuries are inevitable.

Another problem with bodybuilding programming is the obsessive focus on splitting up all the muscles of the upper body, dedicating an entire training day to each, while neglecting the biggest muscles in the body: *the legs*. It makes absolutely no sense to train the lower half of your body only once per week while giving all the smaller muscles so much detailed attention. Despite the fact that you'll end up looking like a top, it's a poor strategy for building muscle, increasing strength, and keeping body fat levels down. The basic movement patterns that train your lower half—squatting, hinging, lunging—produce the greatest metabolic response. Most importantly, having a strong lower half is the best way to protect your body from the most common pain points: *low back pain* and *knee pain*. When "leg day" consists of the same spine-crushing barbell exercises and boring machines week after week, it's no wonder people often skip it.

Progressive Strength Training

One of the most damaging bits of dogma in the fitness world is that you must continuously increase the amount of weight you can squat, deadlift, and bench press. Especially for guys, these are the true tests of strength. If you can't do them well, you're a joke. And if you're not adding more weight to these exercises each week, you're wasting your time. There are more than a few problems with applying this powerlifting-based mindset to everyone. First and foremost, many people lack the mobility and movement control to execute heavy loaded barbell movements safely. They would be better served focusing on exercises that establish proper movement patterns, build core stability, and stress the joints and muscles in ways that build them up instead of tear them down.

Even powerlifters and professional athletes who train daily don't see nonstop linear strength progress. In fact, the most advanced strength athletes plan strategic *deload* periods where they reduce training intensity and volume to prevent injury and improve recovery. They also build in submaximal effort training days in between max effort days for the same purpose. Your connective tissue and central nervous system need recovery periods to prevent breakdown. Demanding that your body add 5 to 10 pounds to each lift every week doesn't make sense. Nor does lifting hard and heavy every workout. A smarter approach involves shoring up weak points first and balancing traditional strength training with joint stabilizing work, mobility training, and corrective exercise.

Exercise Programming

Exercise programming, or lack thereof, is another primary reason traditional weight training is damaging to the average person's body. Most programs are designed exclusively to build muscle and strength, neglecting other important aspects of fitness and longevity. For instance, connective tissue goes through a degradation and regeneration cycle after training, just as muscles do. As cells are damaged and repaired, connective tissue strength increases. But when this process is interrupted before full regeneration is complete, a net accumulation of damage adds up, leading to collagen base degradation.

This is a well-known principle in the fields of physical therapy and corrective exercise, but it is rarely programmed in a way that promotes long-term joint health in addition to fitness gains. To be fair, it's not just a bodybuilding-centric training mindset that leads to imbalances and dysfunction. Every physical activity creates lopsided development. Running, biking, swimming, and every specialized sport from golf to football to jiu-jitsu creates its own set of problems for athletes and hobbyists. Understanding why and how these issues crop up is necessary to prevent and fix them.

Time Commitments

Even if you are sold on the idea of training your body to be more resilient, you might balk at the idea of spending 10+ hours in the weight room each week like athletes and strength competitors. While training several days per week is the best way to make progress and keep your body resilient (more on this later in the section "Injury Prevention Paradox"), most people simply cannot devote that much time to exercise each week. The good news is, you don't have to. In fact, you can build significant muscle, strength, and joint integrity in as little as two days per week. The key is using the right exercises, repetition tempos, and recovery periods to create consistent, positive adaptations.

WHAT MOST PEOPLE GET WRONG ABOUT CORRECTIVE EXERCISE

When you hear the phrase "corrective exercise," visions of boring physical therapy sessions come to mind. But when appropriately implemented, corrective exercise is anything but boring. It's true that most people choose the wrong exercises, but it's not just a matter of exercise selection. It comes down to values and priorities.

Some of the best exercise programs I've come across squeeze a few half-hearted corrective movements into the end of each workout. The idea is to offset muscle imbalances (which are almost always created and made worse by the training program itself). This is the standard approach: keep lifting, work around pain and injuries, and do the bare minimum of corrective exercise necessary to maintain the (broken) status quo. In the end, that's all you're doing—*working around problems.*

But what happens if you flip this line of thinking on its head? Instead of just sprinkling in corrective exercise, what if you based your entire training program around fixing weak links? Not only is this possible while still building strength, muscle, and endurance—it's necessary for many people.

Here are a few undervalued benefits of prioritizing corrective exercise over everything else:

1. **It's the best way to prevent pain and injuries.** Beyond the obvious benefit of correcting problems, corrective exercise principles can be used to prevent injuries and common pain points—even if you don't have a specific injury you are recovering from. This is where the term *prehab* came from—a proactive approach to avoiding injury that uses physical therapy and rehabilitation methods before injuries and dysfunction show up.

2. **It's more mentally stimulating and challenging than a typical "cardio" session or weight training workout.** When you do corrective exercise right, you'll find yourself completely present and in tune with your body. Workouts fly by instead of dragging on.

3. **It produces an intense systemic metabolic response.** Exercise that challenges your ability to coordinate joint and neuromuscular systems causes intense activation of your central nervous system (CNS). In other words, your metabolism will rev up, your muscles will stand at attention, and you'll be sweating bullets. Personally, I've found functional movement training to be much more effective for shedding body fat than mindless treadmill sessions.

4. **It produces greater improvements in total body strength, mobility, and pain-free movement capabilities than *any* other training style.** By definition, corrective exercise shores up weak links preferentially. Most people focus heavily on their strengths. Guys with big arms like to do bicep curls, girls with well-defined glutes like to work legs, whippy endurance types like to run, and thick-wristed brutes like to pick up heavy stuff. But the problem with leaning on your strengths is twofold. First, the more you develop your strengths, the bigger the gap between your strongest links and weakest links. The bigger this gap is, the greater your risk of injury. Second, any progress in your strong attributes is

incremental only. On the flip side, improving your weak points raises the whole system. A chain is only as strong as its weakest link. Nowhere is this cliché more appropriate than in your *kinetic chain*.

5. **It's more fun.** When you really double down on attacking limitations and weaknesses, you won't see incremental improvements. You'll see dramatic leaps in how you look, feel, and move. It's the most satisfying way to approach fitness, despite the fact that most people assume the opposite.

THE FIVE PRIMARY CAUSES OF JOINT PAIN AND DYSFUNCTION

At any given time, about one third of adults in the U.S. are experiencing joint pain or stiffness.[16] That number is growing all the time. A study published in the *Annals of Internal Medicine* revealed that the prevalence of knee pain increased by 65% over a 20-year period from 1974 to 1994.[17] More recent studies confirm this trend isn't slowing down. The number of American adults affected by joint pain and arthritis is expected to jump from an estimated 52.5 million in 2012 to 78.4 million by 2040.[18] Increasing obesity rates, aging populations, and more arthritis diagnoses all play a part.

Underlying this growth trend is bad posture, lack of varied movement, and repetitive use strains. Here are the five most common causes of joint pain and weakness. In virtually zero cases are these factors isolated. Almost always, there is a combination of multiple variables that cause each other and create positive feedback loops. Still, it's helpful to isolate them so you can understand how they affect you. In later chapters, you'll learn how to address each.

1. Posture

Poor posture is the number one nondisease cause of joint pain. It causes muscle tightness, muscle imbalances, increased stress on joints, and compressed nerves. Studies show poor posture, continued over a long period, leads to increased pain and degenerative joint disease risk.[19]

Most injuries also stem from bad posture. You may think you hurt your back picking up a barbell, or a couch, but the injury was actually a cumulative event that started with poor low back posture and culminated in an acute injury while picking something up off the floor. Conversely, good posture supports optimal alignment of joints and reduces risk of pain, repetitive use strains, and injuries. Good posture stems from maintaining a neutral spine—comprised of the three primary natural curves present in any healthy back: cervical, thoracic, and lumbar. From the spine outward, it is maintained by keeping the shoulders, elbows, hips, knees, and other extremities in proper alignment to prevent undue stress.

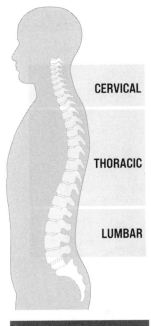

CERVICAL

THORACIC

LUMBAR

FIGURE 1.1

The three natural curves in a healthy spine.

While you've no doubt been told at some point in your life to stand up (and sit up) straight with your shoulders back, you may not have been exposed to the concepts of *static posture* and *dynamic posture*. Static posture is how you hold yourself when unmoving, as in sitting, standing, or sleeping. Dynamic posture is how you hold yourself when walking, running, bending, squatting, reaching, or twisting.

Most people try to correct their poor static posture with conscious effort. You catch yourself slumped over at a desk and sit upright with a straight back to correct it. The tricky part is that consciously changing static posture is rarely enough to create lasting habits, nor does it translate to dynamic posture improvements. That's why despite your best efforts to sit perfectly straight at your desk during the day, your body falls back into bad habits when lifting weights at the gym.

I naturally have a forward curvature of my upper back—a condition called *kyphosis*. It's not severe, but it's still enough to pull my shoulders out of alignment and lead to tight, injury-prone chest muscles. I remember a time when I decided to fix it through sheer will. I spent an entire week walking around with my shoulder blades pinned back. By the end of the week, my back and neck muscles were in knots. I hadn't made any progress. It still felt awkward to stand with my shoulders back, and pressing movements still irritated my upper chest. Why? Because the underlying mechanical problems were still there. My upper back muscles were stretched out and weak, and my chest and shoulder muscles were tight.

To improve posture—static or dynamic—you need both conscious effort and mechanical changes to the musculature that supports proper alignment. That includes targeted strength training and mobility exercise.

FIGURE 1.2

Bad sitting posture vs. good sitting posture.

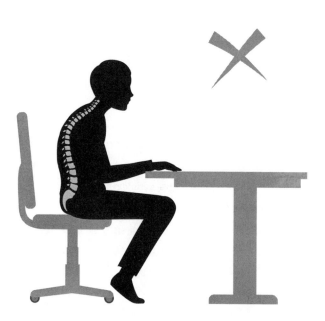
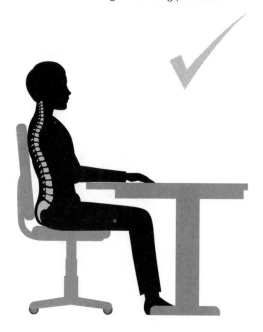

Improving dynamic posture requires retraining the neuromuscular systems that control postural muscles. Your nervous system has been recording and perfecting your movement habits, for better or for worse, since you were born. Altering these lifelong habits is no easy task. But it can be done by (a) moving more and moving in different ways, and (b) establishing new, healthy motor patterns and building strong, stable musculature around problem joints.

By adding more varied movement, you'll train your nervous system to maintain better posture. And by improving the way you sit, stand, walk, and move through daily life, you'll resolve many joint pain episodes without any other intervention. We'll cover this in more detail in chapter 5.

Here are some common static postural faults when sitting:

- The low back rounds, exposing delicate muscles surrounding the lumbar spine to potential strains.
- The head protrudes forward, pulling shoulders and upper back out of alignment.[20]
- Shoulders round forward, causing tight chest and anterior shoulder muscles while lengthening and weakening posterior shoulder muscles.
- Muscles in the buttocks are "turned off," and anterior hip muscles tighten.

2. Movement Quality and Variation

Movement quality describes how effective you are at performing specific exercises and motions. If you exercise with heavy loads and poor movement quality, you are more likely to hurt yourself. It's a simple concept to grasp. But improving movement quality requires unpacking the component parts.

Movement quality is comprised of neuromuscular coordination, joint proprioception, and fatigue management. Let's briefly look at each of these crucial pieces.

Neuromuscular coordination is the ability of your central nervous system to control muscles while executing complex movements. It's essential to address in the early stages of training to prevent bad habits. Some examples of bad neuromuscular habits include rounding the low back when hinging (e.g. during the deadlift), falling forward while squatting, and initiating pushing movements (e.g. bench press, push-up) without establishing proper scapula positioning. Many people mistakenly believe that your levels of coordination are set in stone. You're either born coordinated or not. But that's not true. By establishing joint stability with targeted corrective exercises and frequently practicing the primary movement patterns, you can improve neuromuscular coordination.

Joint proprioception describes your ability to sense the position and movement of your body through space. Many acute injuries result from a proprioceptive fault—your muscles flex or elongate when they should be guarding a vulnerable joint. When you build skill around movements that challenge joint proprioception, your ability to protect yourself from injuries improves intuitively. Most targeted joint proprioception training is performed on unstable surfaces such as wobble boards, BOSU balls, or the inflatable Swiss balls. However, the scientific literature does not appear to support resistance training on unstable surfaces—at least for trained athletes.[21] Unstable environments reduce training loads and force output, which subsequently reduces training benefits. This is why many strength coaches scoff at the idea of instability training altogether. But we shouldn't throw out the baby with the bathwater. Targeted joint proprioception training certainly has its place in the corrective exercise sector. The good news is you don't need fancy instability equipment. Dumbbells, kettlebells, and unilateral movements (targeting only one side of your body at a time) provide plenty of instability while also enabling the use of demanding loads for greater improvements in strength, stability, and functional mobility.

And because all of these mechanisms break down when you're tired, *fatigue management* should be programmed as well. This includes fatigue-proofing important postural muscles that you can't afford to have quit on you. For example, muscles in your upper back keep your shoulders in alignment while pressing, pulling, and carrying heavy loads, ensuring the best biomechanical position for strength and preventing injuries to the rotator cuff muscles. Your upper back muscles should be trained using high repetitions from multiple angles, so they are never your weak link when performing upper body movements. Studies also show that muscular endurance in your low back (the most common pain point) is more important than muscular strength or mobility.[22] When you think about all the supportive work your low back does during the day, this makes sense.

Considering how all these factors play into strength, mobility, and injury risk, it shouldn't be a surprise that our bodies break down when all we do is lift heavy barbells. Or run long distances. Or play a sport that places disproportionate stress on one muscle or joint. Whether you consider yourself a bodybuilder, powerlifter, runner, tennis player, golfer, or simply a fitness enthusiast, broadening your scope of activity helps fend off joint dysfunction. But that is the opposite of what usually happens.

As people age, their scope of activity decreases. They stop playing recreational sports, limit exercise selection to those they deem safe and comfortable, and move through shorter ranges of motion. As injuries and joint pain inevitably crop up, they avoid anything that aggravates their painful body parts—which includes just about everything.

On the opposite end of the spectrum, multisport athletes enjoy better performance success and reduced injury rates than single sport athletes. In the 2018 NFL Draft, 29 out of 32 first-round picks were multisport high school athletes.[23] While well-intentioned parents and high-priced private coaches continue promoting one-sport specialization, the data indicate otherwise when it comes to reaching stardom—and staying healthy. A study commissioned by the National Federation of State High School Associations showed that single-sport athletes are 70% more likely to suffer an injury than are multisport athletes.[24] Why? Because they are at greater risk of suffering repetitive use injuries: elbow pain from throwing a baseball year round, shoulder injuries from extended swimming seasons, and stress fractures to shins and knees from nonstop soccer. They also develop lopsided musculature and narrow movement patterns, further increasing risk of an acute injury.

For you, high school was probably a long time ago, but the principle still applies, no matter your age or fitness level. You don't have to play baseball, basketball, and football to prevent injuries, or to reach your fitness goals. You just have to train your body to be resilient, and keep moving in a variety of ways.

3. Muscle Imbalances

A *muscle imbalance* occurs when one or more muscles in your body are stronger or larger than others. The term is often used to describe aesthetic bodybuilding imbalances, such as a left bicep that's bigger than the right. While everyone has some asymmetry in their muscles, imbalances that alter joint mechanics are the real problem. These types of imbalances alter movement patterns, compromise joint stability, reduce mobility, cause chronic pain, and lead to repetitive use injuries when soft tissues grind against bony tissues. After posture and movement quality, muscle imbalance is the next most common nondisease culprit behind joint pain. In fact, it's tough to separate posture, movement quality, and muscle imbalances because they're all linked together.

Figure 1.3 shows what happens when a muscle imbalance occurs. As you can see, just one component sets off a chain reaction that leads to the development of others. A muscle imbalance alters movement patterns and joint mechanics, which leads to postural faults, excessive compensatory loading on specific joints and muscles, inflammation, pain, and injury. Not only that, you can jump into the cycle at any point. An injury can kickstart the process just as easily as bad posture or a muscle imbalance. It's like a spinning merry-go-round. You can jump on at any point and start the cycle. This is often referred to as the cumulative injury cycle. But because pain is present at every step, *pain compensation cycle* is a more apt term.

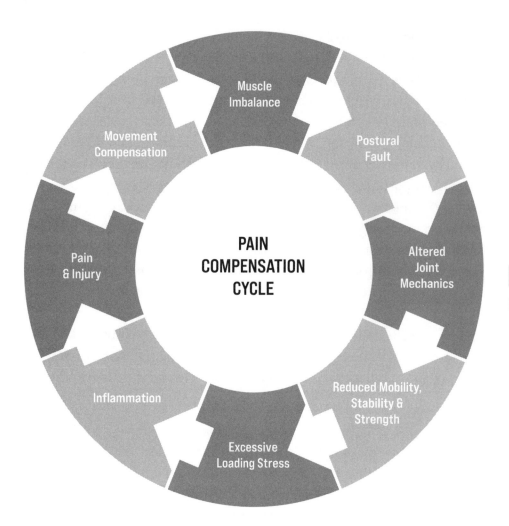

FIGURE 1.3

Pain compensation cycle.

One of the most pervasive myths about muscle imbalances is that you can fix them by stretching. But the research on stretching is not flattering. A 2011 metastudy (study of studies) revealed that stretching has "no significant effect."[25] It gets worse. Stretching before competition or working out impairs performance.[26] And worst of all, studies on stretching for injury prevention show not only that it doesn't help, but that it might actually increase injury risk.[27]

Most of these studies focused on *static stretching*—holding a stretch for several seconds or longer. To be fair, *dynamic stretching*—actively moving back and forth through full ranges of motion—seems to have more merit as a precompetition and athletic improvement tool. Stretching has its place. But mobility training, corrective exercise, and adding more varied movement are much more effective strategies. To resolve muscle imbalances, you must not only fix the actual imbalance but address the underlying cause while simultaneously defending against downstream effects of the pain compensation cycle. It's not an easy problem to solve. But with an understanding of the process, you can break free from the cycle and get off the merry-go-round.

4. Tendinopathy

While joint pain can stem from injuries to ligaments and cartilage, in most cases the source is your *tendons*—the fibrous connective tissue throughout your body that attaches muscle to bone. Because of tendons' role in the force transfer process, they're often the first to break down from overuse, causing inflammation, pain, and cell degeneration. This injury process is called *tendinopathy*. Most tendinopathy cases stem from overuse, while others are caused by a combination of traumatic injury and stressful, repetitive motion.

The myth that tendinopathy is primarily an inflammation problem is the most destructive belief in all of sports medicine. As you'll see later in the book, inflammation is often not the underlying problem. In fact, it is a fundamental part of your body's immune system, designed to heal wounds and defend the body against foreign invaders. In the case of injury, inflammation delivers much-needed oxygen and nutrients to damaged tissue while also clearing out bacteria and dead cells.[28] Treatments aimed solely at blocking inflammation are not the solution to resolving your joint pain.

5. Arthritis, Aging, and Collagen Degradation

Arthritis is the leading cause of joint pain and disability in the United States, affecting 23% of adults—more than 54 million people.[29] It is a disease characterized by inflammation and degeneration of the joints. Because there are more than 100 types of arthritis, and one or more joints can be affected, differentiating between normal aging and arthritic pain is difficult.

The two main types are rheumatoid arthritis and osteoarthritis.

Rheumatoid arthritis (RA) is an autoimmune disorder in which the body's immune system attacks its joint tissue. RA patients often depend on medication and targeted physical therapy to mitigate symptoms.

Osteoarthritis (OA) is the breakdown of cartilage and other collagen structures within joints. Although injuries can expedite the onset of OA, and it worsens with age, it is not considered a normal part of aging. Weight-bearing joints and the hands are most affected, with increased body weight being a major risk factor.[30]

Neither arthritis nor joint pain from aging are death knells to your fitness goals. Experts from Arthritis.org and the Centers for Disease Control agree that staying active is the most important thing you can do to manage symptoms. Anyone with arthritis will tell you, there are good days and bad days. The good days are opportunities to build strength, maintain flexibility, and use your body to its fullest. According to Audrey Lynn Millar, Ph.D, professor of Physical Therapy at Winston Salem State University, staying active also "lubes the joint" you're experiencing pain in, reducing discomfort.[31] But it's not just about managing symptoms. Much of the pain from arthritis and aging stems from collagen degradation.

Other Factors

You may have noticed that sports-related injuries were conspicuously omitted from this list. While injuries do cause pain and will lead to weakness if not healed properly, they are not the main contributors to joint pain. Posture, movement quality, inflammation, and collagen degradation are more common culprits. Besides, most acute injuries have an overuse, posture, or movement fault component that could have been corrected before the injury occurred.

Less common causes of joint pain and weakness are gout, autoimmune disorders, connective tissue disease, and chronic pain diagnoses such as fibromyalgia that negatively impact collagen synthesis and lead to chronic inflammation.[32]

Body weight is another factor that deserves a mention. Studies show overweight women are four times more likely to develop OA than those with healthy weights. Overweight men are five times more likely to develop OA.[33] Each additional pound of body weight adds about 4 pounds of additional pressure on your knees. Only 10 pounds of excess weight puts an additional 40 pounds of pressure on your knees.[30] This is a key reason why reaching your ideal body weight is vital to healthy aging.

KEY TAKEAWAY

Load training is the only therapeutic intervention that addresses all five primary causes of joint pain—posture, movement quality, muscle imbalances, tendinopathy, and collagen degradation. It must be your central strategy for resolving pain now and preventing trouble down the road.

The causes of joint pain are often mixed and muddy, and how you react to pain triggers is modulated by previous injuries, neural sensitivity, and body mechanics.[34] Make no mistake: joint pain is complex. Even the science behind the five primary causes I outlined here is dense. But I want you to be encouraged, because there is a lot you can do to manage pain naturally and fortify your joints for a life of strong, functional movement.

The Anatomy of Pain

The medical system is woefully inadequate for dealing with back pain.
Most patients rarely receive the most important part of the prescription
to get rid of back pain from their doctor—the knowledge and understanding
of their condition required to become their own best advocate.

—Stuart McGill

THE STATE OF PAIN MANAGEMENT

The surgeon tells you that an operation will repair the damaged tissue causing your pain. The pain management doctor tells you it's nerve damage and that prescription pain killers and anti-inflammatories are the best options. The chiropractor tells you the source of your pain is misalignment of bones and joints. The personal trainer tells you it's a muscle strength and stability problem. The yoga instructor says it's your tight hips and weak core muscles. The nutritionist says food allergies and nutrient deficiencies cause your pain. The naturopath tells you that rubbing lavender oil on your temples will provide the relief you're looking for.

Finally, frustrated and exhausted, you search for pain remedies on the internet. You find a company that apparently has found the "one simple secret Holy Grail of pain relief," and all you have to do is make three payments of $99.99 to discover what it is.

The pain management system is frustrating, to say the least. While I've been lucky enough to meet physical therapists, surgeons, sports medicine doctors, trainers, and chiropractors who expertly helped resolve my pain issues, it pays to be your own pain management specialist. Or at least, your own advocate for getting the care you need. You shouldn't perform surgery on yourself, prescribe your own medication, or even diagnose yourself without professional help. But you should understand what pain is, what the common causes are, and the best ways to treat it naturally. Unlike specialists who only look at a thin slice of what is happening in your body, you will be able to see the big picture once you understand how pain works.

THE PURPOSE OF PAIN

Pain is a protective response to tissue injury. It's defined as "an unpleasant sensory and emotional experience associated with actual or potential tissue damage, or described in terms of such damage."[35] It's not only a tissue-specific sensation, it's the product of neurological wiring and has a clear psychological component.

While this wordy definition indicates pain has a specific cause, it leaves out the purpose. Pain is a messenger, with a complex language difficult to interpret. But its underlying message is always the same: "There's a problem here!" That's why for pain caused by tissue damage (*nociceptive pain*), it doesn't make sense to blindly block it.

Pain also serves as a neurologically wired reminder of what not to do. And that reminder can have a lasting impact that keeps you from getting injured again. I once injured my knee just by getting into my car. As I lowered my body and twisted into the driver's seat, I felt a sharp pain in my knee and heard a muffled pop. My mistake was twisting my hip and knee outward as I sat down, while keeping my foot firmly planted on the ground and pointing forward. This stressed the connective tissue in my knee, causing a grade 1 sprain of the MCL ligament. It took several weeks of rest and rehabilitation to get my knee back in shape. To this day, when I get into a vehicle, my foot automatically pivots on its heel to match the external rotation of my knee and hip. It's like my foot is protecting my knee, carefully keeping everything in alignment. One painful moment created a lasting change to my movement mechanics. A positive change.

Pain is not without value, but it's hard to recognize this when you're in pain. Its value lies in guiding you back to health. In the case of tendinopathy and joint overuse injuries, pain is your gauge. Training frequency, load, volume, and exercise selection should all be guided by it.

Whether you suffer from widespread chronic pain or simply have a few beat-up, achy joints from age and overuse, you know that pain takes a toll both mentally and physically. It also takes a bite out of strength gains, energy, and motivation. Pain is a roadblock that will keep you from making progress if you let it. But when you learn to manage pain naturally and effectively, you can find ways through it that allow you to use your body to its full potential.

Let's look at the three main types of pain, how to differentiate between them, and a smarter way to approach pain management.

TYPES OF PAIN

Most pain experts consider *nociceptive pain* and *neuropathic pain* to be the two primary types. The key difference is that nociceptive pain is caused by direct tissue damage, and neuropathic pain is caused by a disease state or nervous system dysfunction. Differentiating between the two helps you determine what course of action is best. Nociceptive pain should be treated like an injury, while neuropathic pain requires more professional oversight and guidance from a qualified medical professional.

Nociceptive pain (nō-si-'sep-tiv) is what you experience when you break a bone, twist an ankle, or smash your thumb with a hammer. The causes range from thermal (heat) to chemical to mechanical.[35] *Nociceptive inflammatory pain,* a subtype of nociceptive pain, is what comes next. The flood of inflammatory cells and increased swelling compresses nerves, causing painful feelings of pressure.[36] This is often described as *throbbing* or *pulsating* pain. Both acute and overuse injuries typically fall into the nociceptive category.

Neuropathic pain is markedly different in its mechanism. It even feels different. While you can't depend on subjective feelings to diagnose yourself, it's helpful to understand what to look for. Neuropathic pain is described as *shooting, tingling, stabbing,* or *burning*—often affecting the lower legs and feet. It can be a chronic feeling or come and go. Everyone experiences one of these sensations from time to time, but if you have ongoing pain that feels this way, you should take it seriously. See a doctor and ask about testing for nerve damage and disease.

A third type, *centralized pain,* occurs when your nervous system amplifies the volume of pain signals. Interestingly, centralized pain often lingers long after the original tissue damage has healed. In many cases of a nociceptive pain response to tissue damage, the lingering pain has nothing to do with the injury. Pain receptors have been sensitized, and sometimes new pain receptors have been formed. This can persist for months or years after the tissue damage occurred. To resolve it, you have to do more than just treat the symptoms. It takes understanding and addressing the root causes of the ongoing pain response. In a sense, typical *nociceptive pain* becomes *neuropathic pain* when the nervous system perpetuates the pain response. The key point here is that pain can have an immediate and specific cause or be a lingering effect of a neuropathic overreaction.

PAIN SENSITIVITY: LISTENING AND INTERPRETING

Neuroplasticity is the ability of the brain to form new connections, especially in response to learning or an injury. In the case of traumatic brain injuries, patients can "rewire" their neural circuitry to restore and maintain normal function. Like a road detour during construction, a damaged brain finds a new path to the destination. This same process of rewiring neural circuitry takes place in the rest of the body as well. It's a fundamental role of the central nervous system that enables us to adapt quickly to our environment and recover from trauma. But like many basic functions of the human body, neuroplasticity can turn against you.

In her book *The Pain Relief Secret*, author and somatic educator Sarah Warren describes how prolonged inflammation leads to pain sensitization and plays a role in the transition from acute to chronic pain: "Adaptations in your brain, spinal cord, and peripheral nerves can outlast the original injury and lead to structure changes, which include the sprouting of new nerve endings and the formation of new synapses between neurons."[37]

When pain caused by inflammation stays elevated for several days, neurons become increasingly responsive to pain signals. This causes flares of nociceptive pain that you might not previously have experienced as painful. Someone gently brushing your hand wouldn't normally hurt. But after slamming your hand in a car door, even a gentle touch will cause you to jerk back. This is called *sensitization*.[34] It's your body's way of protecting an injury from further aggravation, but it can also overreact. As pain receptors continue to upregulate and more inflammatory mediators are released, your acute pain from an injury can transition into chronic pain.

Chronic pain isn't just a nuisance. It blunts your strength and performance through a process called *cortical inhibition*. This is your nervous system's response to injury, where neurons that control muscular force production around the injured area are selectively inhibited. This is another reason why training through joint pain is a fool's errand. By allowing pain to hang around, you're suppressing strength gains. Besides, you'll end up losing any progress you make once your joints start degenerating. And believe me, they will.

The process of sensitization doesn't resolve as fast as injuries do. Upregulated pain receptors, increased nerve endings, and other structural changes to the nervous system can make you sensitized to pain in the future—long after the original injury has healed. Not only that, sensitization doesn't stay isolated to one injured body part. It can affect the way you perceive pain in other areas. This means an injury that produces prolonged inflammation could lead to increased pain sensitivity throughout your body. Not good news. To make matters worse, there are psychological effects of pain and injury that linger. And don't think this is just a problem for the hysterical or overly sensitive. No one is spared from these biochemical processes. They affect all people to varying degrees—from tough-as-nails athletes to recreational exercisers. But with the right knowledge set, you can approach your pain from a more scientific perspective that will keep you on a productive path.

The key is to be in tune with pain sensations while not letting them occupy your mind. This is easier said than done for chronic pain patients or people who have a history of multiple injuries. When you focus too much on pain, you risk making it worse. This is called *catastrophizing*—when fear of additional pain and injury becomes exaggerated. Pain scientists have found that catastrophizing leads to negative outcomes independent of the actual pain.[38] It creates a cycle of overprotective guarding, avoiding movements, and reduced physical activity. Since staying active is one of the most effective pain management techniques, the downward spiral created by catastrophizing can become a self-fulfilling prophecy. You fear that you're going to hurt yourself worse, or that the pain will never get better, so you're less active. Less activity means less joint lubrication, fewer healing mechanisms activated, and more psychological stress.

This downward spiral of pain sensitization and the psychological effects that follow might seem inevitable, but they are not. In the next chapter, I'll show you four tactics for long-term pain relief. But the fact remains, pain must be dealt with in the short term if you want to move and exercise freely. Keep these three ideas in mind as you navigate the murky waters of exercising with pain.

First, be attuned to feelings of *pressure* or *tension* in your joints when exercising. Sensory thresholds increase with age, so you're less likely to feel or be aware of nondangerous stimuli, like a gentle touch to your skin. But your *pressure pain threshold*—the least intensity of pressure you can recognize—decreases with age.[39] This means the older you are, the more attuned you can be to pressure sensations issuing warning signals. Pressure indicates an early inflammatory response, an increase in synovial fluid from joint damage, swelling, or a mechanical problem—like a ligament being in a precarious position.[40] Tension in a muscle or joint usually indicates a lack of flexibility, but it can also mean your tissues are under stress and in danger of tearing. *Let pressure and tension be your guides.* The more often you recognize these sensations, the better you will be at managing pain and preventing injury.

Second, beware of favoring one body part over another. This is easy to do when you are hyperfocused on a painful problem joint. I've fallen prey to this more than once. After a wrist injury, I used wrist wraps while lifting weights to alleviate pain and prevent further damage. I became dependent on them. Over time, my inner elbows degenerated from picking up the slack. I was so worried about my wrists that I didn't see the elbow injury coming. I developed tendinopathy in both elbows that would hound me on and off for over three years.

Third, establish a diagnostic ritual that allows you to search for and locate pain. Don't worry—I'm not asking you to sit mindfully in a quiet room, scanning your body for bad vibes. I'm talking about a series of movements (see chapter 7) that will show you what feels good and what feels off. I've found that when I examine my functional movement capacity along with feelings of pain or tension, it enables me to determine what is just a creaky joint in need of a warm-up and what is a real problem that needs addressing. Acknowledging pain is is the first step toward resolving it.

Jessica Kisiel, exercise physiologist and author of *Winning the Injury Game*, pushes her clients to connect with pain instead of ignoring it:

> Pain has a dual role in your body: communication and protection. It is the body's last resort mechanism to get your attention. You have ignored the subtle signals that your body has sent you: the strange feelings, muscle tightness, reduced range of motion, and so on. To make you take notice and stop your destructive behavior, your body is forced to take harsh action and makes you hurt—terribly. Your pain is trying to help you prevent further or more serious injury.[41]

Slow Down to Build Up

One of the simplest ways to eliminate exercise-related joint pain is to take the momentum out of the movement. This is especially effective for working through tendon pain and learning new exercises. More often than not, you can work through discomfort safely just by reducing the weight and slowing down the repetition speed to at least three seconds during the lifting (concentric) phase and three seconds during the lowering (eccentric) phase. Your body responds in a completely different manner to this type of training. Slow repetition speeds allow you to safely perform previously uncomfortable movements without pain while also strengthening connective tissue.

KEY TAKEAWAY

Ignoring pain is a surefire way to end up injured or in chronic pain. On the opposite end of the spectrum, obsessing about your pain will make it difficult to move forward. As you can see, it's a balancing act. You must view your pain with a more scientific, unemotional perspective. This strategy has three main benefits: (1) it allows you to address underlying problems before serious injuries occur; (2) it shows you what to look for that precedes pain—feelings of pressure, tension, and other strange sensations; and (3) it teaches you to differentiate between counterproductive pain and productive discomfort, a necessary skill for improving fitness.

What to Focus On Instead of Pain Relief

I am not what has happened to me. I am what I choose to become.

—Carl Jung

Pain relief is treating symptoms, not causes. If you do nothing but treat the pain, then the underlying problem is still there. It will rear its ugly head again. Almost always, there is a postural fault, movement habit, or other physiological problem causing your pain. *That* needs to be addressed. Instead of aiming to block pain, focus instead on these four goals: modulate inflammation, resolve and prevent tendinopathy, improve synovial fluid health, and protect collagen health.

1. MODULATE INFLAMMATION

In chapter 1, we talked about how inflammation is a fundamental part of your body's immune system. It's in charge of clearing dead cells away from injury sites, protecting wounds from foreign invaders, and supplying regenerative nutrients for repair. With so many important roles, why would we want to interfere with inflammation at all?

It's a heated debate topic among therapists, sports medicine doctors, and athletic trainers. Everyone agrees that some inflammation is necessary to kick-start healing. Everyone also agrees that too much inflammation is a bad thing. The debate lies in exactly what we should be doing (and when) to manage it. To understand the most practical intervention strategies, let's quickly look at the three phases of inflammation and how they relate to pain.

The Three Phases of Inflammation

When an injury occurs, chemicals are released into the bloodstream and transported to damaged tissues. The influx of blood and nutrients to the injured area causes swelling, stimulates nerves, and presses on pain receptors. This process takes place in three distinct phases: acute inflammation, subacute inflammation, and chronic inflammation.[42] The three phases are the same whether you have local inflammation (in one area of your body) or systemic inflammation (total body).

Acute inflammation

Acute inflammation is the immediate immune response after your body is injured or encounters an infection. Signs of acute inflammation include pain, redness, swelling, joint popping, and range of motion loss. Think about the last time you smacked your knee on something. Within seconds, you noticed redness and swelling. While some of that can be explained simply as tissue damage, most of the physical changes you see are caused by the rush of blood and nutrients your body is pumping to the injury site. It heals wounds and supports tissue growth and repair.

Generally, it's a good thing. It is short-lived, lasting anywhere from a few hours to a few days. Ice packs and nonsteroidal anti-inflammatory drugs (NSAIDs) such as ibuprofen are commonly used to reduce pain and swelling during the acute phase, but your body needs a certain amount of acute inflammation to heal optimally.

Subacute inflammation

Subacute inflammation is the transition period between acute and chronic inflammation. This phase is characterized by normalization of inflammation markers and the laying down of temporary scar tissue upon which more permanent structures can be built. This phase peaks between three and six weeks postinjury but can last several months.

This is a pivotal time period. Successful exercise interventions coupled with practices that keep inflammation in an optimal range will speed up recovery and optimize tissue formations.

Chronic inflammation

Chronic inflammation is low-grade inflammation that lasts for several months or longer—years in some cases. Many practitioners define inflammation lasting more than three months as chronic.

Though chronic inflammation can be an extension of an acute injury, it generally affects people with disease states, poor movement patterns, and high stress levels.

Inflammation: The Good, the Bad, and the Deadly

Inflammation isn't good or bad. In the acute phase, it's necessary to deliver fresh oxygen and nutrients to injured tissues and organs. Even in the subacute phase, some inflammation is necessary to stimulate the healing process. But when inflammation lasts for several weeks, or months, it becomes a problem—increasing risk of disease and joint degeneration.

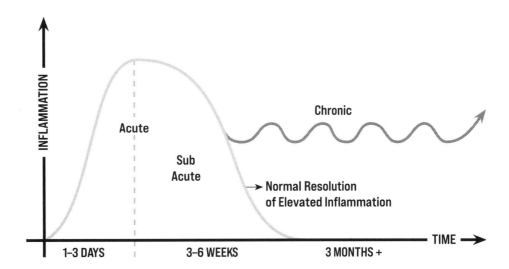

FIGURE 3.1

Three phases of inflammation. (Adapted from Askenase, M. H., & Sansing, L. H., 2016. Stages of the inflammatory response in pathology and tissue repair after intracerebral hemorrhage. *Seminars in Neurology, 36,* 288–297.)

The inflammation theory of disease states that chronic inflammation is the underlying cause of or main expediting factor in most common diseases, including heart disease, cancer, diabetes, arthritis, and Alzheimer's.[43] Over the past few decades, evidence supporting this theory has piled up, aiding our understanding of the biggest scourges of humanity and opening up new treatment options. Opponents of the theory point out that inflammation may be a symptom of underlying health problems, not the cause. Whether or not inflammation is the primary cause of most diseases or not, it's clearly not a good thing to have hanging around.

Chronic inflammation also negatively affects quality of life in the short term, causing chronic pain, weight gain, and depression. Because so much of the media and documentation on inflammation focuses on deadly diseases, this point gets lost, so it's worth repeating. If you have low-grade systemic inflammation, it is damaging your quality of life in virtually every way—the way you look, how you feel, and even how effectively you think. The list of symptoms below makes this point abundantly clear.

Symptoms of Systemic Inflammation

Symptoms are far ranging, including everything from general fatigue to weight gain.[44] Even if you are less concerned about overall health and more worried about your banged-up knees and elbows, pay close attention to this. Studies show low-grade systemic inflammation makes you more susceptible to tendinopathy and joint pain.[45] While most people have one or two of these symptoms, you should seek medical guidance if several of these describe you:

- Weight gain (especially around the midsection)
- Fatigue, brain fog, general lethargy, insomnia
- Joint and muscle pain, spasms, muscle cramps
- Depressed mood and anxiety

- Digestive discomfort (gas, diarrhea, constipation, stomach cramps and pains)
- Skin disorders, including easily irritated skin, persistent redness or puffiness, eczema, and psoriasis
- Frequent infections, colds, and illnesses
- Frequent allergic reactions and allergy symptoms

Symptoms of local chronic inflammation (in a specific region of the body) are more specific:

- Pain, swelling, irritation, or redness lasting longer than six weeks
- Progressive muscle weakness
- Progressive reductions in range of motion

Causes and Risk Factors for Chronic Inflammation

While some of these are out of your control—like genetics and age—you can influence most of these risk factors:

- **Age:** Chronic, low-grade inflammation appears to be a normal part of aging to some degree.[46]
- **Nutrition:** Diets high in refined foods and sugar are associated with greater production of proinflammatory cytokines (substances that trigger an immune response).[47]
- **Obesity:** Obesity and inflammation are inexorably linked due to several factors, including poor lifestyle choices and increased stress on organs and joint systems.[47]
- **Stress:** Accumulating evidence suggests that chronic inflammation worsens stress-induced diseases. The opposite is also true—stress worsens inflammation—which suggests a common pathway for stress-related diseases based on chronic inflammation.[48]
- **Lack of Sleep:** Circadian rhythms (sleep cycles) regulate both our immune systems and inflammation levels. Studies show just one night of sleep loss increases inflammation in the body.[49]
- **Smoking:** Cigarette smoking causes chronic inflammation not just in the mucosal passages and sinuses but in your entire body.[50]
- **OTC Drugs, NSAIDs, Alcohol, and Prescription Medication:** Alcohol and drug abuse is linked to chronic inflammation. But even over-the-counter NSAIDs designed to lower inflammation can have detrimental effects. This is partially due to the inflammation rebound you experience after stopping.[51]

Risk factors for local chronic inflammation also include:

- Previous injury or surgery
- Job that requires repetitive movements (e.g. typing, turning a screwdriver)
- Arthritis

Practical Ways to Lower Total Body Inflammation

Even if you haven't been diagnosed with a chronic inflammatory condition, reducing total body inflammation has an enormous return on investment. Studies show reducing overall inflammation levels improves energy, stabilizes mood and appetite, eases joint pain, and reduces oxidative stress—a key driver of the aging process.[52] Naturally, savvy marketers have cashed in. Health magazines advertise everything from cryotherapy to alkaline water as the new anti-inflammatory breakthrough. It's difficult to determine what really works and what can be practically implemented with so much misinformation. The list below outlines 10 research-backed, practical ways to lower total body inflammation.

1. **Lose weight.** Regardless of how you make it happen, losing weight reduces total body inflammation levels. In addition to easing the mechanical strain on joints (especially knees), weight loss causes a metabolic adaptation that lowers inflammatory markers.[53] This happens both after weight loss occurs and during the weight loss process when calories are restricted. This is the most effective and dependable hack for lowering inflammation. Even if you are only carrying around an extra 10 pounds, losing it makes a big difference. As I mentioned earlier, 10 pounds of weight loss equals about 40 pounds of stress relief on your knees.[54]

2. **Avoid NSAIDs and other anti-inflammatory drugs.** Paradoxically, long-term use of NSAIDs such as naproxen and ibuprofen increases levels of low-grade chronic inflammation. A study published in the journal *Medical Hypothesis* concluded that use of anti-inflammatory agents down-regulates your body's natural ability to manage inflammation.[51] Besides the myriad of negative side effects associated with long-term use of anti-inflammatories, this is another reason why drugs and OTC products are not a viable long-term solution.[55,56] Use NSAIDs and prescription anti-inflammatories only as necessary to relieve (unbearable) pain, swelling, or excessive inflammation. Remember that we need inflammation to heal injuries and microtrauma to connective tissue. Use them for three to seven days if necessary, then stop. A better solution is to avoid NSAIDs altogether and use the anti-inflammatory supplements listed below instead (see item number 10).

3. **Reduce carbohydrate intake.** Compared to low-fat diets, low-carb diets provide better pain relief and anti-inflammatory effects. A study conducted at the University of Alabama at Birmingham showed a low-carbohydrate diet was more effective at reducing pain and reducing oxidative stress markers in patients with knee osteoarthritis.[57] Researchers believe low-carb diets reduce insulin-mediated inflammation.[58]

4. **Follow a low-inflammation diet.** Some foods cause dramatic spikes in blood sugar that raise inflammation levels. Other foods, like the omega-3 fatty acids found in fish, reduce inflammation by increasing the production of anti-inflammatory compounds in the body and decreasing the production of proinflammatory proteins.[59] While there are dozens of popular anti-inflammatory diet plans available, these principles have the most scientific backing:

   - Reduce intake of refined carbohydrates like cookies, cakes, pasta, and baked goods.

   - Reduce intake of processed seed oils like canola oil, margarine, and soybean oil.

   - Eat more healthy fats (focusing on omega-3s).

   - Eat more antioxidant-rich foods (focusing on fruits and vegetables).

   - Use anti-inflammatory spices instead of packaged condiments when cooking and preparing food.

5. **Get moving.** A 2017 study published in the journal *Brain, Behavior and Immunity* showed that just 20 minutes of exercise resulted in a 5% decrease in circulating inflammatory cells.[60] Researchers from the University of California–San Diego School of Medicine, who conducted the study, believe that activating the sympathetic nervous system through exercise triggers an immune response that fights inflammation. According to lead researcher Suzi Hong,

   > Our study shows a workout session does not actually have to be intense to have anti-inflammatory effects. Twenty minutes to half an hour of moderate exercise, including fast walking, appears to be sufficient. Feeling like a workout needs to be at a peak exertion level for a long duration can intimidate those who suffer from chronic inflammatory diseases and could greatly benefit from physical activity.

   Regular exercise is necessary to bring high inflammation levels down, even when you're inflamed and don't feel like moving. The trick is to find ways to exercise without aggravating the injury or causing an inflammatory response that sets you back. As much as you are able, move daily.

6. **Sleep more.** Only one night of sleep loss raises circulating inflammatory cytokine levels.[61] Your body responds to sleep deprivation much like it does to acute stress or trauma, producing a spike in inflammation. When sleep deprivation becomes chronic, so does high inflammation. We all know getting enough sleep is important, but it's tough to make it happen. Matthew Walker, Ph.D, sleep researcher and author of *Why We Sleep,* suggests giving yourself a non-negotiable *sleep opportunity* of eight hours per night.[62] In practice, this means dedicating eight hours between the time you go to bed and the time your alarm goes off. Some nights, you won't fall asleep right away. You'll wake up throughout the night and maybe wake long before your alarm goes off in the morning. You can't guarantee yourself eight hours of uninterrupted sleep, but you can give yourself the opportunity to sleep eight hours every night. This habit trains your body to sleep longer and better over time.

7. **Try yoga or flow-sequenced stretching.** A study published in the journal *Oxidative Medicine and Cellular Longevity* showed practicing yoga lowered inflammation and cortisol, your body's chief stress hormone.[63] If yoga isn't for you, try moving through a series of full body stretches in a flowing sequence each day. This not only makes stretching more interesting, adding an element of skilled learning, it also helps you tie together disparate movements and improve body awareness.

8. **Bathe in a sauna.** The research on sauna bathing for inflammation is sparse compared to the other tactics mentioned here, even compared to many nutritional supplements. But a handful of small studies have shown an inverse relationship between frequent sauna usage and C-reactive protein—a marker of systemic inflammation.[64] Anecdotally, I've personally experienced relief from swollen, inflamed joints after only one sauna session. If you have access to a sauna, it's worth trying.

9. **Use cold therapy when you feel all banged up.** Cold therapy, such as sitting in an ice bath, will help relieve pain and inflammation in flared-up joints. This is less about lowering systemic inflammation and more about calming inflamed body parts. Be wary of any new-age cold therapy devices that don't have substantial evidence for safety or efficacy. Also, limit ice therapy on injured joints because it suppresses important healing processes (more on this later).

10. **Take proven anti-inflammatory supplements.** There are a handful of natural supplements with proven anti-inflammatory benefits. Here's the short-list of anti-inflammatory supplements I recommend:

- **Fish oil:** Numerous studies on the omega-3 fatty acids found in fish oil have demonstrated marked reductions in inflammation levels.[65] Fish oil supplementation also reduces oxidative stress in athletes and supports immune function.[66] The recommended intake for fish oil is 1 gram daily (supplying at least 250 mg of the omega-3 fatty acids EPA and DHA) for general health, and up to 6 grams daily during recovery periods to help with soreness.[67]

- **Turmeric combined with black pepper extract:** Curcumin is the main active compound in turmeric—one of the world's most popular (and scientifically supported) supplements for overall health. In head-to-head studies, turmeric has outperformed ibuprofen for joint pain and function scores (while presenting far fewer negative side effects).[68] Not only does turmeric reduce oxidative stress via its antioxidant effects, it reduces inflammation in osteo-cartilaginous tissue.[69,70] And animal models demonstrate that curcumin can help regenerate damaged nerves after injury. In placebo-controlled human studies, dosages of 200 mg to 1500 mg have been proven safe and effective for pain relief, joint function, and inflammation.[71] Also, take black pepper extract (piperine) with your turmeric. Studies have shown a 2,000% increase (20×) in absorption when turmeric is combined with black pepper extract.[72]

- **Boswellia:** Boswellia serrata is one of the most potent supplements for natural pain relief and inflammation support, partially through its ability to inhibit proinflammatory cytokines.[73] Dosages as low as 100 mg have reduced joint pain and stiffness in as little as seven days.[74] Much of the research on boswellia has been performed on branded extracts, such as Aflapin and 5-Loxin, that isolate specific boswellic acids: namely, acetyl-keto-beta-boswellic acid, or AKBA. These extracts have outperformed generic boswellia supplements in some studies, but research suggests that other boswellic acids have anti-inflammation actions as well.[75] Shoot for 100–150 mg per day of boswellia with high concentrations of AKBA, or take 600–1,000 mg of standard boswellia extract (around 60% boswellic acids).

- **Type II collagen:** Supplementing with type II collagen produces a novel effect in the body: it regulates the immune reaction responsible for intercartilaginous inflammation, which supports the overall healing process and helps manage pain levels. It also has benefits related to collagen production and formation, which we'll cover in later chapters. The recommended daily dosage for isolated type II collagen supplements is 40 mg daily.[76]

While there are other valuable supplements out there, these have a track record of safety and efficacy in peer-reviewed human studies. They also offer other related benefits, such as pain relief, reduced oxidative stress, improved circulation, and more. If you do switch from NSAIDs to natural alternatives, be patient. Most supplement studies show the best pain relief results after several weeks of consistent usage.

Postinjury Inflammation Management

Now you know why acute inflammation is important for healing and why chronic inflammation is detrimental to your health, and you have some practical methods for lowering total body inflammation. But the fact remains: managing inflammation after an injury is tricky. It's more an art than a science. Follow these steps to make sure you effectively manage injury-related inflammation without interfering with the healing process:

Get a professional opinion. I like the phrasing of this: "get a professional *opinion.*" This doesn't mean you have to leap in whatever direction your doctor suggests. Aim to get a diagnosis, an understanding of potential causes, and help establishing timelines for recovery. If you have a doctor or therapist you trust, then by all means follow their advice. But you should still do your homework. *You* are your own best advocate.

Think long term. Studies of athletes who use NSAIDs after an injury show that in the short term, outcomes are improved. They're able to return to competition faster and make quicker improvements in muscular performance tests. But in the long term, they fall apart. Injury recidivism (reinjury of same body part) is 25% higher in athletes who use NSAIDs during recovery.[55] They are able to get pain and inflammation under control sooner, but they return to competition before their injury is fully healed. Weak, malformed tissues make them injury-prone. When it comes to managing inflammation, remember that your goal is not only to get back to 100% but to prevent future injuries.

Don't block inflammation—modulate it. You don't want to completely stop inflammation. You just want to modulate it, which means keep it in the healthy range. To do this, use the minimum effective dose of everything that affects inflammation. That includes NSAIDs, supplements, and even ice therapy.

Manage inflammation by phase. Follow the guide below to help you determine how aggressive you need to be with getting inflammation under control after you suffer an injury.

Taming Inflammation by Phase

Acute phase: Week 1

If possible, avoid anti-inflammatories during the first week after an injury. The use of anti-inflammatory drugs during this phase blunts production of insulin-like growth factor, a hormone that speeds up tissue healing and regeneration.[77] Ice only as needed for swelling and pain. Some studies show that icing immediately after a strain or contusion helps reduce swelling and improves range of motion without significantly affecting healing times. However, icing daily could have negative impacts on healing during the acute phase.

Subacute phase: Weeks 2-7

During weeks 2–7, tissue *proliferation* is in full effect. This means most of the dead and damaged cells have been removed, and new scar tissue is being laid down over the injury. More permanent collagen structures will eventually replace this scar tissue during the *remodeling* phase.

Temporary scar tissue is fragile, so returning to full activity—especially if you perform explosive movements with heavy weight—could cause reinjury. Focus on expanding your pain-free ranges of motion gradually with slow, deliberate movements to help align scar tissue into optimal patterns and reduce abnormal adhesions. We'll cover optimizing connective tissue formations in more detail in chapter 4.

Chronic inflammation: Weeks 8+

Chronic localized inflammation indicates the source of the problem still exists. Continued macrophage activity will lead to the destruction of healthy joint tissue. Joints become tight, deformed, and painful. This is common among osteoarthritis and autoimmune disease patients.[78] If you go to the doctor complaining of chronic joint pain, they will probably prescribe you anti-inflammatory drugs. You may get some relief. But in all likelihood, you just shot yourself in the foot by covering up the problem with an inflammation-blocking Band-Aid.

Even though you may present with inflammatory symptoms several weeks after an injury or overuse strain, inflammation probably isn't the main culprit. True chronic inflammation in joints is a strong indicator of arthritis or an autoimmune response, but in otherwise healthy people the problem is often *inflammation-independent tendinopathy*. Experts in the field of connective tissue injury believe that inflammation and tendon degeneration are different parts of the same injury process. This leads us to the second and maybe the most important concept to focus on *instead* of pain relief.

2. RESOLVE AND PREVENT TENDINOPATHY

The second item on the list is *resolve and prevent tendinopathy*—in that order. It's likely that you already have some level of tendinopathy in your body right now that could lead to injury and chronic pain—even if you don't have any symptoms.

I credit my lack of understanding what tendinopathy really is with 99% of the injuries I incurred for the first 30 years of my life. I was under the impression that acute injuries (e.g. tearing the rotator cuff in my shoulder) resulted from one unlucky accident. I also believed that my chronically painful and weak joints were simply inflamed from overuse. As a young athlete, I turned to cortisone injections and NSAIDs (doctors' suggestions, of course). I iced my arms and knees religiously. I took time off from heavy lifting whenever an old injury would rise back to the surface. Little did I know that every well-intentioned step I took made the problem worse. Now I know better.

Tendinopathy is the most common class of overuse injuries, affecting both competitive athletes and recreational fitness enthusiasts. Most cases present as pain and tenderness near joints. For example, the Achilles tendon near the ankle, patellar tendon just below the kneecap, and forearm tendons near the elbow are all common tendinopathy locations. Tendon injuries often seem to happen suddenly but are usually the result of several microtears that occurred over time. In the past, virtually all cases were referred to as *tendinitis*, which means inflammation of the tendon. And instances where tendon degeneration was apparent were called *tendinosis*. These two conditions were historically viewed as two separate outcomes from the same injury. Today, leading experts are more likely to refer to both conditions as *tendinopathy* instead. It more accurately describes the sliding-scale continuum of tendon injury outcomes.[79]

One of the biggest misconceptions about tendinopathy is that inflammation is the primary cause. For example, the inflammation-based model assumes that a chronically sore knee is caused by inflammation (tendinitis), and that the subsequent tendon degeneration that occurs over time (tendinosis) results from that chronic inflammation. Based on this model, most general practitioners believe that patients who present with overuse injuries require rest and anti-inflammatory medication to promote healing. But more recent studies cast doubt on this philosophy, and experts in the field of tendon health have created a new paradigm.

• • •

Dr. Jill Cook is an Australia-based physiotherapist and one of the world's leading experts on tendon pathology. In the early 2000s, Cook spearheaded and was involved in dozens of tendinopathy studies. Her work includes research on patellar tendinopathy in elite basketball players, muscle development of ballet dancers with hip pain, landing mechanics of athletes with knee pain, prevalence of Achilles tendinopathy in runners, injury rates of alpine skiers, and hundreds more variations of individual injury types in different cross-sections of the population (https://www.researchgate .net/scientific-contributions/Jill-Cook-2052457537). Through decades of research, Cook and her colleagues consistently found evidence of tendinosis (breakdown of the tendon) where inflammation was absent.[80] This research refuted the deeply entrenched belief of inflammation-based tendon degeneration and dogma surrounding the use of NSAIDs for tendon pain.

In June 2009, Dr. Cook and renowned Olympic Games physiotherapist Craig Purdam published an article in the *British Journal of Sports Medicine* that shifted the landscape of modern tendinopathy treatment. The article presented a continuum model for how tendon overuse injuries occur and why pharmacological interventions consistently fall short in long-term tendon injury outcomes.[81] As Dr. Cook's research shows, tendon injuries and pain have a *noninflammatory pathology*. Microscopic analyses of tendon surgical patients show fraying of collagen fibers, weakened collagen cross-links, and scar tissue–like disruptions in the collagen matrix. Tendon repair cells are present, and inflammatory cells are typically absent. This means that tendon degeneration is not simply the result of unchecked chronic inflammation. The degeneration and weakening of connective tissue in overuse injuries has a different cause. This is a key reason why *tendinopathy* has replaced tendinitis and tendinosis when referring to tendon pathology.

Since inflammation isn't always the cause of tendinopathy, it's no wonder why the old recovery methods of rest, ice, and NSAIDs don't perform well in injury studies. Anti-inflammatory pills provide only short-term relief, at best, as do cortisone injections.[82,83] Long-term outcomes are even worse, with anti-inflammatory use causing reduced collagen mass at injury sites and increasing chances of reinjury.[55]

This begs the question: if inflammation isn't the key driver of tendon degeneration, and anti-inflammatory medication only makes the problem worse, what can we do to effectively treat tendinopathy? To answer that question, we must understand what causes tendinopathy to develop in the first place.

Why Does Tendinopathy Develop in the First Place?

Every time you exercise, pick up something heavy, or otherwise stress your joints beyond their normal load volumes, your tendons experience microscopic damage. This is a normal, healthy process and is a fundamental part of developing strength. When the tendon can effectively recover from one training session to the next (or from one stressor to the next), tendon strength and resilience increases. However, when recovery is not adequate, or the tendon damage is too severe, the tendinopathy injury process begins.

Tendinopathy develops (or not) in relation to your tendon load capacity and the corresponding training load applied to your tendons.[84] An optimized load consists of training and stressors that create a healthy amount of adaptation without excessive degeneration. Examples of the "loads" I'm referring to could include your weekly weight training routine, the number of times you bend over to pick up objects off the floor during the day, or how much of a beating your knees take from a long-distance running session. How the body responds to various loads varies from person to person.

Everyone has their own individualized load threshold for tendon adaptation, called the *load tolerance set point*.[85] When you exercise and move at your setpoint, or just slightly beyond it, you experience fitness improvements. When you fail to stress your tendons enough to reach this setpoint, your tendons adapt by reducing their load tolerance. Finally, when you stress your tendons beyond your load tolerance set point, especially when it happens repeatedly, the adaptations can't keep up with the stress and your tendon degenerates.

When the load is extremely far past your tendon's load tolerance (especially if it is already weakened by degenerative changes), the tendon ruptures. This is the traumatic injury type that requires surgery or immobilization in a cast. It seems to come out of nowhere, but it usually doesn't. It is almost always preceded by degenerative changes from inadequate adaptations to daily stressors, bad movement habits, and age. Experts estimate that up to 97% of spontaneous tendon ruptures have some amount of pre-existing tendinopathy.[86]

Tendinopathies commonly start developing in athletes as they reach their early 30s. Years of accumulated stress and declines in tendon stiffness reach a tipping point.[15] It's not uncommon to have multiple tendinopathies develop in your 30s and 40s all at once. Left unchecked, it only gets worse with age. But you don't have to go down this road. Thanks to experts in tendon pathology, we now have a clear understanding of the three separate phases of tendinopathy. With this knowledge, you can appropriately treat each phase, rebuild your broken-down joints, and get back to full function.

The Continuum Model of Tendinopathy

Phase 1: Reactive tendinopathy

The first stage of tendinopathy is the reactive phase. Your tendon responds to rapid increases in load by increasing intratendinous swelling. The tendon becomes stiffer to hold its integrity. Overall, the tendon remains structurally intact with minimal changes to the collagen matrix. At this phase, the tendinopathy is reversible.

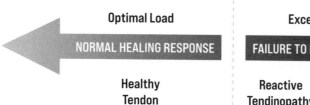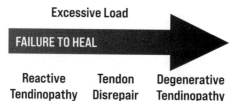

FIGURE 3.2

Continuum model of tendinopathy. (Adapted from Cook, J. L., & Purdam, C. R., 2009. Is tendon pathology a continuum? A pathology model to explain the clinical presentation of load-induced tendinopathy. *British Journal of Sports Medicine,* 43, 409–416, Figure 1.)

Reactive tendinopathy occurs after an acute injury and during the initial phases of an overuse injury. It often shows up when you go from sedentary to active without a ramp-up period. In the case of hard-training athletes, it occurs when training programs are not periodized properly to allow connective tissue to heal.[87] If training loads are reduced, pain and swelling from reactive tendinopathy can resolve in one or two weeks. Early detection and intervention are critical. The longer tendinopathy hangs around, the harder it is to get rid of.

Phase 2: Tendon disrepair

After a few weeks of continued tendon overload, the second stage, the *disrepair phase,* ensues and the tendon's collagen matrix starts to breakdown. This is when the first significant changes in tendon structure happen. Additional tendon thickening occurs, disruption in the collagen matrix architecture becomes apparent (starts to resemble scar tissue), and nerve ingrowth can develop, leading to chronic pain and irritation.[84]

To prevent slipping into degenerative tendinopathy, you need to increase load tolerance and stimulate healing without aggravating the damaged tendon.

Phase 3: Degenerative tendinopathy

Finally, the *degenerative phase* completes the downward cycle by signaling for large-scale tendon cell apoptosis (death) with permanent damage, characterized by intratendinous calcification (calcium deposits within the tendon). Parts of the tendon die off, leaving "holes" in the tendon that are essentially beyond repair. Cross-sections of the tendon become *mechanically silent*—unable to sense loads and respond to them.[84] Risk of tendon rupture is high.

Once you reach this phase, you have dead sections of tendon that do not remodel normally, even with rehabilitative efforts. These dead sections don't cause pain at this phase. Any discomfort felt is likely from healthy tissue surrounding the dead areas becoming reinjured as it tries to compensate for the tendon mass loss. The good news is that sections of tendon can and will build around the dead areas, allowing you to achieve virtually full preinjury function. This is where the phrase "treat the doughnut, not the hole" came from in physical therapy. It means you should focus on the healthy tissue that is being formed around the dead stuff.

As you might have imagined, coming back from degenerative tendinopathy is a long road. Most people don't have the right plan or discipline to follow a progressive program for months. It takes professional oversight and a marathon mindset to battle back from degenerative tendinopathy.

Phase 4: Reactive on disrepair/degeneration

Reactive on disrepair/degeneration (RDD) describes what happens when the healthy tissue beginning to form around the dead holes becomes aggravated. Some discomfort, even swelling and inflammation, is normal as tendons are put through progressively tougher loads and training modalities. Determining how much RDD is healthy versus counterproductive depends on your anatomy, your history, and your specific injury. Unlike true reactive phase injuries, pain and inflammation from RDD can resolve in a few days with the right behavior modifications.[84]

• • •

Now that you have a model for understanding tendinopathy, what can we do about it? According to most forward-thinking physios, there's only one treatment option: *progressive load training.*

How to Resolve Tendinopathy

Severe tendinopathy cases, or those that have been present for several weeks or longer, should be managed by a physical therapist. But you can resolve mild cases of tendinopathy yourself by adjusting exercise habits and building load tolerance in the injured tendon. While your tendon's load tolerance is governed by dozens of variables, including genetics, medication, and anatomy, you can increase it with progressive load training. Not only does intelligent load training reduce pain, it's the only clear path forward to normal tendon function.

In the old days, the first few weeks of tendinopathy were treated with plenty of rest, enough OTC pills to shut down your liver, and some light stretching. Maybe even some electrical stimulation from a TENS unit or massage therapy. I can confirm from personal experience that the conventional approach of treating tendinopathy as an inflammation-based injury doesn't always work. After three years of dealing with severe medial epicondylitis (pain in the inner elbow, a.k.a. golfer's elbow), I was told by a sports medicine physician that my pain was purely caused by overuse and inflammation. He prescribed an anti-inflammatory drug and suggested resting for one to two weeks. Even then, I knew better. But I was desperate, so I went along with it. Two weeks later, the pain had subsided some. But my first light exercise session after the rest period caused my elbow pain to flare up worse than ever. The anti-inflammatory did me no good. And the two-week rest period did nothing but allow my tendon structures to become weaker (confirming, once again, the "use it or lose it" principle of connective tissue health). It would be another three years before I got back to preinjury strength levels.

Tendinopathy treatment shouldn't focus exclusively on controlling inflammation. The primary focus should be on restoring function with progressive load training to trigger cellular healing responses. Studies show this can be accomplished with slow resistance training and gradual reintroduction of sports or lifestyle-specific movements that triggered the injury.[84] The reason exercise is the only logical treatment for restoring tendon function is because tendon injuries follow the *law of mechanotransduction.* It's responsible for structural healing, cleaning up scar tissue, and realigning collagen fibers into more optimal patterns that prevent future injuries.[88] This is a key reason why proactive therapists and trainers start working with postinjury clients as soon as possible to gain back range of motion and strength.

And only load-bearing exercise has the benefit of cellular changes via mechanotransduction. NSAIDs can't do that. Neither can steroid injections. Or icing, electrical stimulation, or listening to healing music frequencies. The only way to get past tendinopathy is to exercise for load capacity and tissue remodeling, using pain as your guide.[89]

A useful framework for thinking about tendinopathy recovery is the EdUReP model.[90] EdUReP stands for Education, Unloading, Reloading, Prevention:

- **Education**: Learn about your tendinopathy causes, outcome expectations, and best practices for recovery.

- **Unloading**: For a brief time period, reduce training load and repetitive activities that cause painful flare-ups.

- **Reloading**: Build up load capacity gradually, starting with light resistance exercise and extremely slow repetitions that do not trigger a pain response (e.g. 3–5 full seconds to lift the weight and 3–5 seconds to lower the weight). Start by performing 3 sets of 10–15 repetitions on two nonconsecutive days per week. When you're able to complete the exercises with minimal pain (3 or less on a scale of 1–10: 0 = no pain, 10 = unbearable pain) and recover fully in between sessions, then increase the resistance by 10%–20%.

  Continue with this progression until you reach a threshold of resistance that only allows you to complete 5 or 6 repetitions with good form.

By this point, you will have significantly increased your load tolerance and joint integrity. As long as your pain levels stay at a 3 out of 10 or less as a subjective pain score, keep increasing the resistance each week.

- **Prevention**: Continue corrective exercise training for at least 8–12 weeks after symptoms resolve and take steps to prevent the underlying tendinopathy.

The last step of the EdURep model—*Prevention*—is the most troublesome. You might feel relief as soon as you stop the offending activity. But that doesn't mean the problem is solved. Studies of Achilles and patellar tendinopathy show that both collagen accumulation and collagen degradation rates are increased after only four weeks of targeted load training. Collagen turnover is elevated at this point, which is a good thing because it means new cells are replacing damaged ones. However, only after 11 weeks of targeted load training does collagen degradation slow down, with collagen accumulation remaining elevated (indicating that most of the clean-up processes have finished and you are accumulating net collagen mass).[91] This is why it is so vital to continue slow-paced, connective tissue-specific training for a full 8–12 weeks after you develop tendinopathy—even if you are no longer experiencing symptoms. In the next chapter, we'll dive into exactly how to maximize connective tissue adaptations to exercise.

How long does it take tendinopathy to heal?

Tendinopathy can take months or longer to fully resolve. Even then, it's common for symptoms to reoccur when your training loads increase or you engage in repetitive activities. Many clinicians suggest returning to your sport or hobby when you can complete regular activities without your pain level going above a 3 out of 10 as a subjective pain score. Tendinopathy recovery requires patience and discipline. You will likely experience some setbacks on your road to full recovery. During these times, take a step back and use the EdUReP model to correct course and prevent the injury from degrading further.

Here, I want to highlight a few important concepts:

1. It's not just about inflammation. In fact, inflammation is likely only a short-term variable during the reactive phase. Any inflammation (and subsequent pain) that follows during the rehabilitation phase should be used as a guide.

2. Early implementation of load management is critical to initiate repair mechanisms. Strength training should commence shortly after the injury or when symptoms occur. Conversely, passive rest will further

reduce load-bearing potential of the injured tendon and inhibit repair mechanisms. Your goal should be to increase your tendon's load tolerance past any levels of stress it will face in your everyday life or training. But do so gradually—only increase resistance 10%–20% from week to week.

3. You shouldn't stretch an injured tendon in the reactive tendinopathy phase. While it's important to maintain pain-free ranges of motion, stretching may increase the injured tendon's compression against bone, further damaging the collagen matrix.[92] Early in the injury phases, self-myofascial release techniques focused on loosening up surrounding muscles can provide some relief and may even increase flexibility (but make sure you target muscles—don't risk aggravating an already upset tendon by mashing on it with massage devices). Stretching can and should be implemented in later phases of tendinopathy recovery, but not while the tendon is still reactive and painful.

4. The joint aches and pains you're feeling right now, at this very moment, probably fall somewhere in the middle of this continuum. Few injuries are absolutely acute. Even traumatic injuries like tearing a rotator cuff in your shoulder are more often preceded by a gradual breakdown of the collagen base over a period of months or years leading up to the injury. This point is backed up by research that shows a "healthy tendon is up to twice as strong as the muscle, making the body of the tendon unlikely to tear before the muscle unless the tendon has already been weakened by degenerative changes."[79]

3. IMPROVE SYNOVIAL FLUID HEALTH

DOROTHY: How did you ever get like this?
TIN MAN: Well, about a year ago, I was chopping that tree—minding my own business—when suddenly it started to rain. And right in the middle of a chop, I . . . I rusted solid. And I've been that way ever since.

— from *The Wizard of Oz*

Historians believe the Tin Man character from *The Wizard of Oz* represented the plight of American steel industry workers. In the 1930s, during the Depression, steel factories shut down. Manufacturing plants were abandoned, and so were the employees. The depiction of the Tin Man so rusted he cannot move illustrates this tragic time. But I see another metaphor: a worker, joints frozen stiff from age and overuse. A condition that progresses so slowly, so persistently, that it seems to take hold in a moment, like rust forming on metal after a rain. And just like the Tin Man needs oil to keep his joints lubricated, you need synovial fluid to keep yours lubricated.

Synovial fluid is the viscous liquid that fills the empty space within your joints, providing lubrication and support. As satisfying as the Tin Man's creaky joints metaphor is, that comparison doesn't explain how synovial fluid works. A more fitting metaphor is tire pressure.

Your joints are like tires, and synovial fluid is like the air that fills the empty space inside. Too little air, and the tire collapses, unable to support the weight of the vehicle. Too much air, and the tire could bulge or even burst from excess pressure. Just like with tire pressure, your joints need a healthy balance of synovial fluid to stay strong and mobile. This is called *hydrodynamic pressure*—the pressure of a liquid within a confined space. If you've ever hydroplaned while driving a vehicle, you've experienced this phenomenon.

When you drive a car on a wet road, hydrodynamic pressure forces water into the gap between the tires and the road. As driving speed increases, so does pressure in the water underneath each tire. This causes a momentary loss of control as your car balances on the thin sheet of pressurized water instead of the road.

As brilliant as this explanation is, I can't take credit for it. David Burris is a mechanical engineering professor at the University of Delaware. In a presentation at the AVS 62nd International Symposium and Exhibition, he used this example to explain how cartilage reabsorbs synovial fluid that leaks out.[93]

Unlike tires, cartilage is porous, and synovial fluid constantly leaks out into the space surrounding the joint. Since loss of synovial fluid leads to increased friction and cartilage thinning, it's partially responsible for joint degeneration and osteoarthritis.

Burris and his colleagues hypothesized that hydrodynamic pressure—created from moving joints—was responsible for driving escaped synovial fluid back into cartilage, preserving fluid balance, and protecting joints from degradation. To test the idea, they slid pieces of cartilage against glass at various speeds, measuring the amount of friction and cartilage erosion. At slower speeds, there was little hydrodynamic pressure, which increased stress on the cartilage. At higher speeds, like what joints experience while walking, the opposite happened. Hydrodynamic pressure increased, like a car hydroplaning on a wet road, and cartilage erosion was minimized. Burris believes that hydrodynamic pressure created from moving joints reduces friction and drives synovial fluid back into cartilage, counteracting fluid lost.

"We know that cartilage thickness is maintained over decades in the joint, and this is the first direct insight into why. It is activity itself that combats the natural deflation process associated with interstitial lubrication," Burris said.

The take-home message is that activity is the driving force behind joint lubrication. This has implications for both how to warm up before exercising and what to do when you're feeling stiff. High-repetition exercise has fallen out of favor in the strength and conditioning world, replaced by low-repetition movements with heavy resistance. It's also been wiped out of warm-up strategy. Strength coaches have rightly transitioned to more scientific methods of preparing athletes for training, using explosive movements and progressive resistance to prepare the central nervous system for max effort. But for stiff joints, high-repetition movements with a deliberate tempo pump your joint capsules full of cushioning synovial fluid.

The Role of Synovial Fluid (SF) in Joint Pain

There are a few different ways SF affects joint pain. If a joint contains too much or too little, or if the SF is full of inflammatory compounds, you're going to feel it.

Inflammatory arthritis is marked by an increased volume of SF with less hyaluronic acid. This makes the liquid too thin and watery, reducing its cushioning effects within the joints.[40] An increase in SF volume alone can cause pain and cartilage damage as well.[94] The joint becomes distended, like a water balloon pumped so full that it starts to bulge. This is why earlier, I said to pay attention to feelings of *pressure*. Pressure indicates swelling and SF disruption, often long before you can see it visually.

In osteoarthritis, SF can act as a reservoir for inflammatory cytokines.[99] When inflammatory cells aggregate in SF, they distend joints, compress blood vessels, stimulate pain receptors, and perpetuate the inflammatory response. This is termed *synovitis*—inflammation of synovial membranes.

Another type of arthritis called post-traumatic arthritis (PTA) is induced by injury. PTA accounts for about 12% of all osteoarthritis cases.[95] Patients with PTA experience increased swelling and SF effusion—leakage into the surrounding tissue. Effusion results in lower volumes of fluid around cartilage and an extremely viscous liquid that is less capable of transporting nutrients. Injuries also disrupt the balance of SF in your joints. In response to an acute injury, SF concentrations can increase up to 20 times greater than normal. You can imagine how this presses on pain receptors.

Things that Damage SF Health

- **Prolonged sedentary periods:** Movement bathes your joints in SF. Sitting at a desk all day, or otherwise not moving regularly, reduces SF concentrations within joints. I notice this particularly in my knees after a long day of writing at my desk.

- **Joint immobilization:** If you use braces or wraps to protect weak joints, make sure you move through full ranges of motion before and after using them. Prolonged immobilization of joints reduces hyaluronic acid concentrations within SF and reduces the clearance of inflammatory compounds.[96]

- **Repeated mechanical stress combined with SF effusion:** Repetitive tasks, especially after an injury or when SF leaks out of the capsule and into surrounding tissues, damages cartilage structures and causes accumulation of inflammatory compounds within SF.

- **Acute injuries:** As already noted, acute injuries cause SF leakage, swelling, and increased viscosity that does not work well as a joint cushion.

The Synovial Fluid Pain Feedback Loop

1. A lack of SF causes joints to grind together, causing inflammation and pain.

2. Increased pain and inflammation lead to reduced mobility. Your comfortable range of motion decreases.

3. Reduced mobility and pain lead to less overall movement. Moving hurts, so you stop. This leads to even less SF, more pain, and even less movement. And so the cycle continues until the pain is beyond your ability to withstand and the condition is totally debilitating.

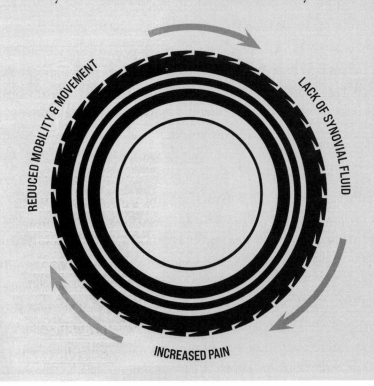

REDUCED MOBILITY & MOVEMENT

LACK OF SYNOVIAL FLUID

INCREASED PAIN

How to Improve Synovial Fluid Health

- **Exercise frequently:** Short, frequent exercise is better for SF balance than long, nonstop sessions. For example, 30 minutes of interval training is better for improving SF in the knees than two hours of nonstop jogging. If you sit in place for long periods during the day, set reminders to stand up every hour to stretch. Flex your knees, squat, twist, bend, and reach. Even if you don't implement a specific stretching method, just moving more in between sedentary sessions will keep your joints in shape. I spend around eight hours per day in front of my computer, with breaks. I have reminders set at three points throughout the day to stand up and stretch my hips, knees, shoulders, and wrists. It makes a big difference. I also have a convertible stand up desk in my office, though I only use it for around an hour per day.

- **Keep moving:** Even if you can't do the exercises you want to, find a way to keep moving. Shoulders too banged up to lift heavy weights? Grab those light dumbbells and elastic bands and work on muscular endurance. Back in too much pain to swing a golf club? Don't lie around, waiting for it to get better. Keep moving. Walk, stretch, do whatever you can without pain, but keep moving. The more you follow this rule, the faster you'll be back to full function. Only movement squeezes SF back into the joint capsule. So don't let yourself become the Tin Man. As exercise physiologists like to say, "motion is lotion."

- **Perform isometric contractions:** An isometric contraction is where you actively hold a muscle at a fixed length, usually performed with resistance. When you perform an isometric contraction, pressure increases within your muscle and joint capsule.[97] This improves load tolerance—the amount of stress a tissue can withstand before rupturing or breaking down—without the risk of movement. It's the safest way to improve both load tolerance and SF health with exercise. In a study published in *The Journal of Physical Therapy Science*, 42 men and women (aged 40–65 years) with knee osteoarthritis followed an isometric exercise program for five weeks. Not only did the experimental group see greater improvements in pain relief and mobility, their strength improvement was also 33% greater than the control group. That's pretty remarkable when you consider the only exercises the experimental group performed consisted of squeezing their leg muscles for 5–10 seconds at a time.[98] Isometric contractions can even reduce inflammatory cytokine levels within SF to help bring down inflammation, allowing the healing process to run naturally.[15]

- **Hydrate before exercise:** We've known for a while that there is a high correlation between subjective pain levels and dehydration. Neuroscience researchers have illuminated why, showing that dehydration causes neurological changes that interfere with medication and even cognitive behavioral therapy.[100] There is also a physiological component. Your cartilage is made of 65%–90% water.[101] When you are dehydrated, your joints grind together, causing inflammation and erosion. Make a conscious effort to hydrate well before exercise and keep sipping water throughout your session.

- **Warm up stiff joints with a deliberate tempo:** Before resistance training, perform a couple of sets of lightweight, high-repetition movements focusing on the body part giving you grief (2–3 sets of 15–25 repetitions). The movement speed shouldn't be explosive but shouldn't be grindingly slow either. Use a smooth, rhythmic tempo. Start with an abbreviated range of motion that does not cause any joint pain. Then gradually expand the range of motion with each repetition until you can complete the full range of motion without feeling stiffness. Perform the exercise in the exact same way you'd lubricate a squeaky door hinge: short, deliberate movements first, then full range of motion as more lubricant (synovial fluid) makes its way into the hinge (joint).

- **Try supplements that increase joint lubrication:** Collagen, hyaluronic acid, glucosamine, and chondroitin are components of the extracellular matrix—the fluidlike mix of compounds that provides structural support for your cells. You may recognize these names as popular nutritional supplements, but they're also fundamental pieces of natural human anatomy. The fabled glucosamine-chondroitin supplement combination has fallen out of favor in recent years, despite showing consistent but underwhelming positive effects on joint health compared to placebos.[102] Collagen and hyaluronic acid have grown in popularity, and for good reason. They show promise for relieving joint pain by up to 30% and improving joint mobility.[102]

4. PROTECT COLLAGEN HEALTH

Maintaining healthy inflammation levels, avoiding tendinopathy, and keeping your cartilage bathed in nutritious synovial fluid will go a long way toward protecting your future collagen health. But time still marches on. With age and overuse, collagen erosion happens. Thinning cartilage structures that once cushioned bone-on-bone connections are no longer thick or flexible enough to do their job. Nerves are pinched between bony tissues, flexibility is lost within joint capsules, and connective tissue becomes brittle.[103]

Fortunately, there are several things you can do to strengthen and protect the collagen structures that make up your connective tissue. In the next chapter, we'll dive into how to increase collagen synthesis for strong, pain-free, age-defying joints. You'll learn the role of collagen within connective tissue, how to produce more of it, how to slow down joint degradation, and exercise techniques for building strong collagen formations.

KEY TAKEAWAY

In the pre-1990s era, it was widely accepted that chronic joint degeneration was strictly caused by inflammation. The prevailing treatments focused exclusively on reducing inflammation: anti-inflammatory drugs, NSAIDs, and corticosteroid injections.[45]

Recent studies cast doubt on the inflammation-based model, as they show that collagen disruption and thinning happens in tendinopathy patients without an inflammatory cause. Collagen degradation and joint pain can also be caused by a lack of synovial fluid.

While the medical world is still divided on the best ways to address chronic joint pain and tendinopathy, taking a four-pronged approach to pain management is your best bet for short-term relief and long-term health. Focus on modulating inflammation, resolving tendinopathy, improving synovial fluid health, and protecting your collagen.

How to Train Your Collagen

Current scientific evidence strongly supports the idea that the development of muscle strength during a training process is not necessarily accompanied by an adequate modulation of tendon stiffness.

... Muscle responds well to a wide range of exercise modalities with an increase of strength. Tendon tissue on the other hand seems only to be responsive to high magnitude loading and repetitive loading cycles featuring long tendon strain durations.

—Mersmann et al., 2017[89]

In 1965, the football coach at the University of Florida hired a team of scientists to create a drink that rapidly replenished fluids and electrolytes lost during games. The first version contained a mixture of water, salt, sugar, potassium, phosphate, and lemon juice. A small group of players tested the concoction and reported feeling sustained energy. Soon, the entire team was gulping down the lemon-flavored beverage during practices and games. Word spread quickly throughout college football that a new performance-enhancing drink was giving University of Florida players an unfair advantage.

The Florida Gators gained momentum over the next few years, edging out the Georgia Tech Yellow Jackets in the 1967 Orange Bowl. During an interview after the game, Bobby Dodd, head coach of the Yellow Jackets, attributed his team's loss to not having the same nutrition as the Gators: "We didn't have Gatorade. That made the difference."

This marked the start of The Gatorade Company, Inc.—a sports nutrition beverage brand now manufactured by Pepsi and distributed worldwide. What we see as a sugar-laden commodity present in every gas station cooler was the most innovative sports nutrition product of its time. From the beginning, the scientists at Gatorade were innovators. Their spirit and culture live on in the Gatorade Sports Science Institute (GSSI)—a think tank made up of dieticians, biochemists, exercise physiologists, and other scientific researchers dedicated to advancing human performance through nutrition science.

Proper hydration and electrolyte balance are still important principles for peak athletic performance, but they are yesterday's discovery. Today, GSSI scientists study the effects of nutrition on the entire human body before, during, and after exercise. Their newer research spans into injury management and connective tissue healing—ways to help athletes get back on the field sooner without sacrificing their long-term health. One such study delved into how nutrient timing and therapeutic exercise techniques can accelerate recovery after soft tissue injuries. The GSSI researchers connected injury recovery outcomes to a key but little-known process called *collagen synthesis*.[104]

Collagen synthesis is a blanket term that describes how your body produces, aggregates, and forms collagen structures. It's an important concept to understand because it directly impacts injury recovery time, tissue repair quality, future injury risk, and overall joint mobility. From an athletic training perspective, collagen synthesis should get the same amount of attention as muscular strength, speed, and performance training. But it doesn't. This is evidenced by the increasingly high rate of soft tissue injuries among athletes.

In high-contact sports such as football, soft tissue injuries (muscle, tendon, ligaments, etc.) account for about 70% of visits to physical therapists.[105] Most of those involve connective tissue rather than just muscle, with at least half coming from overuse injuries rather than sudden acute injuries. According to the Centers for Disease Control (CDC), these figures roughly apply to youth and weekend-warrior adults as well as serious athletes:[106]

- Overuse injuries account for about half of all sports injuries in middle school and high school aged students.

- Since 2000, there has been a fivefold increase in shoulder and elbow injuries among youth baseball and softball players.

- The parts of the body most frequently injured while engaging in sports and recreation activities are the lower extremity (42.0%), upper extremity (30.3%), and head and neck (16.4%).[107]

- More than half of all sports injuries are preventable.

Clearly, joint health lags behind muscular strength, endurance, and performance advancements. As I'll explain, this is a big part of the problem. We're building bigger, stronger muscles. Faster, more powerful athletes. But we're doing it on the scaffolding of stiff, injury-prone joint structures. We need a better way to prevent soft tissue injuries. While many sports medicine professionals still cling tightly to the dogmatic approach of anti-inflammatory drugs, rest, and ice, the science of collagen synthesis provides insight into how we can do better.

Chapter 3 gave you the tools to understand and manage pain naturally. This chapter expands on that, focusing on how you can leverage collagen synthesis to speed up recovery from injuries, improve mobility, and build resilient, pain-free joints. If you're battling through an injury right now, feel like you are injury-prone, or are suffering from joint pain and tendinopathy, understanding and applying the principles behind collagen synthesis can be the difference between getting back to full function and staying on the sidelines indefinitely.

To understand collagen synthesis, we first have to understand what collagen is. We will start our discussion by reviewing the role of collagen in your body, the four stages of collagen synthesis, and how collagen relates to connective tissue health.

What Is Collagen, Anyway?

Despite the typical oversimplified explanations of what collagen is, it's quite a bizarre molecule. In its natural form, collagen consists of three coiled subunits containing exactly 1,050 amino acids. These coils are wound together into a characteristic triple helix structure.

Collagen is the second most abundant substance in the human body (behind water), accounting for about 30% of the total protein. It provides structural support for virtually all organs and soft tissue (including joints).[108] As you age, your body produces less collagen. By age 60, your ability to produce collagen has decreased by 50%, causing aging joints, saggy skin, and lean muscle tissue loss.[109] Thus, it follows that preserving collagen mass in joints and skin is an integral part of healthy aging. It's also why the collagen supplement industry is booming (despite whether the myriad of claims made by supplement marketers are substantiated).

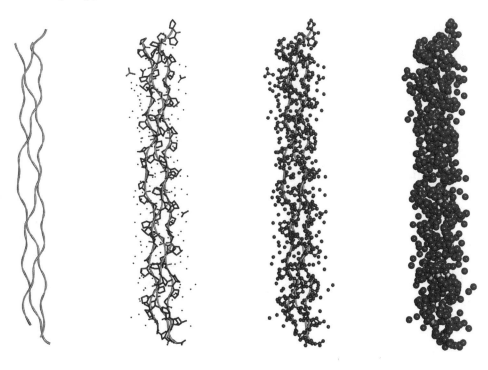

FIGURE 4.1

Triple helix structure of collagen peptides.

Now that we have the obligatory "Collagen 101" lesson out of the way, let's briefly look at the four stages of collagen synthesis. Each one plays a vital role in the growth, remodeling, and accumulation of collagen in your body. Understanding how different environmental factors affect these four stages gives you insight into building healthy joints.

THE FOUR STAGES OF COLLAGEN SYNTHESIS

Collagen synthesis can be broken down into four distinct stages.[110] Without getting (too) lost in the weeds, here is a quick overview:

1. Collagen biosynthesis: the production of collagen in the body

Collagen biosynthesis can be likened to making clay into bricks, which will eventually be used to construct a wall.

Why it matters: Collagen biosynthesis determines how much raw material is produced for your joints to rebuild with and can be directly influenced by nutrition, exercise, and lifestyle factors. Supplementing with collagen peptides made from types I and III appears to boost collagen biosynthesis.[111]

2. Collagen cross-linking: the building of connections between collagen molecules to form collagen fibrils (strawlike chains)

Think of collagen cross-linking as mortaring bricks together when building a wall. It describes the building of connections.

Why it matters: Heavily cross-linked collagen is more resistant to degradation than less cross-linked collagen. And diet influences this process. For example, animal studies show prolonged low-energy diets and low-protein diets may interfere with cross-linking.[112] Studies also show that copper deficiency impairs collagen cross-linking, leading to weak formations that are easily irritated and torn.[113]

3. Collagen fibril formation: the bundling of semi-crystalline collagen chains

Here is where my brick wall metaphor falls apart.... Forget about the wall made from bricks for a second. Collagen fibrils are more like a bundle of straws held together.

Why it matters: The growth, size, and shape of these fibrils are influenced by tissue type, age, and stage of development. These fibrils' composition largely determines how healthy, flexible, and resistant to degradation the soft tissue is. After an injury, fibril formation quality can be enhanced or damaged depending on your exercise habits.

AMINO ACID SEQUENCE

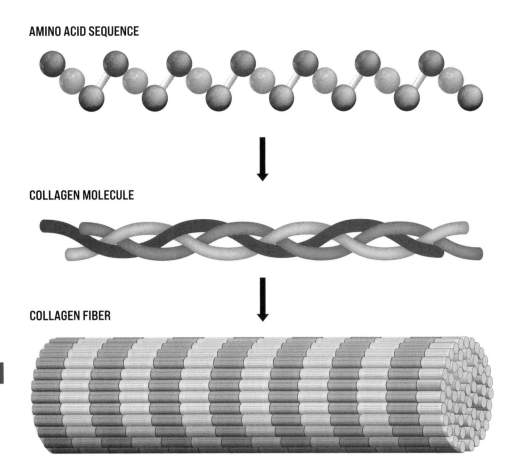

COLLAGEN MOLECULE

COLLAGEN FIBER

How collagen fibers are formed.

Figure 4.2 illustrates the strawlike structure that is formed when collagen is cross-linked with adjacent molecules. This image is more "zoomed out" than the molecular structure image of the collagen triple helix illustration in Figure 4.1.

4. Collagenolysis: the collagen degradation process

Why it matters: It sounds bad, but collagen degradation is an essential physiological process for injury and wound repair.[114] It kickstarts the remodeling of suboptimal collagen formations, which is necessary to repair new injuries and replace scar tissue with healthy tissue.

While some collagenolysis is necessary, excessive collagen degradation causes loss of connective tissue mass and is one of the primary drivers of joint aging and disease. Collagen degradation doesn't just happen with aging, though. A significant portion (up to 15% in animal studies) of newly synthesized collagen is broken down.[115] This is termed *basal degradation*. Because such a significant portion of newly formed collagen is lost immediately, this is a key leverage point for improving joint health.

Now, let's zoom out to better understand how collagen synthesis relates to connective tissue health. The next section reviews the primary connective tissue types and how collagen structures within joints adapt to your exercise habits.

CONNECTIVE TISSUE TYPES AND FUNCTIONS

Your joints and muscles are bound together by connective tissue. Beyond providing structural integrity, connective tissue helps transmit force, protect muscles and bones from injury, shuttle nutrients around, and repair damaged cells. Each has a different role in the muscular force production process, which depends not only on its anatomical structure but also on the collagen content and arrangement. There are five primary types of joint connective tissue:

- **Tendons:** Tendons connect muscles to bones. They're more compliant (stretchy) than ligaments but more rigid than muscles. Tendons are responsible for much of the force transfer through the body during movement.

- **Ligaments:** Ligaments connect bones to other bones. Their primary purpose is joint stabilization.

- **Cartilage:** Cartilage acts as a cushioning barrier within joints and between bones. Unlike tendons and ligaments, cartilage lacks blood vessels and nerves, making it a problematic connective tissue for the body to repair.

- **Intramuscular:** This is connective tissue that runs directly through and between muscle fibers. It helps transfer force from muscles to tendons and vice versa.

- **Fascia:** Fascia is the thin sheath of connective tissue that surrounds muscles. It plays a pivotal role in force transfer between parts of the kinetic chain. Fascia is dense with nerve endings, making it almost as sensitive as skin. This is part of the reason why manual therapy methods like foam rolling and massage have so much support for pain and tension relief.

When a muscle contracts to produce force, energy is transmitted through the muscle and radiated out to intramuscular connective tissue. If you've ever seen a cut of meat with white lines tracing through it, that is intramuscular connective tissue. Generally, meat from older and stronger animals has more connective tissue. It's a stiffer, tougher cut of meat—not ideal for the butcher, but better for the animal (while it was alive) to run and jump explosively with. Conversely, more tender cuts of meat come from animals with relatively little intramuscular connective tissue. Unlike their athletic counterparts, these animals lived a more sedentary lifestyle. It works the same way in your body. If you exercise with heavy resistance, you'll have denser intramuscular connective tissue.

Even though you might think of muscular force as the process of muscle fibers contracting, much of the force production process depends on connective tissue. Upwards of 80% of muscular force produced transfers to surrounding connective tissue.[116] The purpose of this is twofold: it moves energy out of the muscle's way—so it can contract—and it triggers the surrounding connective tissue fibers to bind together to protect them from injury. An important variable that determines how your connective tissue reacts to the force production process is movement speed.

To illustrate why movement speed matters, think about the last time you did a belly flop into a swimming pool. It didn't feel good, did it? Belly flops feel more like being smacked with a giant plastic sheet than falling into a liquid pool. That's because in response to sudden force, water molecules strengthen the tension that connects them, creating a massive surface area capable of knocking the wind out of you.

Now picture yourself standing in the shallow end of the pool. With one arm, you slowly drag your hand horizontally through the water. This time, the water acts more like water. The slow velocity of your hand movement allows the molecules to move individually, rather than joining forces into a belly-smacking sheet of liquid pain.

This is how collagen fibers in your joints work. If you lift weights forcefully or move explosively, your connective tissue tenses up into a rigid sheet. And thankfully so, or your joints would disintegrate every time you moved quickly. But when you move slowly, your connective tissues act more like individual collagen fibers. This is why using slow, deliberate motions while lifting weights helps activate collagen remodeling—breaking apart old junky cross-links, increasing collagen turnover, and allowing your body to rebuild more robust connective tissue structures.[89,117]

After force is transferred through the muscle and intramuscular connective tissue, it moves along the tendon. It's then transferred to the bone, the final stop within the body. Throughout this process, connective tissue plays multiple roles—one of the most important being a shock absorber. It has to be stiff enough to transfer force from muscles efficiently but pliable enough to bend without snapping. The Goldilocks principle applies here: an ideal balance of stiffness and flexibility. There's also variability of stiffness within parts of connective tissue. For example, on the muscular end of the tendon, collagen fibrils are more pliable. On the bone end, they're stiffer and stronger.

Intramuscular connective tissue, tendons, ligaments, and the fascia sheath surrounding muscles are all made primarily of collagen—specifically, type I collagen. As you recall, collagen plays the same role in your joints as bricks that make up a house's walls. Based on this understanding of connective tissue's anatomy and physiology, we can start to assemble a picture of how to build optimal connective tissue structures. We know that connective tissue stiffness is dependent on the total amount of collagen present and the amount of cross-linking. We also know that cross-links increase with power, speed, and heavy resistance training.

Now, this is where things get interesting. *The opposite is also true.* Collagen cross-links can be broken by movements that produce high shear forces between adjacent collagen molecules.[118] Just as your muscles can break down and rebuild stronger with resistance training, so can your joints with intelligent use of connective tissue training principles.

CONNECTIVE TISSUE TRAINING STRATEGIES

At this point, I want to stop and outline a few terms that are crucial to intelligent connective tissue training. You will see these concepts referenced several times throughout the book.

There are three primary types of muscle contractions. Each affects skeletal muscle and connective tissues differently:

1. **Eccentric contraction:** A contraction where the muscle lengthens under load or tension. Think of this as the lowering or lengthening phase of an exercise. For example, the downward phase of a push-up forces your chest muscles to lengthen and simultaneously contract to control the lowering movement. By definition, eccentric contractions occur when the opposing force is greater than the muscular contraction force.

2. **Concentric contraction:** Any muscle contraction where the muscle shortens during the movement. Think of this as the lifting phase of an exercise. When performing a push-up, your chest muscles contract as you push yourself away from the ground.

3. **Isometric contraction:** Eccentric and concentric contractions fall into a broader category called *isotonic contractions*—where muscle length is changed by force applied. An *isometric contraction* occurs when force is generated without the muscle length changing. A classic example is pushing against a wall. You may not move the wall, but you can still exert a massive amount of force against it. Isometric contractions can occur at any point throughout a movement's range of motion. If you hold the bottom position of a push-up with your chest off the ground, that is an isometric contraction that challenges your chest muscles in a fully lengthened position. Holding the top position of a push-up with your arms extended will create an isometric contraction in your shoulders and triceps as they tense up to keep your body from falling to the ground.

When you add the variables of exercise tempo, exercise selection, body mechanics, and rest periods to these three types of contractions, you get a multitude of training strategies that affect muscles and connective tissue in different ways. By understanding how and when to use these training strategies, you can make consistent fitness improvements while also fortifying your joints.

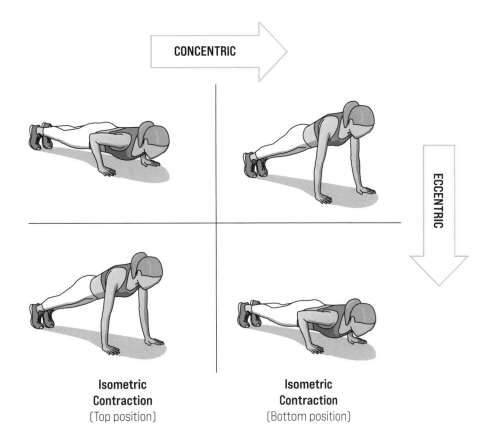

CONCENTRIC

ECCENTRIC

Isometric Contraction
(Top position)

Isometric Contraction
(Bottom position)

Isometric, eccentric, and concentric phases of a push-up.

Isometric Training

This type of training simply utilizes isometric contractions to challenge your muscles and joint systems. The list of proven benefits is staggering. Studies show isometric training does the following:

- Reduces joint pain levels quickly with low injury risk[98,119]

- Reduces cortical inhibition, boosting muscle strength[120]

- Recruits more motor units and creates more force production than traditional resistance training

- Requires less training time to complete

- Prevents reductions in bone density with aging and may increase the mineral content of injured bones[121]

- Improves cardiovascular conditioning and reduces blood pressure[97]

During the initial stages of tendinopathy, isometric training focused on the midrange of the tendon's motion helps reduce pain and build load tolerance without overstressing or compressing the tendon.[120] When normal exercise hurts, isometric exercise is a good way to stimulate muscles and tendons without aggravating the injury. In my experience, it's the most underutilized therapeutic fitness strategy. Why? I would guess it is because isometric training doesn't provide the same psychological satisfaction as flinging weights through space, and it requires intense effort to get the benefits. While isometric exercise shouldn't take the place of regular resistance training, it's a useful training tool that should be part of your routine.

Eccentric Training

This is a form of resistance training that emphasizes slowing down the lowering phase of an exercise to challenge the muscles' ability to elongate, build strength and muscle mass, and optimize collagen formations within connective tissue. It creates more muscular force than any other exercise type. It also produces the largest increases in muscle fiber length, making it a useful flexibility training method.[122] When implemented correctly, it's a relatively safe way to train with weights. Eccentric training has been shown to reduce soccer players' hamstring injury rates by up to 70% and aid in tendinopathy healing.[123]

Heavy Slow Resistance Training (HSR)

HSR utilizes both eccentric and concentric contractions, heavy resistance, and slow repetition speeds. The reason "heavy" is in the name is not necessarily because you're supposed to use heavy weights. It is because the goal of HSR is to progressively increase the resistance with each training session while lowering the number of repetitions performed. Generally, you should start with a light training load that does not trigger a pain response (e.g. 3 sets of 15 repetitions), then progressively increase the weight and reduce repetitions. This gradually builds the load tolerance of the tendon, encourages increased collagen turnover, and relieves pain.[117]

Compared to eccentric-only training, you can produce positive tendon adaptations in less time with HSR. Also, clinical reports show more adherence from clients who use HSR for tendinopathy recovery than just eccentric training, indicating that it's more efficient and enjoyable.[120] In physical therapy practices, HSR is an essential part of rehabilitating damaged connective tissue. But you don't have to wait until you are injured to utilize it.

Synovial Training

Any exercise designed to improve the circulation of synovial fluid in joints is called *synovial training*. When I use this term, I am typically referring to low resistance movements performed with a deliberate speed for high repetitions. As far as I know, "synovial training" is a not a recognized or commonly used phrase in the fitness world. However, I find it a helpful term to use in conversations about connective tissue training.

Energy Load Training

Dynamic exercise that forces your muscles and joints to store energy before quickly releasing it—for example, squatting down before jumping up—is referred to as *energy load training*. As much as I talk about the value of slow repetitions, isometric contractions, and eccentric training, you might think I am against explosive movement training. On the contrary, training your joints to store and release energy efficiently is vital to preventing injuries and building real-world, functional strength.

The most common type of energy load training is *plyometrics*—exercises where muscles exert maximum force in short time periods to increase power. Examples include box jumps, power skipping, and medicine ball throws. The terms *energy load training* and *plyometrics* are often used synonymously, but energy load training has a broader meaning. Essentially, it refers to any exercise where there is a fast turn around between the eccentric contraction and concentric contraction.

Now that we have outlined some specific training strategies, let's look at how each impacts your musculoskeletal system.

SLOW AND HEAVY WINS THE RACE

Muscles are simple creatures compared to joints. While it's not easy to build big muscles, it's relatively simple when you break it down to the fundamentals. The law of progressive overload dictates that when the amount of stress placed on the musculoskeletal system gradually increases, muscle size and strength will increase along with it. Though muscles seem to respond best to moderate training volumes, sets, and rep schemes (e.g. sets of 8–12 repetitions), they can increase in size pretty much to the same extent when training with light, moderate, or heavy loads—as long as the muscles are taken close to muscular failure. Although it's commonly accepted that high repetition training with light loads is the best way to keep joint pain at bay, the research on tendon adaptations to strength training shows something entirely different. As researchers from a tendon health metastudy published in *Frontiers in Physiology* pointed out, heavy resistance training with slow repetitions produces better tendon adaptations:

> Muscle responds well to a wide range of exercise modalities with an increase of strength. Tendon tissue on the other hand seems only to be responsive to high magnitude loading and repetitive loading cycles featuring long tendon strain durations…. High strain rate and frequency modes of loading as, for instance, plyometric exercise, do not seem to consistently stimulate tendon adaptation.[89]

A study of patients with patellar tendinopathy (degeneration of the tendon located just below the kneecap) demonstrated that HSR and slow eccentric training improved short-term and long-term measures of pain, strength, and collagen turnover.[117] In the same study, patients who used corticosteroid injections to manage inflammation and pain showed short-term improvements in pain levels but poor long-term tendon health. Another study of patients with Achilles tendinopathy showed that 12 weeks of slow, eccentric-focused training increased collagen synthesis in injured tissues while not substantially affecting healthy tendons. As the researchers pointed out, this could indicate a relationship between necessary collagen turnover and tendon injury recovery.[118]

The research is clear: slowing down your resistance training tempo is the best way to strengthen tendons and improve collagen metabolism. But it's not just about tendon strain duration. Force production is another key variable for tendon health. For instance, a study from the *Journal of Experimental Biology* measured Achilles tendon adaptations in two different training groups. Group 1 followed an isometric exercise program consisting of 55% maximum voluntary contraction (MVC), or low strain. Group 2 followed a high tendon loading protocol at 90% MVC. At the end of 14 weeks, only the heavy tendon loading group had significant improvements in tendon strength.[124] While heavy training elicits favorable tendon adaptations along with muscle growth, short strain duration exercises (like plyometrics) and light load exercises (like high repetition weight lifting) do not.

Now you can see the problem: light, "safe" training with easy weights and high volume could theoretically produce the same muscular growth results as heavier weights. But your tendons won't adapt to the same degree. This gap combined with repetitive use and chronic joint under-recovery leaves your tendons vulnerable to gradual degeneration. Or worse.

Ironically, many people stop lifting heavy because it hurts. The solution is better programming and better exercise selection that allow for safe, heavy loading and full recovery between sessions. It turns out that lifting heavy isn't just for high-level athletes and strength competitors. It's for everyone who wants to maintain connective tissue health. It's also crucial for maintaining bone mass.

BIG BONES

If you want to get strong, you have to lift heavy. If you are less interested in getting brutally strong but still want to build muscle and maintain a low body fat percentage, heavy lifting is still an important piece of the puzzle. But there's another reason to challenge your body with heavy weights: bone density.

Bone mass peaks around age 30. After that, your bones become increasingly brittle, losing about 1% of their mass each year. As you age, your risk of osteoporosis and bone fractures increases exponentially.[125] There are two ways to prevent a bone health crisis down the road: increase your peak bone mass while you're young, and prevent excessive bone loss as you age.

When it comes to exercise, again there are two primary factors you should focus on. First and foremost, maintain a high level of load bearing movements in your daily life. Walk regularly, look for everyday opportunities to lift and carry things, and live an active lifestyle. Your bones will grow or shrink based on the demands placed on them. Second, practice heavy resistance training each week. In response to lifting heavy loads, your bones send cells called *osteoblasts* to repair minor damage. This damage is a normal part of bone remodeling. Osteoblasts act like plaster for your bones, patching cracks and building them stronger with new collagen formations. Once the collagen mineralizes, it becomes part of your bone, increasing density and mass. While weight training with even moderately heavy weights adds bone mass, studies show heavy weight training (e.g. a weight you can only lift four or five times before failure) initiates the most significant osteoblast response.[6] To be clear, I'm not saying you have to become a powerlifter to maintain bone mass. I'm merely suggesting that you perform at least some maximum effort heavy resistance training regularly instead of only using light weights and high-repetition sets.

BREAK DOWN TO BUILD UP

There's another benefit to isometric, eccentric, and HSR training beyond improving tendon strength and bone mass. These methods also help form optimal collagen fiber alignments within your connective tissue. Healthy collagen formations form a basket-weave pattern, providing a stronger structure for optimal functional movement. Abnormal collagen formations (a.k.a. scar tissue) form crude, overlapping parallel patterns. This type of tissue is weak and injury-prone (see **Figure 4.4**).[126]

During the recovery process, environmental variables such as movement habits, nutrition quality, inflammation levels, and activity can either help or hinder this process. The two main factors are total collagen available for cross-linking and the quality of collagen fibril formation.

If you have nagging joints that seem to get reinjured continually, this is likely part of the problem. Because your connective tissue healed poorly after the original injury, it's weak and prone to minor tears. This creates a repeating cycle of reinjury and inflammation. Until the scar tissue is addressed and replaced with healthy cells (or at least surrounded with healthy cells), full recovery isn't possible.[127]

Another key variable for optimizing collagen synthesis is exercise frequency. In a journal article titled "The Pathogenesis of Tendinopathy: Balancing the Response to Loading," Magnusson and colleagues showed

**HEALTHY
COLLAGEN FORMATION**

**SUBOPTIMAL
COLLAGEN FORMATION**

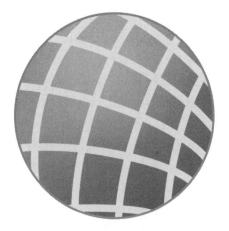

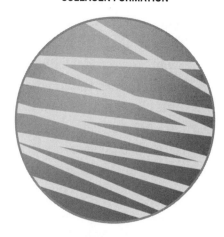

FIGURE 4.4

Healthy collagen
formation vs. suboptimal
collagen formation.

The normal "basketweave" pattern
of collagen formation provides a
stronger, more resilient tissue for
optimal functional movement.

Collagen fibers form a crude,
parallel pattern. This leads
to weak, easily irritated, and
painful tissue formations.

that collagen rebuilding in response to mechanical loading peaks at 24 hours
and stays elevated for up to three days.[128] For body part training, this gives
credence to the idea of waiting a full three to four days between sessions
(e.g. weekly upper body training on Monday and Thursday, and lower body
training on Tuesday and Friday). This ensures that the adaptive response is
not interrupted. Without sufficient rest, net loss of collagen can occur.

Understanding the connective tissue formation process gives us insight
into how to prevent injuries and heal nagging joints marked by junky scar
tissue formations. With this knowledge, you can assemble a training system
that rebuilds and maintains connective tissue structures for strong, functional joints that are resistant to breakdown, irritation, and reinjury.

EFFECTS OF SLOW RESISTANCE TRAINING ON MUSCLES

An argument can be made that slow resistance training is counterproductive for athletes because it's demanding on the nervous system, causes more
DOMS (delayed onset muscle soreness), and could reduce strength if passive
muscle stiffness is decreased too much. While these points are technically
true (at least in the short term), you'd have to push slow movement training to an extreme for these negative side effects to show up. I believe even
athletes who participate in explosive sports will benefit from interspersing
more slow repetition tempos to bolster connective tissue health and safely
increase muscle length in commonly tight muscles. For football players, volleyball players, and other athletes who rely on explosive movements during
competition, training should match the sport's demands: more plyometric

training and speed work with periods of therapeutic slow eccentric training interspersed. Recreational athletes and general population fitness enthusiasts with joint pain will benefit from an approach closer to the other side of the spectrum: more joint-friendly slow rep tempos with plyometric training interspersed at less regular intervals.

Though I've emphasized that slow eccentric movements are under-utilized for connective tissue health, you should not use a slow descent on every movement. In fact, studies show training with super slow movements is not as effective as traditional training with natural movement tempos for strength, muscle, and aerobic benefits. Many coaches see slow eccentric training as an outdated concept for building muscle and improving performance. I agree with that. But as a therapeutic approach, the science is clearly in support of eccentric and HSR training. To be clear, I'm not sure that allowing 10 seconds to lift a weight and 10 seconds to lower the weight has any practical utility (this is the repetition speed used in a commonly cited study against slow resistance training).[129,130] A 3- to 5-second eccentric phase is enough to control the movement and get the aimed-for adaptive response without going to extremes.

Again, you shouldn't rely on slow resistance training all the time. In sports especially, controlling the eccentric phase during fast movements is crucial for injury prevention and performance. Exercises like depth jumps (jumping off a box), squatting with a fast tempo, explosive push-ups, and sprinting train your muscles to lengthen safely and contract forcefully. Explosive movements are clearly superior for activating the larger and more growth-oriented fast-twitch muscle fibers.[131] While you will benefit from focusing primarily on slow, deliberate movements, you should incorporate a variety of movement tempos into your training schedule.

ENERGY LOADING AND THE MUSCLE-TENDON UNIT

If your exercise routine consists only of running or weightlifting or playing a sport, you're setting yourself up for injuries and pain later in life. Even if you implement the recommendations from this book on isometric exercise and heavy slow resistance training, you're still missing one more critical piece of the puzzle: *energy loading*. Without the ability to effectively store energy and release it quickly, your joints will always be at risk. Unless you live in a bubble, it will catch up to you sooner or later—either at the gym or in everyday life. Your ability to prevent injury during quick movements comes down to how effectively your muscles and tendons perform during the *stretch-shortening cycle* (SSC). The SSC refers to an active stretching of a muscle followed by an immediate shortening of that muscle. The faster the stretching movement, the more energy is stored and released during the SSC.

Your tendons' role in the SSC differs based on what activity you are doing and your exercise habits. Athletes who primarily perform short, repetitive, and predictable movement patterns benefit from having stiffer tendons. This allows for a shorter SSC and faster force transfer from bones to tendons. Less energy is expelled and movements are more efficient. Cycling and boxing are two examples of sports that come to mind. On the other hand, athletes who rely on dynamic movements and elastic loading—such as basketball and volleyball players—will benefit from a more compliant (less stiff) tendon.[92] Because stretching a muscle slightly before contracting it allows for greater force production, having elastic tendons becomes a competitive advantage. This is why you can jump higher when you squat down first—it stretches the muscles of your legs, creating elastic energy.

Having a baseline of tendon compliance is not only better for movement performance, it also safeguards you against injuries. To illustrate why, think about the last time you flung a rubber band across a room with your fingers. To get maximum distance, two things had to happen:

#1—The rubber band you chose needed to be stiff enough to create high amounts of elastic energy.

#2—The rubber band had to be flexible enough to allow you to stretch it out before letting it fly.

If the band was too stiff, you wouldn't have been able to stretch it out far enough to fling it effectively. If the band was too old and stretchy, you wouldn't have been able to create enough elastic energy during the stretch to get any distance. It might have even snapped in half if you tried. Your tendons work similarly. You need a healthy balance of stiffness and compliance. Researchers call this *optimal tendon stiffness*.[132] Specifically, you need optimal tendon stiffness at the intersection of your muscles and tendons. This area is called the *myotendinous junction* (MTJ).

More than any other location in your muscular system, the MTJ acts as a shock absorber and spring during explosive movements. When rapid stretch/shorten forces occur that exceed the absorption capabilities of the MTJ, muscle and tendon strain injuries result. Because of its high-stress role, and the fact that it's situated where two different types of tissue meet, it's the most common location for ruptures and overuse injuries.

To really fortify your joints and muscles against injury, you need to help your MTJs by doing two things:

1. **Perform exercises that train the SSC.** Research suggests that energy load training (but not isometric training) increases the tendons and muscles' reaction capabilities during fast stretching movements.[133] This illustrates that while explosive movements are not effective for remodeling collagen structures, they do improve the SSC and increase functional range of

motion. Training your SSC not only helps prevent injuries, it also boosts performance to an almost unbelievable degree. For example, preloading your leg muscles with a quick squatting motion before performing vertical jumps increases jump height by 18%–20%.[134] **Figure 4.5** illustrates how energy is stored and released during the SSC of a vertical jump.

2. **Build neuromuscular endurance.** Fitness training doesn't involve only muscles and joints; nerve signaling (the way nerve cells communicate with each other) is an important consideration as well. The efficiency and endurance of nerve signaling is a crucial element for preventing injury. A study published in the *Scandinavian Journal of Medicine & Science in Sports* showed that repeat sprint training significantly reduces nerve signals to the hamstring muscles.[135] This explains why most injuries occur toward the end of competitions (and the end of a sporting season) rather than at the beginning. When electrical signals to your muscles start to fail and you're still performing the movement, your muscles don't fire properly and your connective tissue absorbs the excess stress. Building endurance of the neuromuscular units that control complex movements effectively shields your body against injury. High-repetition endurance training is a must. Try explaining that to the next heavy-weight-lifting purist you run into at the gym and you'll get a blank stare. But you know better.

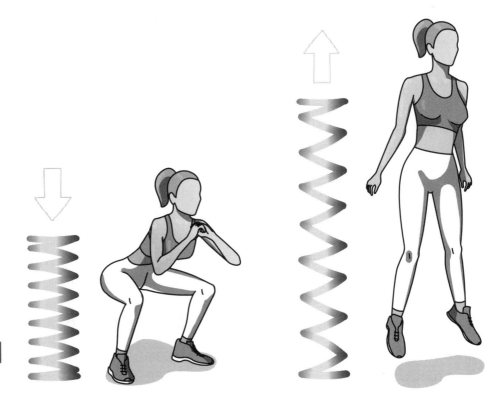

FIGURE 4.5

Stretch-shortening cycle.

YOU'RE MORE PLASTIC THAN YOU THINK

It's generally accepted that tendon, ligament, and cartilage cells turn over much more slowly than muscle cells. Especially cartilage, which is essentially considered a permanent structure with no ability to remodel after age-related erosion or injuries. If you've ever suffered an injury to your shoulder labrum or knee articular cartilage, your doctor and surgeon likely both agreed that the only way to recover fully is through surgery. But a 2019 study published in *Nutrients* casts doubt on this tightly held belief.[136]

In the study, researchers set out to measure the cell turnover rates of various connective tissues. They obtained samples from a small group of patients undergoing knee surgery and measured fractional protein synthesis rates over 24 hours. Surprisingly, they found that basal protein synthesis rates in tendons, ligaments, cartilage, and bone tissue were within the same range as skeletal muscle (1%–2% per day). Further, they found that synovium cells (the lining inside joint capsules that secretes synovial fluid) had higher rates of turnover than other types. They also found that posterior structures on the back side of the knees had slightly lower turnover rates.

The implications are many. The most relevant is that connective tissue structures such as cartilage may be much more plastic than previously thought. The fact that posterior knee structures had lower cell turnover rates provides additional backup to the theory that activity levels affect tissue metabolism. We use the muscles and connective tissue on the front side of our legs more than structures on the back side. Prolonged sitting and lopsided exercise habits that neglect the posterior chain both contribute to this imbalance. The finding is a double-edged sword because it implies faster and more optimal connective tissue adaptations to movement, but also faster and more dramatic declines in connective tissue integrity during sedentary periods (e.g. after surgery or injury).

Although this was a small study that needs further investigation, it should encourage you. Tendons, ligaments, fascia, synovium, and even cartilage structures respond to the physiological inputs we give them. You have much more control over your joint healing processes, strength, and integrity than you realize. This brings us back to the fundamental process behind all these healing mechanisms: collagen synthesis. Now that we have covered the role of exercise, let's look at lifestyle factors that affect collagen metabolism.

LIFESTYLE FACTORS THAT DECREASE COLLAGEN SYNTHESIS

In terms of factors you can control, exercise has the most significant positive impact on collagen synthesis within your joints. But several lifestyle-related variables matter, too. Before worrying about how to boost collagen synthesis, first make sure that you aren't doing anything to hinder it. While some of these are out of your control, you can influence several variables that determine how much collagen your body breaks down:

1. NSAID Usage

NSAIDs such as ibuprofen and naproxen reduce collagen mass at injury sites. A metastudy published in the *Annals of Physical and Rehabilitation Medicine* demonstrated that although NSAIDs effectively relieve joint pain and reduce inflammation in the short term (7 to 14 days), they also delay healing times, increase reinjury rates by up to 25%, and reduce collagen mass at injury sites.

According to this same study, "the adverse effects [of NSAIDs] have clinical relevance, and their possible negative consequences on the long-term healing process are slowly becoming more obvious." The lead author went on to say, "We do not recommend their use for muscle injuries, bone fractures (also stress fractures) or chronic tendinopathy."[55]

NSAIDs are not good for your joints long-term, especially if you take them regularly. If you pop ibuprofen like candy to get through workouts and relieve aches and pains, you're selling your joints short.

2. Steroid Hormones (Corticosteroids)

Doctors commonly recommend oral steroids and cortisone injections as a first line of defense against joint pain. While corticosteroids help relieve pain and inflammation in the short term, they have inhibitory effects on collagen synthesis within connective tissue.[137] Unfortunately, the people who benefit most from steroid hormone usage in the short term (those who need pain relief) are the same individuals who are hurt most in the long term (suffer from a failed healing response in joints).

If you do get a cortisone injection, remember that you still have damaged tissue that is susceptible to further injury even if you are not feeling any pain.

3. Sedentary Lifestyle

A sedentary lifestyle leads to a decrease in total collagen in your body, while resistance-focused exercise increases the collagen formation rate.[138] During injury recovery periods, a reduction in activity leads to a reduction in collagen, further increasing injury risk. And so the cycle continues.

If an injury leads you into a sedentary lifestyle, your problems are compounded by a physiological principle called *Davis's law*. Davis's law states that soft tissues heal according to how they're mechanically stressed.[139] If you stop using a joint, your tendons and ligaments will naturally shorten, reducing mobility and causing severe mechanical problems. In other words, *use it or lose it.*

4. Disease and Genetic Disorders

Over 200 connective tissue and autoimmune disorders impact collagen synthesis, including rheumatoid arthritis, lupus, and Ehlers-Danlos syndrome. Many of these conditions cause the body to attack its own tissues, speeding up collagen degradation.[32]

5. Ultraviolet Radiation (UV Rays)

UV rays, like those produced from tanning lamps, pertain more to skin health than joint health, but it's worth mentioning because of the staggering effect on collagen metabolism. According to an article published in the journal *Amino Acids*, even a one-time exposure to high amounts of UV rays decreases collagen in skin.[140]

6. Age

Collagen production decreases with age. By age 60, your ability to produce collagen has dropped by around 50%.[109,141]

7. Hormonal Imbalances

An imbalance of testosterone and estrogen can inhibit collagen synthesis. Although the research on how estrogen impacts collagen synthesis is conflicting, it appears that low levels of estrogen (especially in aging populations) do inhibit collagen synthesis in joints and skin.[142]

However, too much estrogen also has a detrimental effect on collagen health because it decreases collagen stiffness too much, making it easier for connective tissue to bend and tear. According to Leblanc and colleagues in their study "The effect of estrogen on tendon and ligament metabolism and function,"

> Due to the purpose of the tendon in transmitting as well as storing energy, stiffness is a crucial trait in regards to both of these abilities in that it can have a positive effect on both, as long as it does not exceed a certain range of value on either end.[142]

This means that your tendons and ligaments flourish when there is a balance of stiffness and compliance—enough tension to store and transmit energy without bending too much, and enough flexibility to withstand end ranges of motion without tearing. Likewise, because testosterone is one of the main anabolic (growth) hormones in the body, having optimal levels helps maintain collagen mass in joint structures.

8. Chronic Inflammation

This is perhaps the biggest misconception around collagen health. Acute inflammation, like that experienced right after an injury, is a necessary step for collagen synthesis. It triggers collagen production and helps deliver nutrients to damaged tissue, which ultimately leads to collagen formation.[143] This is yet another reason why blocking inflammation right after an injury is a bad idea. It is only when inflammation is chronically elevated that problems arise. This can happen if inflammation levels stay elevated for several weeks after an injury or if overall systemic inflammation is high for too long. For example, in osteoarthritis, cartilage destruction and inflammation cause type II collagen loss.[144]

9. Poor Lifestyle Choices

Lifestyle choices, including poor sleep habits, smoking, and alcohol abuse, contribute to increased collagen loss and decreased collagen production.[145,146]

10. Nutrient Deficiencies and Extreme Diets

- **Weight loss:** Reduced calorie diets and corresponding weight loss decrease collagen synthesis.[147]
- **Low-protein diets:** Animal studies indicate that low-protein diets decrease collagen formation, likely from enhanced collagen breakdown and impaired collagen cross-linking.[112]
- **Fasting:** An animal study demonstrated that collagen production decreases shortly after fasting begins, and after 96 hours of fasting is reduced by 25% in bone, cartilage, and skeletal muscle. This effect is at least partially attributed to the increase in glucocorticoids released by the body during fasting, which inhibit collagen synthesis.[148]
- **Ketogenic and extreme low-carb diets:** Insulin and somatomedins (insulin-like growth factors) both stimulate collagen synthesis, indicating that ketogenic diets could have harmful effects on collagen mass.[149,150]
- **Vitamin and mineral deficiencies:** Several vitamins are involved in collagen synthesis. A deficiency in any of these impairs the process:
  - ▶ Vitamin A
  - ▶ Vitamin B1
  - ▶ Vitamin B2
  - ▶ Vitamin B6

- ► Vitamin C
- ► Vitamin K
- ► Chromium
- ► Copper
- ► Manganese
- ► Zinc

In sum, just about everything decreases collagen synthesis, right? Low-carb diets do, but so does excess sugar consumption. NSAIDs and anti-inflammatories decrease collagen synthesis, but then again so does chronic inflammation. Could I have just summed this section up by saying "all things in moderation"? Not exactly. But often the solution does lie somewhere in the middle of two extremes. Studies of injured athletes and aging populations reveal some specific tactics you can employ to beef up your collagen synthesis for healthy, supple, injury-proof joints.

FIVE WAYS TO INCREASE COLLAGEN SYNTHESIS

1. Let your body do its job.

In response to injury and tissue damage, your body naturally triggers collagen biosynthesis. You don't have to do anything to make that happen. Other than get hurt, of course. Use ice and pain meds only during the first week after injury for pain management or to control excess swelling. Don't try to quash inflammation just for the sake of quashing it.

After the first week, keeping inflammation in the healthy range becomes more important for aiding the healing process—especially as you return to normal activities and exercises that could trigger ongoing inflammatory flare-ups.

2. Use common sense and moderation when it comes to lifestyle choices.

Avoid smoking, drug use, and high alcohol intake (keep it to two drinks or fewer per day). Get some natural sunlight, but don't allow your skin to become red and burned. Get seven to nine hours of sleep per night. Limit your intake of NSAIDs and other steroid hormones, including cortisone shots.

If you must take NSAIDs such as ibuprofen and naproxen for an injury or pain, only use them for a week or less before weaning off or switching to a natural supplement with proven anti-inflammatory benefits. Eat, move, and rest in a way that supports optimal testosterone and estrogen levels. That includes lifting weights to build muscle and strength, consuming plenty of protein from testosterone-boosting foods such as eggs and grass-fed beef, and avoiding excess body fat gain.[150,151]

3. Try deep tissue massage and manual therapy.

Deep tissue massage can improve collagen synthesis—especially during the midterm rehabilitation phase of injury recovery. It helps break up scar tissue and aids the remodeling necessary to lay down optimally formed collagen fibers. However, massage is contraindicated during the acute phase of injury because your body needs time to develop new tissue without further aggravation.[152]

I've used self-massage to treat several injuries, including a pulled groin muscle and elbow tendinopathy. I can confidently say that consistent self-massage made a significant difference in my recovery time. In the case of elbow tendinopathy, I was stuck with the same pain and weakness for months. Once I started doing manual massage therapy on the muscles surrounding the elbow, it finally loosened up and my symptoms subsided. Then, I was able to do the necessary corrective exercise work without severe pain.

Recommendation: Don't use deep tissue massage or self-massage techniques in the first 1–2 weeks after an injury. Wait until the initial inflammatory response has subsided. Do use massage, manual therapy, and other manual techniques such as foam rolling to loosen up stiff tissues before a corrective exercise session.

4. Eat collagen-boosting foods.

When it comes to food, it's less about finding secret superfoods that boost collagen synthesis and more about giving your body the raw material it needs to build from.

Here are a few specific foods that support collagen synthesis:

- **Citrus fruits:** Vitamin C plays a crucial role in collagen biosynthesis.
- **Oysters, shellfish, and seafood:** These seafood dishes are rich in zinc and copper, two minerals that support collagen synthesis.
- **Leafy greens:** Spinach, kale, and other leafy greens are rich in antioxidants like vitamin A and vitamin C that support healthy inflammation levels and help regulate enzymes responsible for collagen breakdown.
- **White tea and green tea:** White tea and green tea are believed to help prevent enzyme activity that speeds up collagen degradation, protecting your collagen formations.[153]
- **Protein:** It's common to experience spontaneous reductions in calories consumed after an injury occurs. Your overall activity levels have decreased and your appetite has too. You might even eat less on purpose to avoid weight gain. This can be problematic if your protein intake decreases. If you find yourself in this predicament—trying

to maintain body fat levels, muscle mass, and strength following an injury—a good solution is to increase the percentage of protein in your diet. Get more calories from protein and less from fat and carbohydrates. By consuming roughly the same amount of protein that you usually would, you'll be protecting muscle mass, which will translate to a shorter path to full recovery.

5. Use supplements proven to support collagen synthesis.

- **Whey protein:** A study published in the *Scandinavian Journal of Medicine and Science in Sports* demonstrated that subjects who used whey protein isolate along with resistance training saw greater increases in tendon mass.[154] Consume at least 20–40 grams per day, ideally within one hour of exercising the joints you'd like to bolster. If whey and dairy-based products upset your stomach, like they do mine, try a plant-based protein supplement or essential amino acid supplement.

- **Pea protein + rice protein:** Although whey is considered the gold standard of protein supplementation, pea proteins promote similar strength and muscle adaptations when taken in conjunction with resistance training.[155] Pea protein is slightly inferior, largely because it's low in the amino acid methionine. You can remedy this by taking rice protein with it, which contains a healthy proportion of methionine per serving. Look for a brand of plant protein that contains both pea and rice protein in the ingredients section of the product label, with pea protein as the primary protein source (ingredients are listed in order of greatest quantity).[155]

- **Essential amino acids (EAAs):** While protein supplementation has more historical research backing than amino acid supplements, EAAs may provide the same or better results than whey protein with more economy. Studies have shown that EAA supplementation stimulates more muscle protein synthesis (MPS) than the ever-popular branched chain amino acid (BCAA) supplement, and as much MPS as whey protein.[156] EAAs have the added benefits of lower insulin spikes and easier digestion. Finding a palatable EAA supplement is a challenge due to its grainy texture and bitter flavor. One option is to add EAAs to a protein blend, which studies indicate is superior to protein supplementation alone.[157] Shoot for around 7 grams of EAAs immediately after working out if you decide to go this route.

- **Vitamin C + collagen protein:** An eight-person, placebo controlled study published in the *American Journal of Clinical Nutrition* showed that taking vitamin C along with collagen protein doubled markers of collagen synthesis in ankle joints. Collagen protein and vitamin C supplements taken individually also have regenerative benefits.[158–160] A study published in the *Journal of Sports Science and Medicine* showed that 5 grams of collagen peptides significantly improved injured ankle joints' perceived function and decreased ankle sprain risk after a three-month follow-up.[111] Even a metastudy that compiled data from more than 60 scientific studies concluded that supplementing with collagen effectively "stimulates collagenic tissue regeneration by increasing not only collagen synthesis but minor components (glycosaminoglycans and hyaluronic acid) synthesis as well."[159]

- **Type II collagen:** A study published in *HealthMED* showed that supplementing with 750 mg of a natural collagen matrix comprised of 93% type II collagen stimulated collagen synthesis within cartilage tissues. Isolated type II collagen supplements with dosages as low as 10–40 mg per day have also shown benefits for inflammation and joint pain.[76,161]

COLLAGEN AS A NUTRITIONAL SUPPLEMENT

Collagen has been grossly overmarketed for conditions ranging from gut health to beauty to appetite control. Its popularity is based mainly on its cheap manufacturing cost, making it a cash cow for supplement companies. But there is solid research behind collagen for supporting injury recovery, joint health, and skin elasticity. Certain types, taken at certain times, do appear to optimize collagen synthesis by stimulating the production of connective tissue cells involved in building and repair.[111]

There are several types of collagen in your body, but upwards of 90% is made of types I, II, and III.[108] Most collagen protein supplements are made primarily from types I and III. These two are responsible for the mechanical loading and healing properties of tendons and ligaments. Type II collagen is the primary component of joint cartilage and the most bioavailable version when taken orally. It requires a much smaller dosage than types I and III.

Collagen protein supplements and type II collagen supplements are both good for your joints, but they have different mechanisms of action. Collagen protein benefits your joints by kick-starting collagen production and supplying the building blocks of healthy joints. Type II collagen supplements have a novel "oral vaccine" effect that builds immune cell tolerance, reduces autoimmune reactions, and relieves inflammation-based pain.[162] Think of collagen protein as a joint builder and type II collagen as an anti-inflammatory pain reliever.

While type II collagen is almost always in capsule form, collagen protein is usually a powder that makes its way into shake mixes, coffee creamers, and other food-based supplements. This creates further confusion about whether or not collagen protein is a viable meal replacement. It is not recommended to replace dietary protein with collagen protein because it lacks the essential amino acid L-tryptophan and is low in other vital amino acids like L-leucine and L-lysine. However, studies show you can safely consume as much as 36% of your daily protein from collagen while still maintaining indispensable amino acid balance requirements.[163] If you consume 150 grams of protein per day, you could consume upward of 50 grams of collagen protein without creating amino acid imbalances in your body. But you only need 5–15 grams per day (depending on the type) to get the joint, bone, and muscle health benefits.

It's worth mentioning that nutrient timing appears to be important for supplying your joints with collagen. Unlike muscles, connective tissue cells have limited blood flow, so they depend on pulling fluid from the joint capsule. You'll recall from our discussion of how synovial fluid works that joints act like sponges, soaking up surrounding liquid for lubrication. This implies that nutrients need to be already present in synovial fluid stores to be utilized by joints during exercise. It also illustrates why preworkout nutrition and hydration is vital for joints—not just muscles.

Preworkout recommendation: To increase collagen synthesis, tissue regeneration, and joint recovery, supplement with 5–10 grams of collagen protein 30–60 minutes before exercise. Choose a supplement that lists "hydrolyzed collagen," "collagen hydrolysate," or "collagen peptides" to mirror the supplements proven effective in studies. Adding 100–200 mg of vitamin C to your preworkout routine further supports tissue repair and healing rates. Type II collagen supplements appear to be preferentially effective at reducing cartilage inflammation in dosages as low as 10 mg per day.[161] For added joint inflammation support, you could also supplement with type II collagen immediately before training.

Which is better: collagen protein or type II collagen?

While the studies supporting usage of undenatured type II collagen are often referenced in arguments to claim it is superior to "cheaper" hydrolyzed collagen proteins, there's much more to the story. The two types have completely different modes of action.

Undenatured type II collagen supplements (primarily derived from chicken cartilage) work through immunomodulation effects. When you consume it regularly, your body views it as a safe protein, reducing the immune response (i.e. inflammation) that attacks it as a foreign substance.

In patients with rheumatoid arthritis, a disease in which the body attacks its own cartilage structures, this is especially effective for reducing chronic pain and inflammation.[162] Type II collagen has also proven useful for inflammation and pain relief in healthy people. One study showed that healthy, exercising subjects suffering from joint pain were able to work out longer without getting sore when they consumed type II collagen.[76]

Essentially, type II collagen produces an anti-inflammatory effect that preferentially benefits joint cartilage. Some type II collagen supplements also have other building blocks of connective tissue attached to them, like glucosamine and chondroitin. Consuming these compounds may further help with the rebuilding process.

Collagen protein (a.k.a. hydrolyzed collagen, collagen peptides, collagen types I and III) has a different effect in the body. The collagen protein supplements you see on health food store shelves have usually been hydrolyzed (broken down by enzymes) into short chains of amino acids called *peptides*. It's a common misconception that the hydrolyzation process breaks collagen down into its constituent amino acids, which would render it no more or less effective than amino acids from meat or dairy. In fact, the hydrolyzation process performs the same role as your digestive system—breaking the collagen down into shorter peptide sequences that are more readily absorbed by the body. These peptides have strong bonds that create a specific physiological effect in the body when absorbed intact.

When consumed as hydrolyzed collagen, around 10% of the collagen peptides are absorbed intact, stimulating collagen production in the body.[111] This creates more raw material for your joints to rebuild with and optimizes the tissue formation process. Critics of collagen supplementation are quick to point out that it scores lower than other protein sources on amino acid composition tests. But this is a moot point when it comes to joint health. It's not about the amino acid profile—it's about the physiological response your body has when it is absorbed intact.

(NOTE: There does appear to be significant variance in the quality of collagen proteins on the market, which explains why some collagen supplements produce significant positive effects while others show lackluster results in studies.)

The other ~90% of the peptides not absorbed intact are eventually broken down into amino acids and utilized in the body in much the same way dietary protein is. Researchers believe the high glycine and proline content of collagen provides readily available building blocks for connective tissue and other cells of the body, which may even have a muscle-sparing effect by leaving more essential amino acids available for muscle protein synthesis.[163]

KEY TAKEAWAY

Type II collagen has anti-inflammatory and protective effects on joints. Collagen protein supplements play a role in the building and repair of connective tissue, especially injured or degenerated tissues. Both have been shown to reduce joint pain and can be utilized separately or together, depending on your goals.

CHAPTER 5

Movement: The Original Mobility

In industrialized societies, tendon and ligament (collectively referred to
here as sinew) ruptures are occurring with greater frequency. In developing
countries where more individuals are involved in life-long physical labor
and regular exercise, sinew ruptures remain relatively uncommon.

— Jennifer Paxton et al., 2012[164]

It is my professional opinion as a biomechanist that movement is
what most humans are missing more than any other factors, and
the bulk of the scientific community has dropped the ball.

— Katy Bowman, author of *Move Your DNA*

The Hadza Tribe of Tanzania is one of the last surviving hunter-gatherer
societies. Unlike the rest of the world, which is dependent on industrializa-
tion and agriculture, the Hadza live much like our ancestors did two million
years ago. They spend most of their days hunting and foraging for food,
walking long distances, climbing trees to pick fruit and get a better view
of distant land, collecting edible plants, and digging for tubers and other
root vegetables. They hunt animals with handmade bows and arrows, gather
honey from beehives, and build shelters from grasses, branches, and mud.

As the modern world continues to creep in, edging out 90% of traditional Hadza land in the last 50 years, researchers and environmentalists are
working to help the tribe continue their traditions while also learning from
them. According to their own history, the Hadza have lived in their current
environment, next to the Serengeti plains in East Africa, since their beginning. This is also near the location where one of the earliest hominid species,
Homo habilis, lived 1.9 million years ago. While anthropologists are quick
to point out that we shouldn't assume Hadza life mirrors early human life
dating back hundreds of thousands of years, their hunter-gatherer lifestyle
gives us a glimpse into our past and a better understanding of how other
prehistoric human tribes lived.[165]

In the early 2000s, a group of anthropologists led by David Raichlen began
collecting movement data on the Hadza. Forty-four Hadza tribe members

agreed to wear GPS units as they foraged, hunted, and walked through their lands. After 342 foraging trips, a pattern of movement emerged known as the *Lévy walk*.[166]

Named after French mathematician Paul Lévy, the Lévy walk is a pattern characterized by short, sporadic movements within a small geographical area, combined with longer bouts of travel at less frequent intervals. As a written explanation, it doesn't make much sense. But when you look at the Lévy walk on a charted GPS map, through the lens of a hunter-gatherer, its utility becomes clear.

Imagine you are a hunter-gatherer tribesman. You know there is a patch of berries within walking distance, a thick forest nearby, and a few other potentially resource-rich spots around you. On a typical foraging bout, you would trek long distances to stop at these hot spots, taking time to pace around and harvest fruit, tubers, and other plants. Then you might take another short trip after discovering a grove of fruit trees nearby, taking time to gather food before continuing your foraging journey.

It's a commonsense way to approach foraging. It doesn't require maps or high levels of cognition and memory, and it has the added benefit of minimizing oversampling from one location due to its mostly random nature. On a topographical map, the Lévy walk appears as random, circular squiggles connected with longer, straight line paths.

Because humans are the most intelligent foragers on the planet, you might think that more intricate foraging systems would be used. But the

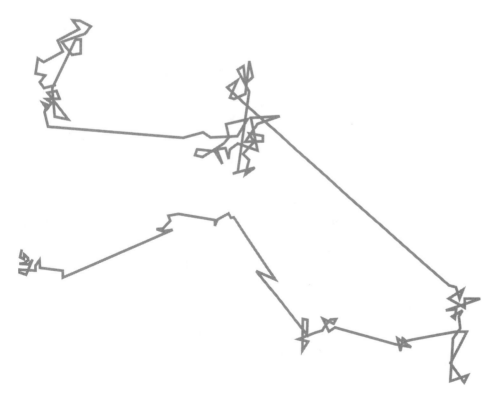

FIGURE 5.1

An example of the Lévy walk (bird's-eye view). (Adapted from Raichlen, D. A., Wood, B. M., Gordon, A. D., Mabulla, A. Z., Marlowe, F. W., & Pontzer, H, 2014. Evidence of Lévy walk foraging patterns in human hunter-gatherers. *Proc Natl Acad Sci U S A, 111,* 728–733.)

Hadza study demonstrates otherwise. What makes this finding interesting is that the Lévy walk mimics the foraging patterns of virtually every animal on the planet, from insects to fish to primates.

Studies of modern human movement patterns mirror the Hadza findings. Whether on a college campus or traipsing around Disney World, people adopt the Lévy walk to forage and explore. It appears to be an innate pattern of human behavior.

The Lévy walk epitomizes natural movement. It's varied in form, intensity, and distance, with an element of randomness. It exemplifies a wonderfully diverse array of movement that nourishes the human body and gives us insight into what is missing most from our modern, sedentary lifestyles.

WHY MOVEMENT TRUMPS EXERCISE

We're getting lazier, it's just a matter of time .... *Yeah, I want delivery and I'm going to need someone to feed me. No, no I'll be in the tub. Yeah, key is under the mat. Chip chop chip.*

— Jim Gaffigan, *Beyond the Pale*

You and I live in a time when movement is optional.

Instead of foraging for food, we can get everything we need for the week in one trip to the grocery store. Or, we can just have the food delivered. Most modern jobs require virtually no movement other than repetitive typing, clicking, and staring at computer screens. Vehicles, elevators, and strip malls cut down the required amount of walking steps to near zero. All these inventions and conveniences have driven society forward. But at what cost? And what should we be doing differently to tap into our movement-oriented roots?

The most practical solution, it would seem, is to exercise more. The truly disciplined of us aim for an hour of exercise several days per week, performed inside a gym devoid of sunlight after sitting at a desk for eight hours. For most people, that's as close to a healthy day of movement as it gets. Long, sedentary stretches of time spliced with short periods of intense movement. As I'll explain in the next section, this pattern of behavior inevitably leads to injury.

While the right kind of exercise helps build and maintain muscle, keep body fat low, and improve joint health, exercise only goes so far. Nonexercise movement—what you do most of the day when you're not at the gym—is much more powerful. That's because your body adapts to what you do *most of the time*. This is another reason why stretching fails to provide lasting changes to flexibility and mobility. The two minutes you spend stretching your legs each day is a drop in the bucket compared to what you do with the other 1,338 minutes. You could stretch for 20 minutes daily, and it would still only account for around 1.4% of the day. When you consider that most people sit for 11–12 hours each day, it's not hard to see why stretching— and even exercise—falls short when it comes to correcting the problems our modern lifestyles have created.

As you might recall from earlier chapters, the law that drives the way your body responds to movement is called *mechanotransduction*. In her book *Move Your DNA*, biomechanist Katy Bowman explains how mechanotransduction dictates what happens to your body as a result of movement habits:

> Motions that used to be incidental to living (read: occurring all day long) and cellular loads that used to be built into everyday life have been doled out—to computers, machines, and other people moving on our behalf. There is no way to physically recover the specific bends and torques, no way to recreate one hundred weekly hours of cell-squashing in seven, and no technology, at this time, smart enough to override nature.[167]

The thing most people miss—even health professionals—is that the benefits of movement go far beyond just increasing heart rate, building strength, or improving mobility. Every time you move, muscle and joint systems circulate blood and oxygen and expel waste products. On a cellular level, varied movement is what creates, maintains, and reinforces physiological health.

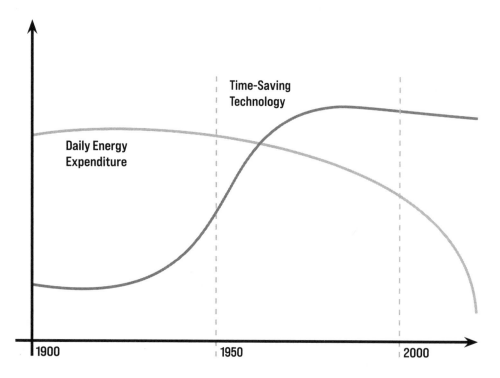

FIGURE 5.2

Changes in movement habits over time. (Adapted from Vogels, N., Egger, G., Plasqi, G., et al., 2004. Estimating changes in daily physical activity levels over time: Implications for health interventions from a novel approach. *Int J Sports Med., 25,* 607–610.)

WHAT WE CAN LEARN ABOUT MOVEMENT FROM TREES

Biosphere 2 is an artificial Earth science system constructed inside a dome made of steel tubing and glass frames, designed to be completely self-sustaining (1987–1991). The original purpose was to help scientists understand how our planet's living systems work together. One of the most fascinating and unexpected findings was the role of wind in a tree's life. Before reaching maturity, many trees in the biosphere snapped under their own weight. Researchers learned later this was caused by lack of *stress wood*—a wood that forms in place of normal wood as a response to external forces. This necessary mechanical acclimation was lacking in the biosphere trees, preventing them from surviving.

There's an underlying principle at work here. Stress creates resilience. Lack of stress creates weakness. In the case of the biosphere trees, the stress they were missing was wind. Wind doesn't just blow in one direction, or at one speed. It's constantly changing directions, slowing down, speeding up—creating an infinite array of forces for the trees to counterbalance against. Ironically, the lack of varied movement and counterforce is what felled the trees.

Just as you can't mimic the wind by pushing against a tree for a few minutes, you can't mimic natural, varied human movement through isolation exercises for muscles or repetitive aerobic training at the gym. On the contrary, popular exercise methods often exacerbate the problems caused by a lack of varied movement instead of mitigating them.

The Danger of Isolation

Overdependence on isolation exercises (e.g. bicep curls) and repetitive movements put you at risk of injury in three distinct ways:

1. Exercises that isolate only one or two body parts build muscle strength in a small area while neglecting adjacent muscles. The gap between strong areas and weak areas is where injuries occur.

2. Limited movement variation creates strength and coordination through limited ranges of motion. If you're strong through the top 80% of a joint's range of motion (ROM) but have virtually no training through the bottom 20%, your injury risk is increased.

3. Isolation movements by definition target only the prime mover muscles—the ones that directly cause the desired motion. This leaves out the supporting cast of stabilizer muscles that are necessary for safe, functional movement in the real world.

While isolation exercises can be part of a successful training program, the core of your training should involve compound movements that challenge multiple muscle groups and joint systems together.

Now, let's look at what happens to the two primary goals of mobility training (injury prevention and pain relief) when we add more varied movement into our lives.

MOVEMENT, LOAD VOLUME, AND INJURY RISK

In order to be awarded the Special Warfare Operator Naval Rating and the Navy Enlisted Classification 5326 Combatant Swimmer (Navy SEAL), candidates must undergo more than a year of intensive physical, mental, and battle-ready training. The extremes of fatigue and torment that would-be SEALs have to endure is difficult to comprehend. It's not just grueling physical conditioning—it's pushing through mentally demanding tasks on virtually no sleep. Running in combat boots with bleeding, chafing, infected feet. Carrying heavy loads despite dislocated joints and ruptured tendons. Swimming through dark, shark-infested, freezing cold waters—for hours. Being tied up and tossed into a pool as part of "drown proofing" training. Remaining a team player and helping the person next to you even though every instinct and molecule of energy you have has been spent on self-preservation. Beyond the physical and mental conditioning, it's learning the ins and outs of some of the most challenging warfare skills, including underwater demolition, parachuting, and weapons training.

Despite the impressive performance feats, I find myself marveling most at the resiliency a SEAL's body must have to survive training without traumatic injury. The truth is, overuse injuries and acute injuries do contribute to the high candidate dropout rate. Those who make it through must be genetically superior, with superhuman, unbreakable joints, right? While genetics does play a role in predisposition to connective tissue and muscle injuries, it's what happens before initiation that prevents debilitating injuries on Day 1 of training.

The Navy makes it clear that SEAL training isn't designed to get you in shape. You must be in excellent condition and pass the Physical Screening Test before even being considered a SEAL candidate. The importance of preparing physically to enter SEAL training can't be understated. In Marcus Luttrell's book *Lone Survivor*, he describes how a "farm boy from the backwoods of East Texas" came to be a SEAL:[168]

> In fact, my natural-born assets are very average. I'm pretty big, which was an accident at birth. I'm pretty strong, because a lot of other people took a lot of trouble training me, and I'm unbelievably determined, because when you're as naturally ungifted as I am, you have to keep driving forward, right?

Marcus describes in detail his pre-SEAL training regimen, which didn't start a few months before formal training. It started years prior when he was still a kid in East Texas. Marcus spent the summers, along with his twin brother Morgan, under the tutelage of his father—swimming, racing, and diving through a lake near their home. They were taught discipline and survival. It was at about age 12 when Marcus realized "beyond doubt" that he was going to become a Navy SEAL.

Later in their teen years, Marcus and Morgan began more intensive training under a former Green Beret sergeant named Billy Shelton who lived close by. Shelton operated a full-scale pre-SEAL training program for teenagers—complete with weightlifting, 12-mile runs, and obstacles performed while carrying concrete blocks overhead. At Shelton's advising, Marcus had studied martial arts to master unarmed combat starting in grade school. By the time Marcus and Morgan were ready to enter formal SEAL training, they had a decade of preparation under their belts. The insanely high volumes of running and resistance training wouldn't be a shock to their system. The resilience of their muscles and load capacity of their tendons had already been forged years before being assaulted by SEAL training on the beaches of Coronado.

Load Management

Conventional wisdom suggests that to avoid injury, you should reduce training volume and play it safe. Avoid overtraining. Especially as you age and accumulate sprains and strains that inevitably crop up throughout your body. There is also a common misconception that strength and conditioning (performance) and physiotherapy (injury recovery and prevention) are on opposite ends of the spectrum. In reality, they are two sides of the same coin. To understand how movement relates to injury risk, let's look at another extreme on the spectrum of human movement.

Tim Gabbett is an Australia-based sports scientist with Ph.Ds in human physiology and applied science of professional football. Gabbett's work focuses on injury prevention, specifically in elite athletes in the NBA, MLB, NCAA, and Olympic Games. He has published over 200 peer-reviewed articles and is considered by many to be the world's foremost expert on load management. Gabbett's ground-breaking research is changing the way professional athletes prepare for competition. In his research, he describes a phenomenon called the *injury prevention paradox*, which states that high-volume training has a protective effect against injury. And that while overtraining is a common cause of injury, undertraining is just as common.[169]

According to Gabbett, the most important concept for injury prevention is the *acute:chronic workload ratio* (ACWR). The ratio is determined by measuring the difference between acute workloads—how much physically demanding activity an athlete faces over a period of seven days or shorter—and chronic workloads—the amount of work an athlete completes over a period of four weeks or longer. For example, a weekend tournament that includes several competitions is the acute workload. The one- to two-month period of training surrounding the competition is the chronic workload.

A three-year study of English Premier League football players showed that spikes in the ACWR are associated with 5–7 times greater injury rates—either during the high-intensity periods or the days afterward, as fatigue sets in.[170] To minimize injury risk, athletes should strive to keep the ACWR down by matching their preparative training to demands faced during competition. Using tracking devices and high-tech software programs, trainers can predict their athletes' injuries with startling accuracy.

This model flies in the face of commonly held beliefs about what causes injury. Despite popular opinion, noncontact injuries are not caused by overtraining but by inappropriate programming. It's the rapid increases and fluctuations in training loads that cause injury. Athletes accustomed to higher training volumes have fewer injuries than athletes training at lower volumes. Just as overtraining causes tendon degeneration from lack of recovery, undertraining leads to reduced connective tissue load capacity and reactive tendinopathy. Consistent, intense training is the best way to prevent injury.[171,172]

The research on ACWR explains why weekend warriors often sprain their shoulders with one overhead serve of a tennis racket, while elite athletes can complete hundreds of repetitions, day after day, without injury or tendon degeneration. Also, novice athletes tend to have imbalances between the development of their muscles and tendons, with muscles being more

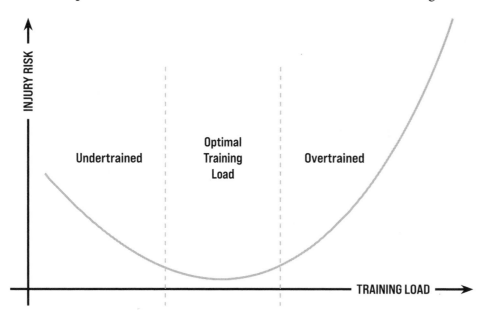

FIGURE 5.3

Training-injury prevention paradox U-shaped graph. (Adapted from Gabbett, T., 2016. The training-injury prevention paradox: Should athletes be training smarter and harder? *British Journal of Sports Medicine, 50,* Figure 1.)

developed and tendon health falling behind. This muscle-tendon imbalance is a major risk factor for tendinopathy.[89]

Think back to the last time you were injured. It probably happened right after you started a new sport, exercise routine, or significantly changed your movement habits. It could be as simple as going from three strength training sessions per week to five per week. Perhaps you took up jogging and immediately ran three or four miles per day instead of slowly ramping up to longer runs. In all these scenarios, your connective tissue load capacities are not up to snuff, so they break down.

Key Takeaway

The take-home message for athletes is that exposure to increased loads during a training cycle reduces injury risk during the sprints of game play (and over the next several days as the negative effects of overreaching set in). A higher level of fitness means lower risk of injury. The take-home message for nonathletes is similar. *This is the most important injury-prevention lesson in the book*: being sedentary all week and then playing golf or tennis on the weekend is the easiest way to get injured and develop joint pain. Even within daily time periods, being sedentary all day and then exercising intensely for one hour will lead to injury. It might show up as tendinopathy, or it might be an acute tear or sprain. But it will happen.

I'm not saying to randomly perform cartwheels and jumping jacks when you're standing in line at the coffee shop. Though it's not the worst idea. The point I'm trying to drive home is that by managing your chronic load levels through regular movement—especially movement that reinforces or works in opposition to your lifestyle—you'll prevent injuries and build strength and movement mastery in the process. The more you use a particular joint, the more important it is that you expose it to a variety of stressors (reread this sentence—it's that important).

Injury prevention training boils down to two things:

1. Reduce the acute and chronic stress placed on at-risk tissues (common injury areas or weak points) through periodization of intensity and proper movement mechanics.

2. Increase the stress a tissue can tolerate prior to failure. This is accomplished through building overall muscle mass and strength, connective tissue resilience, sports- or lifestyle-specific corrective exercise, and fatigue management (you're more prone to injuries when you are tired).

Gabbett leaves us with one more important piece of the puzzle regarding high fitness levels: *get there as safely as possible*. This means, apply the principle of progressive overload in a controlled manner. To minimize risk of injury, limit weekly training load increases to 10%–20%. For example, going from a four-day training week to a five-day training week is a 14% increase in total volume (assuming you perform the same number of repetitions).

When you start any new exercise modality—be it weight training, running, bike riding, or a sport—start slow. Train the new modality no more than twice per week for at least four to six weeks (ideally with two to three days of rest between). This will give your connective tissue time to heal between sessions and increase load tolerance. (Remember, collagen synthesis levels within joints stay elevated for three full days postexercise.)[128] You can then bump up the training frequency to three days per week for another four to six weeks. This rule applies whether you're a couch potato or dedicated fitness junky.

I recall a time (not too long ago…) when I was exercising a few days per week with a mixture of weight training, running, and swimming. I decided I was going to start jumping rope to build more agility and lower leg strength. Like a moron, I jumped right into intense, 10-minute rope skipping sessions *daily*. After several days, I started developing pain in my right Achilles. When I aggravated it further a few weeks later, my physical therapist confirmed that I had a nasty case of insertional Achilles tendinopathy—one of the most difficult overuse injuries to treat. It took months to overcome. And it could have been prevented if I had eased into jumping rope with once or twice weekly sessions instead of assaulting my Achilles daily.

Common sense will be your best guide when it comes to increasing volume. But well-planned periodization and intelligent programming will ensure you progress safely. These methods aren't just for professional athletes. You can use the same periodization techniques the pros do without the fancy spreadsheets and apps monitoring your biomarkers. It just takes an understanding of how and when to adjust training goals to maximize progress while minimizing risk of tendinopathy, injury, and burnout.

MOVEMENT AND PAIN RELIEF

Back pain. It's the mother of all pain. Physical therapists, chiropractors, and pain management doctors will tell you that back pain is the most common complaint from patients. As anyone who has ever injured their back knows, you use it for everything. Which means virtually everything makes it hurt worse—from bending over to coughing to lying in bed. When I looked up the online search volume for various body parts plus the word "pain," the number of searches for *back pain* totaled more than the search volume of *knee, neck, shoulder, foot, elbow,* and *wrist pain* combined.

There are hundreds of conventional and alternative therapies for back pain, with varying degrees of research behind them. Surgery, steroid injections, nerve blocks, acupuncture, chiropractic, massage…the list goes on and on. But one of the most proven back pain therapies is free. All it requires is two legs and some space to move around.

In a study published in the journal *Aging*, researchers at UCLA School of Medicine demonstrated that *walking* is just as effective for back pain relief as conventional pain treatment methods like heat, cold, massage, and relaxation techniques.[173]

In another study published in *Annals of Internal Medicine*, osteoarthritis patients assigned to a walking program experienced a 27% decrease in pain. During a poststudy follow-up, researchers also found that the walking group used pain medication less frequently.[174]

There is no more underrated and research-backed therapeutic tool than walking. It reduces back pain, and body pain in general, through dozens of mechanisms. Studies show that walking does the following:

- Increases circulation of natural opioids in the body[175]

- Reduces pain sensitivity[176]

- Stimulates production and circulation of synovial fluid within joints[177]

- Improves lumbar (low back) function[178]

- Strengthens foot muscles, creating a more stable and pliable base for the hips, back, and neck (especially in minimalist shoes)[179]

- Reduces perceived pain levels, improves blood pressure, and strengthens feelings of personal power[180] (if you walk with upright posture instead of slumped)

- Reduces bone density loss with age, helping to prevent osteoporosis and reduce osteoarthritis pain[181]

- Is a surprisingly effective weight loss and weight management technique, which in turn keeps overall compression forces on joints down[182]

- Increases blood flow to spinal muscles, improving oxygen and nutrient delivery required for cellular healing[183]

- Speeds up elimination of cellular waste products through the repeated contractions of various muscle groups throughout the body[183]

- Reduces the levels of the stress hormone, cortisol, which has a correlative relationship with subjective pain levels[184]

- (Barefoot walking) Improves body awareness and wound healing, reduces inflammation, and helps prevent chronic inflammatory diseases[185]

Walking doesn't just help relieve back pain—it targets the central causes of pain. And as you can see from the many studies on walking and pain relief, the benefits are not limited to the locomotion of walking. It's movement in general that increases circulation of natural opioids, reduces pain sensitivity, stimulates synovial fluid production, and supports cellular health.

Walking is the clearly the most underrated natural pain reliever. But in head-to-head studies, another natural pain management method was even more effective: *retro walking*.

Retro walking is exactly what you might have guessed—walking backward. It takes more neuromuscular coordination than forward walking. It also stresses muscles differently, requiring more work from the quadriceps muscles on the front of your legs. But most of all, it's challenging because it requires you to move your body in an unusual way.[186] This is why retro walking performs so well in studies compared to forward walking. It's divergent. It squeezes and pumps muscles that you don't normally use, delivers oxygen to soft tissues that aren't normally well circulated, and stimulates a physiological response through mechanotransduction that forward walking doesn't.

Everyone should walk. And though I don't advise retro walking down the sidewalk, for safety reasons, the research on retro walking drives home the point that everyone should include varied movement into their daily lives. Especially if you have chronic pain, nagging injuries, or stiff joints.

How Varied Movement Reduces Guarding and Pain

Guarding is the tensing of muscle and shortening of posture to protect an injured, inflamed, or painful body part. It's an overlooked pain-related behavior that plays a major contributing role in age-related mobility and activity declines. Studies show that patients who can reduce guarding behaviors experience lower levels of pain, anxiety, and distress. Because guarding has a psychological component (fear of injury and pain), exposure to novel movements helps retrain the nervous system. Varied movement is the best way to show the central nervous system that it's OK to relax and to move around without tensing up.[187]

HOW TO WEAVE MOVEMENT INTO YOUR LIFE

Movement is the original mobility training. It helps prevent injuries, reduces pain, and maintains range of motion. But for those of us without jobs that require varied physical activity, it can be tough to weave it into everyday life. Here are some practical ways to add movement to your days:

1. Establish a walking habit.

Carve 20 minutes out of your day for a walk. Though it can seem like finding a dependable chunk of time to walk each day is next to impossible, it's doable if you're willing to cut some fat and inject some discipline.

Put it this way: if you were audited by a time management expert, do you think she could find a spare 20 minutes in your daily routine to use for walking? I bet so. Most people spend way too much time watching TV, glued to their devices, and dragging their feet when switching tasks.

Find 20 minutes. Preferably early in the morning or right after work. Enlist a walking buddy if you want. Commit to walking for 20 minutes each day for one week straight. Then decide if it's a habit you want to keep. Remember all the proven benefits of walking. It doesn't just nourish your body; it also encourages the cleaning of mental clutter.

One more thing: don't assume walking is for people who can't do other forms of exercise. The ultrafit and competitive athletes will benefit just as well.

2. Place movement cues in your environment.

If you looked around my office, you'd notice a Theraband FlexBar for wrist and elbow exercises sitting next to my keyboard. You'd see elastic exercise bands hanging from a bookshelf. Two small kettlebells and a yoga wheel lying on the floor behind my chair. And a TRX suspension training strap hanging on the wall next to the door. This might look like clutter to some people, and it might seem over the top to others—especially in a work environment I've dedicated mostly to writing—but for me, it works. I don't use these tools to "work out" per se; I use them for movement snacks—short, unplanned movement sessions, often only lasting a minute or two.

I squeeze and bend the Flexbar as I'm reading emails or thinking through a problem. I hang from the TRX strap when my shoulders feel tight. I stretch my back against the yoga wheel after sitting for long periods. And I use the exercise bands and kettlebells randomly throughout the day to get some blood flowing. It not only gives me varied movement that I know my body needs, it keeps my mind fresh and my energy levels elevated.

All this crazy environmental manipulation follows the well-established behavioral principle of *stimulus control*—the phenomenon of a stimulus increasing the probability of a behavior (because of a history of that behavior being reinforced in the presence of the stimulus). It's an effective trick you can play on yourself. And you don't necessarily have to scatter fitness equipment throughout your home to take advantage of environmental movement cues. You could put your walking shoes on the top shelf of the shoe rack, where you see them every time you go outside. Get a standing desk if you work at a computer. Create space in your family room so there is room to lie down and stretch. Keep a Frisbee or ball next to your dog's leash. Get your bike down from the rack and fill up the tires so it's ready for a ride at a moment's notice.

Build an environment for yourself that encourages movement, and by default you will move more.

3. Countertrain against movements you habitually perform.

Golfers identify as golfers. It's what they love to do, and it's what they think about all day when they're not golfing. If they go to the gym, you can find them practicing their swing in between sets, doing weighted rotations that mimic the club swing movement, and performing wrist curls to increase club speed. This training strategy adds more volume to movement patterns that already get disproportionate amounts of repetition.

The golfer would benefit more from doing exercises that counteract overused muscles and movement patterns: antirotation core strength exercises like planks, wrist extensions to counteract all the wrist flexion, and rotator cuff exercises to stabilize overused shoulders. Ironically, the ability to stabilize and engage core muscles will improve driving distance better than swinging a dumbbell through the air. And that can be accomplished by practicing basic movements such as the squat, hip hinge, upper body press, and upper body pull.

Countertraining in this way isn't just a smart strategy for preventing injuries; it improves overall fitness and physical ability. The more rounded an athlete you are, the better you will be at movements that require full body integration. Look for opportunities to add movement to your daily routine that counteract muscle imbalances created by your lifestyle.

4. Move in the morning.

Another way to think about adding more movement is to reduce the stretches of time where you are sedentary. For most people, the biggest opportunity to do that is to move first thing in the morning. After a full night's sleep, you have been sedentary for 8–10 hours. Again, if you are like most people, your morning consists of sitting down to eat breakfast, sitting in a car to drive to the office, and sitting at your desk. Instead of extending the sedentary time period, break it up with some movement first thing in the morning. This isn't a workout—it's just going through the motions to give your body some nutritious movement.

Perform a few repetitions of exercises that target the major movements: body weight squats and hip hinges and upper body pressing and pulling with light resistance bands or dumbbells. You won't feel like doing this right when you get out of bed. Do it anyway, just for a few minutes. If you can establish this habit, you'll wonder how you ever started your day without it. Your body and mind will feel much sharper and you'll have fewer kinks in your muscles and joints.

5. Play.

Kids have an intuitive sense for exploring varied movement. Just look around at any playground and you'll notice a remarkably diverse set of movement opportunities. Monkey bars for hanging. Ropes for climbing. Swinging tires, spinning wheels, jumping platforms.

But play isn't just for kids. In his book *Play: How it Shapes the Brain, Opens the Imagination, and Invigorates the Soul*, author Stuart Brown makes a convincing case that play has an essential role in learning, happiness, and creativity. Even for adults.

Play trains us to be adaptable. To think outside the box and move outside the box. If you don't have play in your life, find it. It could be pick-up basketball at the park, ultimate Frisbee on weekends, or bowling with your kids. Don't be an "adult" who is too serious to participate in silly games, standing in the corner with your arms crossed. Look for opportunities to *play*.

6. Try new exercise routines.

You probably don't identify as a specific type of athlete. But you're still at risk of movement staleness. Most people who exercise do the same thing, day after day and week after week. While planning corrective exercise and periodizing training is a good idea, simply mixing up your workouts can be just as effective and rewarding. If all you do is lift weights, try a boot camp class. If you're into yoga, purchase a training package and get instructions on how to build strength. Look for opportunities to challenge your body in novel ways.

7. Plan activities, trips, and vacations around varied movement.

For me, vacation isn't sitting on a beach sipping piña coladas. That sounds like a nightmare. I would only last about 10 minutes before boredom, anxiety, and feelings of guilt for being such a bum took over. No, vacation to me is getting *out of my head* and *into my body*. That's why I always plan one or two intensive activities when traveling.

During a trip to Dillon, Colorado, I spent most of my time hiking and walking mountainside trails. I remember my hip flexors and butt cheeks getting sore in places I'd never felt soreness before. During my first trip out of the country, to Costa Rica, I spent several days surfing. My neck muscles were sore from bridging up on the board, and the musculature around my ankles ached from walking up and down the sandy beaches. These activities challenged my body in novel ways, causing fatigue and muscle soreness. But overall, my joints felt great during and after both trips.

8. Plan idle time.

Another problem with lack of movement is that we rarely take true idle time. We don't move enough, but we're also in constant motion—if not physically, then mentally. We fidget with our phones, stare at computer screens, and death-grip our steering wheels as we battle traffic. This type of low-level tension eats away at our minds and bodies.

When you move more, your body demands real rest. Real idle time. And because you don't feel guilty about being a couch potato, you're more likely to give in. This is what natural movement and natural rest look like—lots of low-intensity movement, some intense physical exertion, and periods of complete rest.

9. Leverage everyday activities.

The most irritating kind of injury comes from doing something that shouldn't cause injury. Mowing the lawn, a project at home, picking something off the floor. But all too often, these are the exact things that get people hurt. It's not supposed to be this way—even with advanced age. When you train with optimal posture and alignment, learn to stabilize your core, and use correct form when performing movements like hinging at the hips, squatting, pulling and lifting—you can translate those movement patterns to real life.

Now, a movement or project that would typically cause pain serves as a type of fitness supplement, reinforcing proper mechanics. Hobbies like golfing, going for a hike, or even doing chores around the house are no longer activities that ache your joints but varied movements that give your body the exact physiological nourishment it needs to stay healthy and pain-free. Getting to this level takes a three-pronged approach: (1) mastery of the basic human movements with focused load training, (2) posture awareness, and (3) translating correct body position and movement quality (from exercise training) to everyday activities.

Nonexercise Activity Thermogenesis (NEAT)

Nonexercise activity thermogenesis basically refers to all the usual activities and bodily functions that burn up calories. Chewing your food. Digesting your food. Walking. Breathing. Even thinking. All these activities require energy. More energy than you might think.

In fact, once you see the math equation behind caloric balance, you'll see that NEAT is the most underrated fat-burning tool we have. While most people focus on keeping their caloric intake under control and exercising more, NEAT is the real unsung hero of getting (or staying) trim and fit.

Studies show NEAT accounts for only about 15% of daily energy expenditure in sedentary individuals. But in more active people, NEAT can account for up to 50% of daily energy expenditure. For a person who requires 2,500 calories per day to maintain their body weight, increasing NEAT from 15% to 50% creates a difference of 875 calories burned.[188] That's *twice* the number of calories burned from jogging at a moderate pace for one hour straight. So, if you're looking for a way to boost weight loss efforts or to more easily maintain a healthy body weight, focus on NEAT. Here are the most impactful NEAT-related tactics you can employ right now:

1. **Eat more protein.** Protein has a higher thermic effect of feeding than any other macronutrient. Around 20%–35% of the calories you consume from protein are burned up during the digestion process.

2. **Build some muscle.** Muscle is more metabolically expensive than body fat. The more muscle you have, the more calories you'll burn each day—even at rest. Having more muscle also improves your body's ability to regulate blood glucose levels after meals, which has been linked to reduced body fat levels.[3]

3. **Increase workout intensity.** Adding more daily activity like walking is a good idea, but adding more intensity to your exercise routine will make a bigger impact on your metabolism. This is due to *excess post-exercise oxygen consumption.* After an intense weight training session or circuit training routine, your body burns calories at a higher rate for several hours after the exercise session has ended.

4. **Move more.** Look for opportunities to increase nonexercise movement throughout the day: taking the stairs instead of the elevator, walking while talking on the phone instead of sitting down, or standing instead of sitting when possible.

Science-Backed Mobility Training

If you can't fly, then run. If you can't run, then walk. If you
can't walk, then crawl. But by all means, keep moving.

—Martin Luther King, Jr.

Now that we've established why adding more varied movement has to be a priority, we've earned the right to talk about mobility. Mobility training is a hot topic in fitness. Compared to several years ago, today it's much less common to see gym rats marching into the weight room and immediately performing high-intensity sets of bench presses or squats. Now, fitness fanatics spend countless hours stretching, mobilizing, stabilizing, massaging, and foam rolling before even thinking about picking up a weight or stepping onto a treadmill. Why? Because experts say limited mobility reduces athletic performance, causes pain, and leads to injury. Some studies support this. Collegiate athletes with tighter ligaments and muscles are more prone to injury, leading researchers to conclude that preseason flexibility programs "may decrease injuries."[189]

The idea seems reasonable enough: stretch your muscles to improve flexibility, which will help prevent injury and improve overall performance. But in practice, mobility training is often a colossal waste of time. Depending on when and how you implement mobility training, it can even increase injury risk and reduce muscular force potential. Besides, muscle and strength imbalances are more likely than limited mobility to cause injury. A 2016 study published in *BMJ Open Sport & Exercise Medicine* found no relationship between mobility and injury risk, and that "strength asymmetry was statistically significant in predicting injury."[190] This is not to say that it's OK to be so tight that you can't bend over to tie your shoelaces. Limited mobility is a problem. But it's only one piece of a larger puzzle.

Neuromuscular coordination training, or agility training, is even more effective for preventing injuries. In one study, professional female soccer players who underwent structured agility training achieved a 400% reduction in injury rates.[191] Practicing jumps, throws, and other total body coordinated movements is surprisingly effective for keeping athletes healthy.

The last few decades have spawned numerous alternative approaches to mobility training with questionable legitimacy, but they have also given us solid research and principles we can use to build more mobile, injury-proof bodies. There's a right and a wrong way to approach mobility training. It starts with understanding what mobility is and why we should care about it in the first place.

MOBILITY VS. FLEXIBILITY

Mobility is defined as the "ability to move or be moved freely and easily." In the world of sports and fitness, it means the ability to move your joints through full, effective ranges of motion. Mobility is closely related to flexibility, but there's a key difference.

Flexibility is the ability of a *muscle* to stretch *passively* through a range of motion. Mobility is the ability of a *joint* to move *actively* through a range of motion.

Let's look at hamstring function to illustrate this difference. Your capacity to reach down and grab your toes with straight legs illustrates *flexibility*. It's a passive movement, maintained by holding a stretch. Conversely, your ability to hinge at the hips and pick up a weight off the floor (efficiently and without injury) illustrates *mobility*. It requires actively moving a joint system (your hips) through a full range of motion.

The idea of stretching to improve flexibility has fallen out of favor in much of the fitness world, and for good reason. A vast body of research on injury recovery, athletic performance, and pain management has obliterated nearly every argument for stretching in the traditional sense. But many people, even fitness professionals, are sticking to their guns—stretching daily, despite any measurable benefits, and recommending their clients do the same. Does stretching have a place in your fitness routine? Let's look to studies on flexibility and leading experts in injury management, physiotherapy, and biomechanics.

THE SCIENCE OF STRETCHING (IS NOT FLATTERING)

We've all heard that stretching helps lengthen muscles, reduce joint pain, and prevent injuries. But the science behind stretching doesn't hold up. A 2011 metastudy revealed that stretching has "no significant effect."[25]

I think this presents the most accurate and relevant finding—in general, traditional stretching routines have few significant benefits. Studies of runners, soldiers, and soccer players have come to this same conclusion. But when you drill into specific research on performance and recovery outcomes, the future of stretching as a fitness tool looks even more bleak.

A physical therapy study published in the journal *Sports Medicine* concluded, "Strong evidence exists that stretching has no beneficial effect on injury prevention."[27] Not only did the researchers clearly state that stretching is not effective, they also debunked the commonly held belief that making tendons more compliant is advantageous in the first place. The practice of stretching is ineffective for injury prevention, and the underlying intention of stretching for injury prevention might not even make sense.

Another metastudy published in the *British Journal of Sports Medicine* summarized the findings of 3,462 results from the research archives of PubMed, EMBASE, Web of Science, and SPORTDiscus. Researchers found favorable, or at least hopeful, outcomes for virtually every injury prevention technique studied. Except for stretching. Even strength training showed better results.[192]

Though the science of stretching for injury prevention doesn't hold up, many people stretch before a competition to warm up and boost performance. But this idea doesn't hold water either. A research review published in the journal *Medicine & Science in Sports & Exercise* gathered findings from 106 articles on stretching for muscle performance. They found that holding stretches for greater than 60 seconds consistently decreased muscular force potential. Shorter duration stretches of less than 60 seconds were not shown to compromise maximal muscle performance significantly. This study indicates that prolonged static stretching before working out is a bad idea, and that shorter duration stretches may be OK, though likely without significant benefit.[25]

This is not to say that you shouldn't warm up at all. One of the most studied warm-up routines in the world is FIFA's "11+" routine—which consists of isometric holds, agility drills, balance training, and game-play simulations. Studies of female soccer players have demonstrated that this type of warm-up reduces injury rates by around 30%.[193] Passive stretching is conspicuously vacant from the 11+ warm-up.

There's a disconnect here. We know that limited mobility is a problem. But efforts to fix it with stretching have failed miserably in studies. What's the reason for this gap? It's a complex debate that probably won't be settled anytime soon. However, two concepts give us insight into how to think about stretching and what we should be doing instead:

1. **Stretching makes you better at stretching.** Although most researchers agree that static stretching alone isn't an effective warm-up or injury prevention technique, some studies still show that stretching increases range of motion. The explanation for this is simple: an increased tolerance to the sensation of stretching. It's not that your muscles or tendons become looser—you simply get used to the uncomfortable feeling of stretching and are willing to push the range of motion farther. Studies going back to the 1980s and earlier have demonstrated this.[194]

2. **Muscles lengthen most effectively (with the least joint stress) when they are contracted while being lengthened.** A 2010 study published in *Manual Therapy* divided subjects into three groups to assess different modes of lengthening hamstring muscles: stretching, strength training in lengthened positions, and the control group (no intervention). While both experimental groups showed an increase in stretch tolerance, only the strength training group produced a shift in the torque-angle curve, which suggests an increase in muscle length. Stretching did not produce any changes to the torque-angle curve nor did it improve flexibility. As researchers pointed out, the effects of stretching can be explained by "increases in stretch tolerance."[195]

You can more effectively lengthen a muscle when it is contracted versus when it is relaxed. As counterintuitive as this sounds, you can feel this principle at work. Here's a quick experiment to illustrate.

From a standing position: bend your knees slightly and relax your calf muscles and ankles. Now, shift your body weight onto one leg, allowing your knee to drift forward over your foot. Keep pushing your knee forward gently until you feel tension near the back of your ankle. Take a mental note of how your ankle and calf muscles feel in this position, then return to a neutral standing position.

Now, again shift your weight onto one leg and assume the same ending position with your knee forward of your foot. This time, curl your toes and contract your foot muscles as if you were trying to squeeze the floor. Now where do you feel the tension? You likely felt it migrate up into your calf and maybe even your hamstring. The tension is no longer solely in your connective tissue, but also in your muscles.

The concept of muscles lengthening most effectively when contracted has major implications for how we should think about mobility. First, it shows us that contracting a muscle during a stretch is gentler and safer because it takes the tension off your tendons and ligaments. Second, it shows us that loaded stretching (where a weight is added to the stretch), full range of motion resistance training, and end range isometric contractions are more effective methods of lengthening muscles than passively yanking on joints with boring, static stretching routines.

I stumbled into this concept personally after straining my hamstring muscle. For my entire life, I've had trouble bending over and touching my toes. I'm just not a naturally limber person. Despite years of static stretching, my flexibility was still pathetic. After straining my hamstring (don't even remember what harmless activity caused it), I focused on improving eccentric control and end range of motion contractions. From what I had read at the time, lack of control during the eccentric phase of knee flexion was often the culprit behind hamstring muscle strains. I leaned on two primary exercises: machine lying leg curls with a five-second eccentric phase and physioball leg curls with isometric holds in the end range position (knees straight). After a few weeks of training, the pain in my hamstring died down to a dull twinge, allowing me to continue my normal exercise routine. Unexpectedly, my hamstring flexibility improved dramatically. I noticed immediate improvements in hamstring function during deadlifts, kettlebell swings, and other hip hinge exercises. I was only able to improve my hamstring range of motion after consistently practicing *loaded* stretches.

WHAT YOU NEED TO KNOW ABOUT MUSCLE IMBALANCES

Another reason why stretching doesn't work for most people is that it targets the wrong problem. Muscle imbalances and limited ranges of motion are often compensatory effects the nervous system puts in place to protect you from injury. Take having tight hamstrings as an example. If you have not trained your low back to hinge correctly, your core muscles are weak, or your hips are unstable, your nervous system will slam on the breaks when you try to touch your toes. It knows that if you extend all the way down to maximum hamstring muscle length, you'll be open for all sorts of injuries. This is called *protective tension*. In this scenario, short hamstring muscles aren't the problem. It's lack of strength and stability through the midsection. For most people—especially nonathletes—this is often the case.

The best solution to fixing a muscle imbalance also depends on the body part. Tight chest muscles and shoulders respond well to dynamic mobilizations that move through the entire range of motion. Tight calves and Achilles tendons respond well to loaded stretches and isometric holds. Tight forearms and wrists respond well to nerve gliding and dynamic stretches. As you can see, there are a variety of choices for corrective exercise modalities. The key to choosing the correct course of action is knowing which muscles to strengthen, which to lengthen, and the best way to accomplish that without aggravating problem areas.

How Do Muscle Imbalances Develop?

Muscle imbalances develop for a host of reasons:

- Poor posture
- Repetitive movements
- Poor exercise technique
- Imbalanced strength training
- Injuries
- Neurological disorders
- Pain compensation response

- Overuse of isolation exercises
- Lack of neuromuscular coordination
- Sedentary lifestyle
- Overall lack of general fitness and strength
- Genetic and structural deviations (e.g. scoliosis)

While the initial trigger of a muscle imbalance is difficult to pinpoint, the downstream effects are predictable: muscle imbalances compromise the mobility-stability relationship of joints, which leads to dysfunctional movement patterns, which leads to joint system breakdown. Again, refer to the pain compensation diagram (page 22, Figure 1.3). Notice how the cycle is a closed loop—each action reinforces the subsequent action.

Types of Muscle Imbalances

Muscle imbalance is a sort of ambiguous term in the sports training world. There doesn't seem to be a consensus on clear boundaries and definitions, partially because there is a lot of overlap. But for functional application, there are just five basic types you should know:

Agonist-antagonist imbalance

Alterations to agonist and antagonist muscle groups represent the most common type of muscle imbalance. In this scenario, the prime mover muscle (agonist) is used disproportionately more than its opposing counterpart (antagonist). This causes the prime mover muscle group to become *hypertonic*—which means shortened, strengthened in a limited range of motion, and easily activated during movement. This imbalance also decreases neural activity to the opposing antagonist muscle groups, which subsequently becomes stretched out and weak. This is known as *latency*.[196]

Overused agonists become *hypertonic* (short, tight, easily triggered), and underused antagonists become *latent* (inhibited, overstretched, weak).

The agonist/antagonist imbalance frequently happens to the chest and upper back regions. Your chest and anterior deltoids shorten from sitting with shoulders hunched forward. If you favor pressing exercises over pulling exercises, your upper chest muscles become even stronger and tighter compared to those in your upper back. This results in short, painful chest muscles that are prone to irritation and a destabilized shoulder girdle.

The solution is threefold:

1. Improve strength and stability in latent antagonist muscles (e.g. your upper back).

2. Improve mobility and reduce tension in your hypertonic agonist muscles (e.g. your chest).

3. Reinforce goals #1 and #2 above with postural and corrective exercises that help rebalance the agonist/antagonist relationship during movement.

Only when you address all three aspects can you correct the imbalance. This is one reason why generic stretching programs fail to produce results, and why strength training without smart mobility training leads to muscle tension, pain, and injury. One needs the other to be effective.

Length-tension relationship imbalance

The length-tension curve is a model that represents the force-generating capability of muscles when held at different lengths. While the agonist/antagonist imbalance describes the relationship of opposing muscle groups, the length-tension imbalance describes how an individual muscle's length affects its force generation capabilities. Let me demonstrate.

You know intuitively that muscles generate the most power when the motion begins from an optimal joint position. If you are throwing a baseball, you won't be able to generate much power if your elbow is completely flexed, as if you were about to throw a dart. Likewise, if your elbow is fully extended, you won't be able to throw with much power either—it would be an awkward slinging motion instead of a typical overhand throw. However, when you begin the throwing movement with your elbow at about 90 degrees, you're able to create much more force and throwing speed.[197]

FIGURE 6.1

Optimal length-tension relationship of the elbow joint for throwing a baseball.

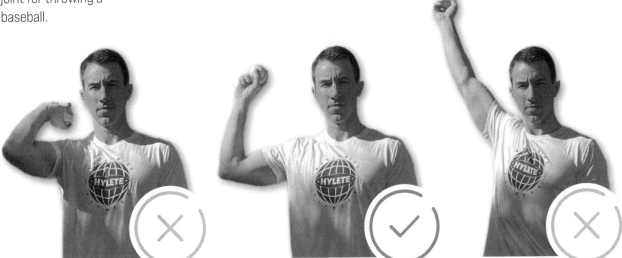

Muscles that have shortened from overuse or poor posture, such as the chest muscles and hip flexors, demonstrate greater force-potential in contracted positions—but not in normal positions. If you've ever seen a weightlifter moving an impressive amount of weight through a comically short range of motion, you've seen this principle at work. It's problematic for two reasons:

1. It incentivizes weight lifters and athletes to favor shortened ranges of motion. Even if you don't consciously emphasize a shortened range of motion where you feel stronger, your body naturally gravitates to it as a path of least resistance.

2. It increases injury risk because there is a large gap between force potential in the limited ROM and full ROM.

Example: Bicep tendon ruptures often occur during pressing movements near the bottom of the repetition. The imbalanced lifter can comfortably handle the weight in their sweet spot—the top portion—but their bicep tendon is not prepared to handle the load while at the bottom of the repetition.

Shortening of muscles can happen over the course of a few weeks from inactivity, such as using a wrist brace (wrist extensors) or prolonged periods of sitting (hip flexors). Lengthening beyond optimal levels also happens overtime when held in elongated positions. For example, if you spend several hours reading in bed each day with your head propped up on a pillow and your neck cranked forward, it will gradually lengthen and weaken the neck extensor muscles that hold your head in place. Similarly, if you sit with shoulders rounded forward for most of the day it will lengthen and weaken your posterior shoulder muscles.

I listed these examples to demonstrate that there are problems at both extremes of the length-tension spectrum, and that there's an optimal length-tension relationship ratio for force production and injury risk. In the case of shortened muscles, mobility training that increases muscle length helps restore optimal length-tension ratios.[198] So even though stretching doesn't perform well in studies, the idea of passive muscle lengthening does have some merit when viewed through the lens of optimizing the length-tension relationship of specific muscles. But again, stretching alone isn't the answer. Strategic strength training must be part of the equation.

Beyond addressing shortened or elongated muscles with corrective exercise, working through full ranges of motion helps prevent length-tension imbalances and helps your body recognize potential injuries before they happen due to greater proprioceptive awareness.

Force-couple imbalance

Muscles work in coordination with one another to achieve joint movement and stability. In physiology, this relationship is referred to as a *force-couple*.[199] For example, to achieve a neutral spine position, several muscles activate to form balanced tension around your hips: abdominal and erector spinae muscles pull upward on the pelvis, while hip flexors and hamstrings pull downward. Depending on which joint system is moving and how it is moving, muscles have various roles:[200]

- *Agonist*: primary driving force
- *Antagonist*: works in opposition to agonist for balance
- *Synergist*: secondary muscle that assists the primary movement
- *Stabilizer*: contracts along with agonist to help maintain joint integrity

This is why it's helpful to construct exercise programs based on movement systems rather than muscles. It's also why overuse of isolation exercises can lead to another type of muscle imbalance called a *force-couple imbalance*.

Force-couple imbalances occur when one or more muscles within a joint stabilization system fail to do their job. Shoulders are notorious for having force-couple deviations. During shoulder flexion and abduction, the deltoids move the arms up and away from your body while the rotator cuff muscles exert compressive forces to keep the shoulder joint in place. Poor posture, too much bench-pressing, and overactive deltoid muscles leave the upper back and rotator cuff neglected. This leads to an increase in dislocating and destabilizing forces during shoulder movements, which increases risk of injury, shoulder impingement, and joint degeneration.

This is a complex imbalance that requires adjustments on several fronts: exercise programming, posture, and movement training. Well-timed isolation exercises to strengthen the neglected muscles are useful, as are movements that challenge the stabilizers preferentially to rebalance force-couple relationships around the joint. The best ways to avoid developing a force-couple imbalance are to add plenty of varied movement to your life, use compound exercises that challenge stabilizer and antagonist muscles, and limit the use of isolation movements for overdeveloped prime mover muscles (e.g. lats, deltoids).

Synergistic dominance

Synergistic dominance is when the secondary assisting muscles carry out the primary function of a weakened or inactive prime mover.[196] This is common in people who have experienced traumatic injuries and have developed compensating movements to work around pain and movement limitations. A typical example is when the gluteal muscles fail to act as primary movers during squatting, hinging, and walking. This can happen from sitting all day—which essentially turns off your butt muscles—or from tight hip flexors that keep your butt from firing correctly (via the *law of reciprocal inhibition*). In this scenario, the hip flexors and hamstrings must step up as prime movers of hip extension. Not only does this reduce force capability, it overworks synergist muscles that aren't designed to be prime movers, leading to overuse injuries.

Side dominance imbalance

Unless you're genuinely ambidextrous, you are either right- or left-side dominant (right- or left-handed). This is entirely natural and doesn't always cause problems. But when one side becomes disproportionately stronger, more developed, or mobile, it creates movement faults that can lead to injury. Deviations to posture in the shoulders and hips can also create extra tension on the spine. The simplest way to prevent this is to add plenty of *unilateral movements* to your training routine—exercises performed using one arm or leg at a time. By forcing your weak side to keep up with your strong side, you'll close the strength gap and develop a more balanced body.

Stretching, Oversimplified

Now you can see why stretching is an oversimplified solution to a complex problem that involves far more than just tight muscles. In some cases, increasing flexibility even exacerbates the muscle imbalance. Corrective exercise should involve addressing postural faults, mobility limitations, neuromuscular coordination, pain, and injuries. Despite the bleak results of formal studies, stretching to mobilize tight muscles has its place—but it should only play a small, strategic part in a much broader strategy. It should be used primarily as a tool to correct muscle imbalances and help you get into better positions during sports and weight training.

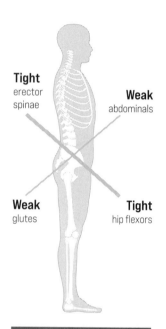

FIGURE 6.2

Lower cross syndrome.

Common Muscle Imbalances

- **Lower Cross Syndrome:** Lower cross syndrome is characterized by tight hip flexors and hip extensors, and weak abdominals and glutes (butt muscles). This is one of the most common major muscle imbalances, primarily caused by sitting and ineffective exercise methods that don't properly engage the glutes and core muscles while mobilizing the hips.

- **Upper Cross Syndrome:** Upper cross syndrome is characterized by tight muscles in the chest and upper trapezius region along with latent neck flexors and upper back muscles. This is also usually caused by poor posture like slouched sitting and tilting the head downward (as if looking at a phone).

- **Shoulder Internal/External Rotation:** This condition is usually part of upper cross syndrome, but it's worth calling out separately. The internal rotation muscles around the shoulder (e.g. chest, lats) are commonly stronger and hypertonic compared to the muscles that externally rotate the shoulder (e.g. infraspinatus, teres minor, lower

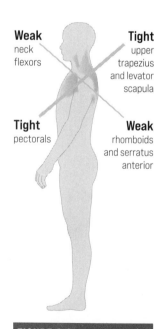

FIGURE 6.3

Upper cross syndrome.

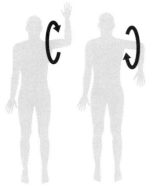

External Rotation | **Internal Rotation**

FIGURE 6.4

Shoulder internal/external rotation.

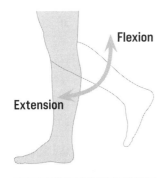

Flexion

Extension

FIGURE 6.5

Knee flexion/extension.

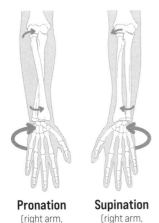

Pronation
(right arm, palm down)

Supination
(right arm, palm up)

FIGURE 6.6

Forearm pronation/supination.

trapezius). This constant internal rotation tension puts the shoulder in a painful, disadvantageous position.

- **Knee Extension/Flexion:** The quadriceps muscles (anterior thigh muscles) are commonly stronger than the hamstrings (posterior thigh muscles). This can lead to knee injuries and hamstring tears when the hamstrings are forced to contract faster than they can effectively lengthen.[201] More hamstring training volume with exaggerated eccentrics helps counteract this imbalance.

- **Forearm Pronation/Supination:** The muscles of the forearm that internally rotate your palm downward (as in pouring a drink out on the ground) are almost always strong and hypertonic compared to forearm supinators (rotating the palm up). In both exercise and everyday life, you're much more likely to use and develop your pronators. This is a common cause not only of wrist pain but elbow and shoulder pain as well.

FOUR PRINCIPLES OF EFFECTIVE MOBILITY TRAINING

You don't have to be an expert in diagnosing and fixing muscle imbalances, although understanding them goes a long way toward course correcting when you experience bumps in the road. A well-thought-out mobility training plan will help you prevent and fix muscle imbalances, while also reducing pain and increasing performance. Instead of blindly stretching all your muscles in an effort to become super flexible, use these four strategies for building a mobility program that makes sense.

1. Make it goal specific.

Gymnasts need flexible hamstrings and strong core muscles. Kickboxers need mobility and strength in their groin muscles for kicking. Surfers need thoracic (midback) extension and endurance in their neck extensors for bridging up on their boards while paddling out. Baseball players need a stable shoulder girdle and strong upper back to prevent throwing motions from tearing their rotator cuff apart. People who spend much of their day in front of the computer need to have good posture and an active posterior chain to prevent desk slouching from destroying their back. In each case, mobility training involves general range of motion competency with lifestyle-specific training.

You shouldn't yank on every muscle and joint that feels tight. Nor should you endlessly foam roll all the sore parts of your body until you're covered with bruises. Smart mobility training involves aiming at specific goals, and those goals should be based on what you are trying to accomplish. Professional athletes have high-paid trainers and physiotherapists to look after them. Their full-time job is tuning and optimizing their bodies. That's likely not the case for you. So while I highly recommend working with a qualified professional to assess your posture and movement, you have to be your own advocate. No one knows your body quite like you. Understanding how your lifestyle contributes to specific muscle imbalances and how to employ strength and mobility training to correct those imbalances are vital skills for staying healthy and making progress toward your fitness goals. If you're going to spend time on mobility training, make sure it aligns with your goals and your body's specific needs.

2. Prioritize stability over mobility.

One of the best ways to get injured is to stretch a joint that's already unstable. Before worrying about improving *mobility*, make sure you have a baseline level of joint *stability*.

Your first priority should be building stability around the lumbar spine and muscles of the core. Once you have sufficient stability around your core, you can safely expand mobility and start focused movement training. This process takes time and repetition and must be carried out sequentially to reduce the risk of muscle imbalances and injuries.

There's a saying physiotherapists often use: "Proximal stability leads to distal mobility." *Proximal* means nearest the most interior aspect of your body. *Distal* means farthest away from your core. In other words, achieve stability around your trunk and you'll be able to more effectively expand the functional range of motion in your legs, shoulders, and arms. Another more vision-inducing phrase is "You cannot fire a cannon from a canoe." Without a solid base, nothing on the exterior will work right. You now know that mobility restrictions are often caused by protection tension from the nervous system—not tight muscles—so you can see how this saying rings true. When you have a weak link, or a body part you know is not working correctly, the natural tendency is to attempt to stretch your way out of it. It's counterintuitive, but the best approach is to build stability from the core outward before worrying about increasing range of motion. Focus on stability first, then mobility.

3. Straighten before strengthening.

Because posture is what you do most of the time, it is often at the root of joint pain, muscle imbalances, and injuries. On top of that, it tends to worsen with age. If you don't address posture, you'll be continually slapping Band-Aids on the problems caused by it. It's a game you simply can't win. But you can't just fix posture by consciously holding yourself differently. It takes structural changes to musculature and neural wiring. It requires a combination of training your body to maintain better posture and consciously working to hold yourself in better positions. While at work, you catch yourself slouching and consciously adjust, making a small improvement in static posture. While exercising, you train muscles and movements that improve dynamic posture, and you see a little progress from week to week. It's a painstakingly slow process, but it works. And it's worth it.

Postural assessment is beyond the scope of this book. It's highly individual and requires an experienced eye. Besides hiring a professional to assess your movement, you should also work with a professional to evaluate your posture and provide recommendations on what muscles to strengthen and what muscles to lengthen. I try to do this at least three times per year, adjusting my exercise program to fit. Work with a qualified professional such as a sports medicine physician, physical therapist, or other certified corrective exercise specialist. Tell them you would like a functional movement screening, postural assessment, and written plan for optimizing your posture.

Just don't get too caught up in minor asymmetries. Everyone has subtle posture deviations. Perfection is not the goal here. While I recommend getting an assessment from a third party, you will benefit from studying models of what good posture is and adjusting your body to match it. In the next chapter, I'll walk you through routines you can perform right now to improve posture.

4. Mobilize in multiple planes.

The three planes of human movement are the sagittal, frontal, and transverse planes.[202]

- **Sagittal plane:** forward and backward movements (divides body into left and right halves)

- **Frontal plane:** side to side movements (divides body into front and back halves)

- **Transverse plane:** rotational movements (divides body into upper and lower halves)

Strength training and mobility exercises typically train the sagittal and frontal planes with basic forward and backward movements and side-to-side movements (e.g. pushing, pulling, raising arms, lowering arms). But faulty movement patterns and injuries most commonly occur in the transverse plane. Rotation of the hip, twisting of the knee, and circumduction (circular movement) of the shoulder all involve rotational motions in the transverse plane. It's no coincidence that the transverse plane is the most neglected.

Also, you need the ability to move effectively through all three planes in coordination. This is where most athletic movement takes place, as well as everyday activities like unloading groceries from a car or getting out of bed. For this reason, every mobility training program should include *multiplanar movements*—those that pass through more than one plane. Improving skill in these complex patterns will make your body more resilient to injury and tie together strength and coordination of multiple body parts, improving overall athleticism and functional movement capability.

Some basic examples of effective multiplanar loaded movements are:

- one arm pulling with lower body rotation (imagine starting a lawnmower)

- cable wood choppers (similar to a throwing movement, but with arms extended using cable resistance)

- side lunges with simultaneous reaching to the ground

These movements have the added benefit of building core strength in a more functional way than crunches or sit-ups. While I'm not against resistance training exercises that use heavy loads while moving through the transverse plane, I've found that adding body-weight multiplanar movements to warm-up routines is a safer method. This allows you to practice trunk rotation movements while reducing injury risk since you are not holding heavy weights. Your spine is designed to twist, but it doesn't like to twist under heavy loads.

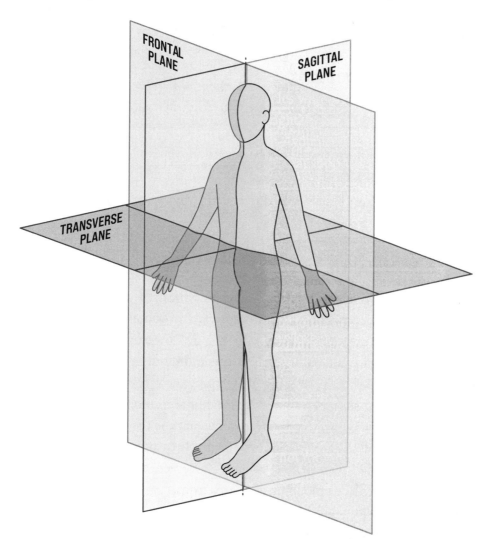

FIGURE 6.7

Three planes of motion.

TYPES OF MOBILITY TRAINING

Despite the endless options for increasing range of motion proficiency, mobility training boils down to four basic categories. Each has its place in an effective mobility training program. The exercises mentioned in this chapter are described in detail in chapter 11, "Mastering the Movements."

1. Static Stretching

Let's face it. The research supporting static stretching is lacking. But that doesn't mean you should kick it to the curb completely. It just means you have to be smart about what muscles to focus on, what stretches you perform, and when to perform them. Holding stretches for long periods before competition or heavy weightlifting is a bad idea. But stretching after competition or training—or as part of a comprehensive mobility routine—certainly has merit. Lengthening hypertonic (short, tight) muscles can help fix muscle imbalances, reduce muscle tension, prevent injuries, and help you establish better posture and positioning during movement.

Dr. Stuart McGill is considered by many to be the world's leading expert on low back pain. He has published more than 240 peer-review journal articles on pain, injuries, and functional fitness. While Dr. McGill has long been vocal about how overusing static stretching can deaden muscles and diminish peak strength, even he advocates static stretching to rebalance muscle asymmetries.[203]

The best time to use static stretching is after a workout, or any other time of day when you will not be performing high-intensity exercises soon after. I find that focusing on one stretch per day—targeting common hypertonic muscles—allows me to make quick progress without hours of mindless stretching. Focusing on just one stretch per day also increases adherence, both in my own training experience and for clients I've worked with. If you give yourself a list of 15–20 stretches to perform at the end of each workout, you won't stick to the program for long. But anybody can sit down for a couple minutes and complete one static stretch. Because you'll only focus on one at a time, the exercise you choose must provide the biggest bang for your buck. It should help improve postural faults, involve multiple major muscle groups, and be a stretch you can make noticeable progress on from week to week.

Here are some examples of high ROI (return on investment) stretches that lengthen muscles prone to tightness, while also adding an element of core stability training:

- Glutes and hip abductors ► Pigeon (page 215)
- Hip flexors and hamstrings ► Cossack Squat (page 210)
- Lats and thoracic spine ► Anchored Lat Stretch (page 222)

How long should you hold a stretch?

There are as many theories on how long to hold a stretch as there are number of stretches. Studies show holding an elongated position for 10 minutes or more can stimulate increases in protein content within the muscles, effectively improving the length-tension relationship and possibly even giving you more muscle base to build strength upon.[204] But this is highly inconvenient and simply unrealistic for most people. At a bare minimum, static stretches should be held for at least 10 seconds. This is just long enough to activate the golgi tendon organ (GTO) response within your muscles. The GTO is responsible for inhibiting muscle spindle activity, designed to avoid injury. When activated during a stretch, it allows your muscles to relax just enough to extend beyond their resting length.[205]

An effective method that combines static and dynamic stretching is the 10-10-10 method, made popular by the physical therapists and mobility experts at GMB Fitness (https://gmb.io). Here's how it works:

- Gently move into the stretch and hold for 10 seconds.

- Move in and out of the stretch for 10 repetitions, gradually pushing yourself into a more elongated position with each repetition.

- Again, hold the stretch for 10 seconds, this time pushing the limits of your flexibility slightly more than the first 10-second hold.

I find this method to be more mentally stimulating than holding a stretch for two to three minutes. It also allows you to feel the tension and weak points of the movement before pushing the limits of your flexibility. And it provides a satisfying, measurable way of organizing stretches into sets. If you feel compelled to use static stretching for pain relief, cooling down, or just stretching tight muscles because it feels good, try performing one to three sets of the 10-10-10 method. You can use this stretching method either before or after a workout.

Loaded stretching is another form of static stretching that works wonders on stubbornly tight muscles. By using additional loads from weights, your muscles absorb the tension instead of your tendons and ligaments. Not only is this more joint friendly, studies show it's a more effective way of lengthening muscles than static stretching.[195] If you've never used loaded stretching before, use a light weight and end the stretch if you experience excessive discomfort or feel that your joints are in a precarious position. Here are some loaded stretches that target common hard-to-stretch muscles:

- **Loaded Calf Stretch:** Using a calf raise machine, barbell, or holding dumbbells (choose a weight you can complete at least 10 repetitions with), move into the fully extended portion of the repetition. Be sure to keep some tension in your calves to focus the stretch on the muscles rather than the joint articulation. Hold the stretch for 10–45 seconds.

- **Scapular Pull-ups (Active Bar Hanging, page 223):** Using your own body weight, hang from a pull-up bar with your feet off the ground. Create a small amount of tension on the bar by pulling your scapula back and down. This will engage and lengthen your upper back muscles and obliques and take some pressure off the ligaments in your shoulders. Hold the stretch for 10–45 seconds, with periods of gently relaxing your scapula muscles then contracting them again.

- **Incline Dumbbell Fly Holds (page 236):** Using an incline bench and a set of dumbbells you can complete at least 10 repetitions of incline flies with, move into the lowered portion of the repetition. Keep your palms facing each other and elbows slightly bent. Be careful not to extend the stretch beyond your normal range of motion. You should feel the stretch in your upper chest and anterior shoulders. Stop the stretch if you feel discomfort in the middle or rear of your shoulder, which indicates the stabilizer muscles in your rotator cuff are being overstressed. Even in the fully stretched position, you don't want the weights hanging against your shoulder capsule. Keep some tension in your chest throughout the stretch, holding the bottom position for 10–45 seconds.

- **Lying Dumbbell Pullover Holds (page 248)** Lie across a flat bench on your back—you can lie with your body along the bench, or perpendicular to it. Place your feet flat on the floor for stability. Hold the dumbbell with hands cupped around one end and reach your arms back over your head with elbows slightly bent. Keep your abdominal muscles tight to avoid arching your low back—your thoracic spine and shoulders will provide much of the joint movement. When you feel a stretch in your upper back (lats), pause and hold the stretch for 10–45 seconds before pulling the weight back over your head, finishing with the weight directly above your chest.

- **Loaded Thoracic Extensions:** Using a TRX trainer or other suspension training strap, grab the handles with both hands while facing away from anchor strap position. With elbows bent, lean forward until your arms extend behind your head and you feel a stretch in your upper back, upper chest, and obliques. Use your body weight and lean into the stretch, focusing on lengthening your thoracic (upper back) spine and maintaining a tight core. Hold for 10–45 seconds.

- **Bulgarian Split Squat Holds (page 262):** Using a flat bench or box and a set of dumbbells that you can comfortably perform 10 repetitions of lunges with, move into the Bulgarian split squat position (rear leg elevated on a bench, around hip height; front leg on the ground with knee around 90 degrees; upper body in upright posture). Lunge forward and downward until you feel a stretch in your rear hip flexor. Hold for 10–45 seconds, then alternate legs.

- **Isometric Romanian Deadlift (page 265):** Using a barbell, dumbbell, or kettlebell, hinge forward at the hips with knees slightly bent until you feel a stretch in your hamstrings. This is effectively the lowering portion of a Romanian deadlift. Stop the movement when you cannot reach toward the ground any farther without your low or upper back losing their natural arch. Hold the bottom position for a few moments while keeping your core tight—3–5 seconds. Then extend your hips and stand back up to complete the repetition.

- **Goblet Squat Holds (page 260):** As you reach the bottom range of motion during a squat while holding a weight in front of your chest, hold the bottom position for 3–5 seconds before completing the repetition. During the hold, focus on squeezing your glutes and preventing your low back from slouching.

Counting Your Stretches

If you find counting the seconds to be monotonous, try counting your breaths instead. This has the added benefit of ensuring you're breathing deeply and properly. For a 10-second stretch, count five deep breaths (allowing 2–3 seconds per breath).

2. Dynamic Stretching

Dynamic stretching involves actively moving through a full range of motion. It solves many of the problems that static stretching creates and is superior in a few ways. Unlike static stretching, it increases blood flow to muscles.[206] When used before training in small doses, it doesn't negatively affect performance. It's a better diagnostic tool than static stretching because you're able to feel your joints and muscles better, locating tight spots and weaknesses more easily as you move through the motion. It more closely matches what you'll experience in the real world. And it gives you more opportunities to mobilize the entire joint system versus just creating tension on one piece of tissue during a static stretch.

Mindfully moving through ranges of motion, gradually lengthening the target muscles with each repetition, is also much more intuitive and engaging. I've been able to make faster improvements with dynamic stretching than static stretching simply because it's more enjoyable and I'm more likely to be consistent with it. I have a quick mobility flow that I go through each morning, and again before each workout. Over time, my ability to hold stretches in more elongated positions has improved, despite not spending much time performing static stretches.

Much of the benefit of dynamic stretching is neurological. It's not just about stretching your muscles to elongate them. The frequency of practicing specific motor patterns is largely responsible for improvements in your range of motion. In terms of warming up or preparing for a specific movement, dynamic stretching is clearly superior to static. Here are some dynamic stretches you can perform before exercising or any other time of day to improve flexibility and prepare your body for movement (see chapter 11, "Mastering the Movements," for instructions on each):

- Cossack Squat (page 210)
- Hinge to Squat (page 218)
- World's Greatest Stretch (page 220)
- Band Pass Through (page 225)
- Swimmer's Stretch (page 227)
- Thoracic Extension on Foam Roller (page 229)

Advanced Dynamic Mobility Techniques

The three subtypes of dynamic stretching are ballistic stretching, PNF (proprioceptive neuromuscular facilitation) stretching, and active isolated stretching.

- **Ballistic stretching** is an extreme form of dynamic stretching using bouncing movements to push muscles beyond their normal range of motion. It's widely considered high risk and should only be used under the supervision of a qualified therapist (if at all). Ballistic stretching does have a major strength; because the muscle is contracting while the tendon is elongated, it decreases connective tissue stiffness, allowing for a greater adaptive response within the tendon and more elastic energy to be stored before explosive movements. Static stretching does not have this benefit.[92] However, you don't necessarily have to use ballistic stretching to get this benefit. Eccentric training and dynamic stretches where the muscles stay active throughout the movement also improve tendon compliance.

- **PNF stretching** involves both stretching and contracting a target muscle in an alternating sequence, typically with the aid of a partner.

The contract-relax technique reduces neural inhibition and increases passive ranges of motion. Studies show PNF stretching is more effective than ballistic stretching. And because it requires the aid of a trained professional, it's generally safer. PNF stretching should only be implemented under the tutelage of a qualified professional.[207]

- **Active isolated stretching (AIS)** is a hybrid stretching technique that uses short static holds of no more than two seconds for multiple repetitions—usually 10 at a time. The theory behind this technique is that it allows the target muscles to elongate without triggering the stretching reflex or reciprocal contraction of the opposing muscle group. Proponents of AIS claim it's safer than static stretching and still provides the athletic enhancements without causing decreases in blood flow to the target muscle. At least four studies have confirmed that AIS leads to the same increases in flexibility as static stretching.[8] Anecdotally, I can confirm AIS works well as a warm-up or a quick (and comfortable) way to improve range of motion. The key is to avoid fast movements and overstretching. These elicit the stretch-reflex, which reduces the effectiveness of AIS.[208] Instead, move toward the end of your natural range of motion during the stretch and stop before you feel discomfort. Hold for two seconds, relax, and repeat for a total of 10 repetitions. Complete this cycle two or three times. You'll notice that your range of motion increases throughout the repetitions even though you aren't actively pushing it beyond your normal ROM.

While there is research supporting some of these more advanced stretching techniques, especially after surgery, most people can accomplish their mobility goals by using controlled, dynamic stretches.

3. Manual Therapy

Manual therapy is a catch-all category for all the massaging, rolling, and myofascial release techniques that aim to increase mobility by manually loosening up stiff, painful tissues. Techniques like foam rolling and electric percussion massage are more popular than ever with elite athletes and gym goers. There is evidence that massage reduces soreness and improves blood flow. But the main benefit of manual therapy from a mobility perspective is how it reduces muscle hypertonicity and produces short-term increases in flexibility—a useful tool to utilize before stretching and full ROM movements.[209]

High tensile forces placed on muscles trigger something called *autogenic inhibition*.[210] Autogenic inhibition is when the excitability of hypertonic muscles is reduced, inhibiting the typical rebellious responses you get from those tight muscles when trying to stretch them. The sensory receptor responsible for all this activity is the golgi tendon organ (GTO)—the same receptor mentioned earlier in our discussion of static stretching. GTOs are located in the junctions between your tendons and muscles. Their job is to inhibit muscle contraction and prevent damage when high amounts of force or tension are placed on the tendon. In effect, the GTO relaxes the muscle. This is useful not only for injury prevention but also for manipulating tight muscles.

Some studies indicate that GTOs could be responsible for why manual therapies like foam rolling help relax muscles and increase flexibility—especially when applied to muscle knots (*trigger points*) and tight soft tissues.[211] But the underlying mechanisms of how manual therapy works are still unclear. In a metastudy on foam rolling published in *Frontiers in Physiology*, researchers stated that the most plausible explanation for why it improves flexibility and subsequent performance could be the effect on pain modulation systems.[210] This makes intuitive sense. If you've ever practiced foam rolling, you know that it feels good (at least after you're done mashing on tight muscles, anyway). It seems to loosen things up, allowing you to move and stretch with less pain.

Despite the lack of agreement in the fitness community regarding the utility of manual therapy, studies show it increases flexibility (at least in the short term), enhances recovery, and helps reduce compressive forces on surrounding joints.[212] Respected therapists use it in their practices. And compared to other mobility tools, it seems to have little or no downside. If you find foam rolling or other manual therapy techniques help you, then there is no harm in adding them to your preworkout or postworkout routine. If you have painful tendons and stiff joints, using manual therapy to loosen up the surrounding muscles can be an effective way to take the pressure off aggravated joints.

Popular manual therapy techniques: from least to most aggressive

1. Self-massage
2. Foam rolling
3. Percussion massage (electric massage device)
4. Myofascial release
5. Deep tissue massage (from licensed massage therapist)

What is myofascial release?

Myofascial release is a technique that involves applying sustained pressure to regions of connective tissue that restrict motion and muscle function. The theory is that pressure applied allows the fascia (band of connective tissue surrounding muscle) to elongate, reducing resting tension and allowing muscular systems to operate normally. For muscle knots, you can use self-myofascial release by applying constant gentle pressure to the sore area using your hand, a lacrosse ball, foam roller, or other therapeutic tool. Practitioners generally aim for five minutes of gentle pressure with short breaks throughout the session.

4. Functional Movement Training

There's a lot of debate around what *functional training* means. To me, functional training for athletes is any training that helps them with their specific sport. For nonathletes and general fitness enthusiasts, it's exercise that improves functions of their daily life. I don't think there's a need to complicate the definition further. Regarding what exercises to perform, that *does* get more complicated.

Functional movement training doesn't usually look like mobility training, but that's exactly what it is. It's essentially training your body to move effectively through challenging ranges of motion with unconventional loading techniques. It challenges your muscles, joints, and neural systems in ways that improve movement efficiency. The functional exercise crowd does get made fun of, probably because diehard functional movement people spend too much time standing on inflatable balls and performing silly exercises that have no translation to real life. Every gym has a few patrons like this. They spend their entire workout doing functional training, with no visible results to show for it. On the opposite end of the spectrum are the purists who posit that only the deadlift, squat, and bench press are necessary for strength and physique enhancement. Both radical approaches are not ideal.

Like any type of mobility work, functional movement training can be a waste of time if you don't do it right. But when executed correctly, it will do wonders for injury prevention and performance. When it comes to functional movement, follow these five principles for maximum mobility benefits:

1. **Train movements, not muscles.** This is the golden rule of functional movement. Train your body to push, pull, squat, hinge, and carry objects more effectively.

2. **Expand your functional ROM.** Injury expert Tim Gabbett prepares his athletes for the worst-case scenarios they'll face in competition. That involves preparing the athletes for movements that push them outside their comfortable ranges of motion. If there are movements you struggle with, you are likely coming up short at the beginning or far end of the movement. Try reducing the resistance and slowing down the movement until you have mastered the end ranges of the exercise.

3. **Train your body to stabilize in various load positions.** Most exercises considered to be functional involve intensive core stabilization during movement (e.g. throwing a medicine ball sideways) or while holding

static positions (e.g. the plank). The ability to stabilize is at the center of functional movement. It protects you from injury, increases power capacity, and improves movement efficiency. Functional movement is not always about movement, either. What does not move is just as important. For example, exercises like the single leg deadlift and single arm dumbbell row challenge your antirotation capabilities—your ability to prevent your hips and spine from twisting out of alignment when faced with external rotation forces.

4. **Train all the classifications of muscles.** Don't rely on machines and easy isolation movements during your workouts. Focus on compound movements that engage not just the prime movers of the exercise but also all the supporting cast of stabilizers. Corrective exercises are generally meant to bring supportive muscles up to speed with the prime mover muscles.

5. **Train muscles and joints to work in coordination.** Remember that some studies have demonstrated agility training to be more effective for preventing injuries than flexibility training. Effective functional movement training teaches your muscles and joints to work in unison.

5. Postural Training

Postural training isn't generally considered "mobility training" because it deals with how you hold yourself at rest. But it should be. Because your mobility can only be as good as the posture it originates from. In the next chapter, we'll look at common postural faults and a checklist you can use to keep your body in alignment at all times.

Corrective Routines

**All human beings should be able and willing
to perform basic maintenance on themselves.**

— Dr. Kelly Starrett, founder of The Ready State
and author of *Becoming a Supple Leopard*

"Good posture" is an ambiguous term. You know it generally means standing up straight and not slouching, but you likely don't have any actionable way to check and fix your postural faults. Before going over a checklist you can use to immediately improve posture, let's look at what good posture is. Good posture refers to proper alignment of the body along the three weight-bearing joints. This is referred to as *neutral position*—where your body is balanced around an imaginary vertical line that runs from the crown of your head to the middle of your feet.

The three weight-bearing joints are the ankle, knee, and hip. The shoulders aren't considered one of the primary weight-bearing joints, but they do support the upper thoracic spine and your head. Which is no easy task. The simplest way to ensure your body is in neutral position is to place the crown of your head and the three weight-bearing joints in a straight vertical line.

In a seated position, you can use the same markers, except that the chain of postural points ends at the hips. The knees, lower legs, and arms are pretty much out of the equation. Their positioning depends on the height of your chair and the setup of a desk if you have one in front of you.

COMMON POSTURAL FAULTS

Postural faults are rarely isolated to one body part—especially when the spine is involved. Your body naturally tries to correct postural faults in one joint by compromising another. For example, forward head protrusion is often the result of upper back rounding (kyphosis), which itself is usually the result of low back overextension (lordosis). Lordosis is commonly caused by tight hips… which is usually caused by movement habits and muscle imbalances.

Another example: if you have ever seen someone jogging with bowed legs caused by advanced osteoarthritis, you know how painful it is to watch.

In order to jog without suffering a knee injury, the bowlegged runner must tilt their hip sharply to the left as they land each left foot stride. This allows them to temporarily align their knee and foot for impact with the ground. On the next stride, they tilt their hips sharply to the right to bring the right knee and foot into alignment. This produces a stiff, waddling motion. While stiffness may be a problem, it's a compensation their body has put in place to protect their knees from further damage.

Some postural faults, like the knee deviation example, are caused by disease states or other abnormalities. Any posture problems that stem from surgeries, injuries, diseases, or other congenital issues should be treated by a medical professional. Get a professional opinion if you're unsure. But most postural faults are caused by lifestyle and muscle imbalances and can be improved. Here are some of the most common postural faults:

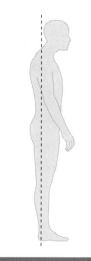

FIGURE 7.1

Forward head protrusion.

Forward Head Protrusion

Forward head protrusion is when the head's resting posture is moved forward, away from neutral position. Forward head protrusion puts stress on the muscles in the back of your neck and pulls the thoracic (upper back) spine out of alignment. This can cause neck pain, headaches, and other downstream negative effects on the spine. It also causes weakening and stretching of the muscles in your upper back and your shoulder blade retractors—the muscles responsible for keeping the shoulders in the optimal back-and-down position.

Kyphosis

Kyphosis is excessive forward curvature up the thoracic spine, giving the appearance of hunchback posture. It's common in osteoporosis patients and people with poor sitting posture. Kyphosis can cause shoulder impingement and pain, forward head protrusion, and muscle imbalances between the upper chest and upper back muscles. People with kyphosis usually have hypertonic chest and anterior shoulder muscles and latent upper back muscles.

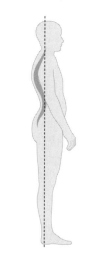

FIGURE 7.2

Kyphosis.

Lordosis

Lordosis is increased curvature of the lumbar spine. People with lordosis have the appearance of sticking their butt out backward and belly out forward. It's usually combined with forward pelvic tilt. Lordosis can cause low back pain, kyphosis, and excessive pressure on the spine that could eventually limit one's ability to move. Lordosis is often caused by tight hip flexors and weak external obliques.

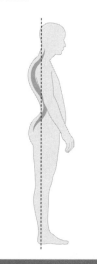

FIGURE 7.3

Lordosis.

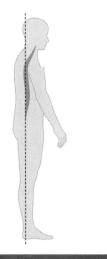

FIGURE 7.4

Flat back.

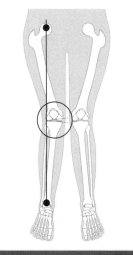

FIGURE 7.5

Knee valgus.

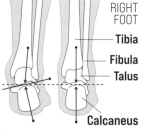

FIGURE 7.6

Foot overpronation.

Flat Back

Flat back is the opposite of lordosis. It's characterized by the front of the pelvis being tucked in. Instead of having a natural S-shaped curve, the back is flat. This causes instability and weakness in the upper spine, leads to forward head protrusion, and reduces the efficiency of the glutes and muscles around the pelvis to control lower body movements. People with flat back find it difficult to stand or walk for long periods of time. Flat back is usually combined with posterior pelvic tilt and shortened abdominal muscles.

Knee Valgus

Knee valgus is when the knees collapse inward. This stresses the ligaments of the inner knee and ankle. It usually presents along with overpronation of the foot and poor side-to-side hip mobility. Knee valgus during explosive movements like jumping can result in traumatic injuries to the knee. More commonly, it results in tendinitis and pain while walking or twisting at the knee joint. Knee valgus is often caused by limited ankle mobility, weak glute muscles, and lack of stability around the hip and knee.

Foot Overpronation

Foot overpronation is when the arch of the foot collapses, and the foot angles inward excessively. Instead of the weight of your body being balanced between the heel, sole, big toe, and pinky toe regions of the foot, the weight falls on the inside edge. This causes knee valgus and increases the risk of knee injury. It can also lead to shin splints, plantar fasciitis, Achilles tendinopathy, and low back pain. Foot overpronation is often caused by weak foot muscles from overdependence on cushioned shoes. This postural fault usually involves changes in the musculature of the foot and the ankle.

Are all postural deviations fixable?

Not all postural deviations are fixable. Diseases, injuries, and natural variations in anatomy create postural deviations that should not necessarily be fixed. If you're concerned about a postural deviation, perform this test: move your body into what you view as optimal posture (more on this in the next section). If you can hold the position for 10 to 15 seconds without pain, it's likely something you can fix. If not, you should get further guidance on how to address any underlying injuries or abnormalities.

THE POSTURE CHECKLIST: TOE TO HEAD

Use this checklist to quickly assess your posture and return it to neutral position. It will seem like too many steps to remember or use consistently when you first read through it. But it only takes a few passes before this sequence becomes second nature. As you scan your body from the toes up, it will be easy to remember which body part is supposed to be in what location. Use this checklist as often as you remember to. The more you consciously adjust your posture to neutral position, the easier it will be for your body to maintain it when you're not thinking about. Like any skill, it takes repetition and time to master.

This is different from establishing an athletic stance, where your feet are shoulder width apart and your knees are bent, ready to leap or run. The aim here is to minimize joint stress.

STANDING POSTURE CHECKLIST

1. Stand with your feet pointed forward, placed directly under your knees. Knees should be straight, but not locked out to the point of hyperextension.

2. Squeeze your foot muscles and toes just enough to feel the weight of your body balanced evenly between your heel and the balls of your feet.

3. Align your hips directly over your knees. For most people, this means shifting your hips a few inches forward by creating tension in the glutes.

4. Tighten your transverse abdominis (TVA), the deep stabilizing muscle of your abdomen, by pulling your belly button inward toward your spine with your lower stomach muscles. Your lower body and foot contact with the ground should feel solid now.

5. Pack the scapula—looking straight ahead, straighten your arms toward the ground and spread your fingers wide. Rotate the thumb side of your hands away from your body so your palms are facing forward. Pull your shoulders back until you feel a pinch between your shoulder blades, then lower your shoulders toward the ground. This is the back-and-down position of a fully retracted scapula.

6. Lengthen your neck toward the ceiling as if a string were pulling your head upward, then tuck your chin inward enough to feel slight tension in the posterior muscles of your neck.

7. Scan your body from the head down to your toes, then back up again, taking note of how each joint system feels.

8. Relax all the muscles involved as much as possible while still maintaining your joint position.

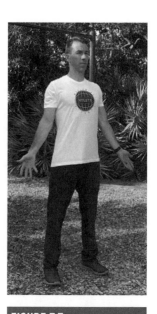

FIGURE 7.7

Standing posture.

9. Bonus—Adjusting Pelvic Tilt: After achieving neutral posture, turn sideways and examine your hip position in the mirror. If you're not wearing a belt, imagine you are. The belt should be near parallel to the ground. Not tilted too far forward or backward.

Practice using the detailed checklist a few times, then switch to the quick mental cue list below. If you can remember "feet, knees, hips, shoulders, head," I'm betting you'll be able to quickly recall where each body part is supposed to be. It is, after all, natural.

Standing Quick Mental Cue List

1. **Feet:** pointed forward.

2. **Knees:** directly above heels.

3. **Hips:** on top of knees—squeeze your glutes and activate your TVA.

4. **Shoulders:** pack the scapula back and down.

5. **Head:** pull up toward ceiling, tuck chin slightly.

SITTING POSTURE CHECKLIST

The average American spends 8 to 10 hours per day sitting.[213] That's more than the average amount of sleep people get each night. For young adults and teens, time spent sitting is even higher, mostly due to increases in computer usage. Riding in vehicles, commuting, television, and other sedentary hobbies are also to blame. Sitting for long time periods increases risk of obesity, high blood pressure, stroke, and heart disease, inspiring the catch phrase "Sitting is the new smoking."[207] It's also one of the primary causes of muscle imbalances, postural faults, and the ensuing joint pain and instability. Based on these stats, it's even more important to get your sitting posture right than your standing posture right. Use this checklist to establish good sitting posture as soon as you plop down in the chair, and again whenever you catch yourself slouching throughout the day:

1. After sitting down, move your knees into a 90-degree angle with your feet planted firmly on the ground. Shift forward slightly so that some weight is redistributed from your butt to your feet.

2. Adjust the angle of your upper body so that your head is directly on top of your hip line.

3. The natural tendency is to round your low back into a slouch, so straighten your low back line by squeezing your glutes and tightening your TVA.

4. Activate the scapula—Pull your shoulders back until you feel a pinch between your shoulder blades, then lower your shoulders toward the ground (back-and-down scapula position).

5. Lengthen your neck toward the ceiling as if a string were pulling your head upward, then tuck your chin inward enough to feel slight tension in the posterior muscles of your neck.

6. Scan your body from the head down to your toes, then back up again, taking note of how each joint system feels. You should feel weight evenly distributed among your butt, back of thighs, and feet on the ground.

7. Relax all the muscles involved as much as possible while still maintaining your joint position.

8. Bonus—Get up and move around every half hour. Stand, walk, and stretch to increase circulation and prevent muscle shortening.

Sitting Quick Mental Cue List

1. **Feet:** planted firmly on the ground.
2. **Knees:** bent to 90 degrees.
3. **Hips:** directly underneath head.
4. **Shoulders:** pack the scapula back and down.
5. **Head:** pull up toward ceiling, tuck chin slightly.

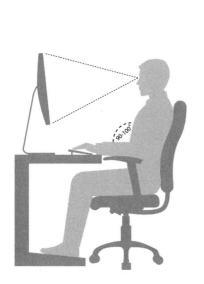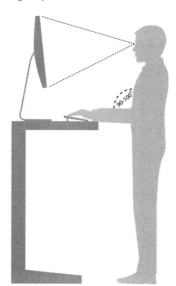

FIGURE 7.8

Optimal sitting and standing desk setup.

The Ergonomics of Computer Work

Chronic sitters spend most of their time in front of the computer. To maintain good posture, you must have the right environment. This is where smart construction of your work setup is key:

1. **Chair height:** Your chair should be set to a height that enables you to displace some of your body weight from your butt to your feet. This prevents your spine from bearing the full load of your upper

body. Your chair height should also allow your hands to rest just below the height of your elbows to reduce wrist strain.

2. **Desk height:** Your desk setup should enable you to place your monitor, keyboard, and mouse in optimal positions: the top of your computer slightly above eye level and computer monitor at least an arm's length away.

3. **Monitor height:** The middle of your monitor should be at eye level. This will help prevent you from tilting your head up or down, reducing neck strain. If you use a laptop, consider getting a laptop stand and external keyboard and mouse. It's nearly impossible to maintain good posture while working on a laptop due to the downward angle your neck has to assume.

4. **Keyboard:** Your keyboard should be set at a height close to your naval. This enables you to work with elbows at around 90 degrees. A common cause of elbow and wrist pain is setting your keyboard too high. This forces the small muscles in your forearms to flex in an already shortened position. If you suffer from elbow or wrist pain, you should seriously consider getting an ergonomic keyboard with keys that are angled out slightly. It's strange at first, but after you get used to it, you'll find it's easier to type and feels better on your arms.

5. **Mouse:** Traditional computer mouses force your arm into a pronated position, causing strain to the inner elbow and wrist tendons. Repetitive motions with your mouse can quickly cause repetitive use strains that lead to medial epicondylitis (tendinopathy of the inner elbow, a.k.a. golfer's elbow). If you have elbow or wrist pain, consider getting an ergonomic mouse that keeps your wrist in a neutral position—thumb toward the ceiling.

6. **Standing desks:** After getting a standing desk to reduce my sitting time, I realized how much I enjoy sitting. It's more comfortable, and I can get better work done than when standing. Still, I recommend getting a standing desk that you can raise or lower easily. The best way to use a standing desk is to give yourself periodic breaks from sitting throughout the day—even if it's only standing for 10–15 minutes per hour.

7. **Other tips:** Place a small pillow or rolled up towel behind your low back when sitting to remind you of what good posture is. Choose a pillow or towel just thick enough that you'll feel pressure against your low back when slouching. Using a lumbar support tool allows you to maintain good posture without the constant muscle tension and focus required to do so on your own.

THE WALKING POSTURE CHECKLIST

There is an unexpectedly large body of research on the effects of posture *while walking*. Beyond the obvious recommendations of walking with upright posture to reduce stress on your neck and low back, there are also significant psychological effects. Most people walk hunched over, staring at their feet or at the gravel in front of them instead of being aware of their surroundings. Walking like this is bad for your posture, bad for your eyes, and even bad for your mental health.

Conversely, walking with upright posture decreases blood pressure, reduces subjective pain levels, and improves several psychological metrics (stress levels, personal assessment, and confidence).[208]

If this sounds silly to you, or if it just seem trivial, don't rush judgment. Next time you're out for a walk, take notice of how you hold yourself. Stand up straight, with your shoulders back and your head positioned above your body instead of protruding forward in front of it. Notice how the sidewalk in front of you snakes and bends to fit the contours of the road. If you're in a crowded area, notice how much easier it is to make eye contact with people. If you are next to a road, notice how you can easily determine who is paying attention behind the wheel and who is on their phone, liable to swerve and plaster some unsuspecting pedestrian. Let your eyes relax, gazing into the distance. After all, our eyes need a break from all the near-sighted computer work, too.

Then, take notice of how you feel. Unlike staring at the ground in front of you, looking forward enables you to think forward—to connect with the world and the people outside of yourself, instead of just focusing on the dirt beneath your feet. While you can put this into practice on a city street when shopping or running errands, the benefits really become evident when you go for an extended walk—at least 15 or 20 minutes.

Use this simple checklist to get even more benefits from walking:

1. While walking, bring your hips forward so they are directly underneath your head. This prevents upper back rounding.

2. Fix your gaze straight ahead of you, not on the ground. Keep your eyes focused on the farthest objects you can find.

3. Use your whole foot when striking the ground. Most people are heel-toe walkers, slamming their heel into the ground with each step, sending a shockwave through their hips and low back and creating opposite force friction. Instead, try landing more toward the middle of your foot with each step. If you experience heel pain or Achilles pain when walking, shorten your stride to further reduce compression forces.

4. Bonus—Walk barefoot or using minimalist shoes (flat soles that do not have a thick cushion). Assuming your feet are healthy enough to do this, it's an effective way to build foot strength and ankle stability. After a lifetime of spraining my ankles repeatedly during sports, my ankles felt stiff and brittle. They were my weak link when running, squatting, and doing one-legged exercises. I tried crazy stuff—foot curls, picking up objects with my toes—but nothing worked as well as learning to walk in minimalist footwear.

The first few times I tried it, the muscles around my ankles and in the middle of my feet were extremely sore. It also felt awkward. But after a few weeks, it started to feel natural. I could feel the muscles in the arches of my feet and throughout my toes contracting and springing forward with each step. My feet felt strong. They stopped hurting when I went for long walks. My ankles became more stable, and my balance was noticeably better when performing lower body exercises. I was skeptical at first—after all, it sounds like one of those new-age health techniques that turns out to be detrimental to your health. But it works. Recent studies support it as a practice for strengthening foot muscles as well. A 2018 study published in *Medicine & Science in Sports & Exercise* demonstrated that eight weeks of walking in minimalist shoes significantly improved foot muscle strength. Some test subjects saw improvements in as little as four weeks.[208]

Beyond strengthening tendons and muscles, there's a proprioceptive benefit from learning to walk without thick footwear. Your feet can send more accurate signals to your brain about the landscape you're on. This improves coordination and balance. It also helps you establish even foot pressure—helping to reduce ankle and knee injuries caused by walking with overpronated feet or excessive heel striking. And it teaches your body to walk in a way that more naturally suits your anatomy.

Another option is to walk in flip flops or open-toed sandals. Pay attention to the patterning of your feet the next time you walk in a pair of flip flops. You will notice that your toes naturally contract just before striking the ground with each step. This prevents the sandal from flying off your foot and reduces the "clop" sound as your foot lands. If you walk with lazy feet, it's noisier. So you get instant feedback. Flip-flop walking is a great way to train your feet to stay active and a good introduction to minimalist footwear. As with minimalist shoes, you should start slow and work your way up to longer distances gradually.

I still use traditional walking and running shoes at certain times—you won't see me hiking through the mountains in thin sandals or slip-on shoes. I'm not a diehard barefoot walker. I simply look at walking with minimalist shoes, or barefoot, as a therapeutic technique. I encourage you to do the same.

Word of caution: start slow. If your feet are used to cushioned shoes, you can easily injure the tendons in your ankles, feet, and toes. Start slow and do not walk long distances in minimalist shoes more than two times per week. Discontinue walking with minimalist footwear if you start experiencing prolonged pain in the back of your ankle, an indication that your Achilles tendon is overstressed. Start with just a few minutes at a time. You will be using muscles and connective tissue that haven't been stressed since you were a barefoot kid running around the neighborhood. Also, avoid running long distances in minimalist footwear. It's a growing trend, but recent studies show high rates of shin and ankle injuries. One study of 99 runners using minimalist footwear reported 23 injuries at the close of the study.[214]

MORNING MOBILITY ROUTINE

If you are like most people, your morning routine involves an alarm clock, coffee, and stumbling toward your first obligation of the day. If you think about this from a varied movement perspective, it's a problem. Your body has just been completely sedentary for 7–9 hours. If you launch straight into the day's tasks after waking, you could be looking at another 8 hours without really using your body. That means you may spend 15–17 hours of a 24-hour period where you don't squat, reach over your head, lunge with one leg, pull something, or rotate your torso.

While a dedicated few hit the gym early in the morning, go for a walk, or do some other exercise, most people don't. Even hardcore morning fitness junkies are likely missing out on one of the highest ROI mobility tactics: *a morning mobility routine.*

There are a handful of mobility strategies I've employed over the last few years that have been real game changers. Adding more varied movement is near the top of the list. So is the switch to dynamic stretching from traditional static stretching. But my morning routine has made more of an impact on my pain levels and joint mobility than anything else. Unfortunately, it's also one of the toughest habits to implement. Not because it's difficult, but because mornings are crazy busy for people and the last thing they feel like doing is moving their bodies more than necessary.

In my experience, people get excited about this idea and then let it fall away like a New Year's resolution. They forget just how busy and unpredictable their mornings are. Or they overestimate their motivation levels in the morning. But once they establish the habit, they never go back. The benefits are profound and immediate. To me, starting my day without a quick movement routine is like starting the day without caffeine. I'm that serious.

Because this habit is so easy to push to the side, even for the disciplined, we're going to use a streamlined version you can complete in about five

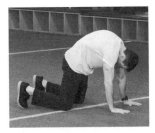

Cat-Cow

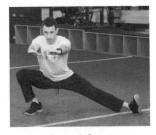

World's Greatest Stretch

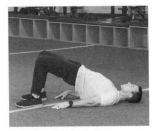

Glute Bridge

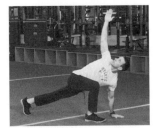

Hinge to Squat

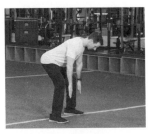

Cossack Squat

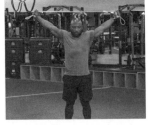

Band Pass Through

minutes. Anyone can carve out five minutes from their morning. Follow this routine for one week. Then take stock of the benefits. I bet you'll notice more energy, less muscle tension, and fewer aches and pains.

There are two basic parts to the morning mobility routine: a series of dynamic stretches to grease your joints and loosen up commonly tight muscles, and a circuit of lightweight resistance exercises. Detailed instructions for the exercises listed below can be found in chapter 11, "Mastering the Movements."

Body-Weight Mobility Sequence

Perform these exercises in sequence. Add movement to each one by pulsing in and out of the last 50% or so of the range of motion in a controlled manner, similar to the active isolated stretching method discussed earlier. Do this for five repetitions with each movement. Then hold the final position for five seconds—just long enough to establish a solid position. Again—pulse five times, hold for five seconds (two or three deep breaths).

That's it. Then move on. Also, don't neglect the transitions. This type of flowing sequence is superior to separated stretches because it challenges your ability to move smoothly from one to the next, adding an extra element of stability and full-body coordination. Once you get used to the movements, this sequence takes only two to three minutes to complete.

- Cat-Cow (page 217)
- World's Greatest Stretch (page 220)
- Glute Bridge (page 212)
- Hinge to Squat (page 218)
- Cossack Squat (page 210)
- Band Pass Through (page 225)

Weighted Mobility Sequence

After spraying WD-40 into a creaky, rusty old door hinge, do you yank on the door as hard as you can for 30 seconds? No, you work the door hinge back and forth smoothly several times until the lubricant permeates through the hinge and the creaking stops. That is essentially what we are doing with this weighted mobility sequence—except instead of a door hinge, it's your joints. And instead of WD-40, it's your synovial fluid.

After finishing the body-weight sequence from the last section, you'll move directly into the weighted sequence below using a light pair of dumbbells, kettlebells, or elastic bands. Start with a set of 5–15 pound weights (each). If you're recovering from an injury, you could go even lighter. If you're a highly tuned machine of an athlete and the weights feel comically light, that's OK. The goal isn't to build muscle or break a sweat—it's to mobilize your joints. The light weights serve three primary purposes:

1. The weights create a micro-loaded stretch at the end of the movement, allowing you to get into more elongated positions.

2. The weights help counterbalance your body weight, improving mechanics and helping you get into better positions during exercises like the goblet squat and Romanian deadlift.

3. The weights add an element of skill—giving you the ability to noticeably improve your mechanics and range of motion from week to week.

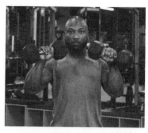
Dumbbell Zottman Curl

You don't want to perform the movements explosively, but you also don't want to move the weights grindingly slow. Aim for somewhere in the middle— a deliberate tempo, taking one or two seconds to lift the weight and one or two seconds to lower the weight. Pause just long enough between repetitions to avoid bouncing out of the bottom of the movement. Pay attention to your exercise tempo, but don't be a perfectionist here. Focus on form, and the speed of the movement will take care of itself.

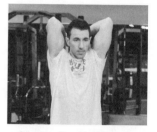
Standing Dumbbell Pullover

Remember, you aren't trying to stress your muscles or build strength. Your goal is to get your blood pumping, increase synovial fluid production, improve neuromuscular coordination, and expand your functional range of motion under loads. Once you get used to the movements, the weighted sequence will only take two to three minutes to complete. I selected these specific exercises to address common movement limitations (e.g. scapula upward rotation), tight muscles (e.g. hamstrings), and underdeveloped muscles (e.g. forearm supinators). Perform 10 repetitions of each exercise listed below:

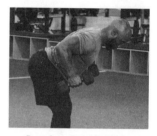
Bent Over Dumbbell Row

- Dumbbell Zottman Curl (page 251)
- Standing Dumbell Pullover (page 256)
- Bent Over Dumbbell Row (page 243)
- Dumbbell Romanian Deadlift (page 265)
- Dumbbell Goblet Squat (page 260)
- Dumbbell Pronation/Supination (page 254)

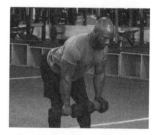
Dumbbell Romanian Deadlift

For the first week, keep it simple. Resist the temptation to add more exercises and repetitions. Make it easy on yourself so the habit sticks. Then see how you feel about your new morning routine after a week. At that point, feel free to add other mobility exercises or stretches. You can also spend more time moving in and out of the dynamic stretches that feel tight or awkward or use heavier weights for the weighted mobility sequence. Also, you don't have to do this as soon as you roll out of bed. It could be after your shower, just before breakfast, or between other parts of your morning routine. The key is to place it somewhere in your existing routine.

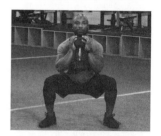
Dumbbell Goblet Squat

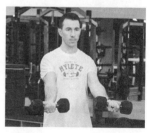
Dumbbell Pronation/Supination

If you are traveling or wake up somewhere where you do not have weights, do the exercises anyway. Get creative and use a paperweight or elastic band. Alternate holding it in one hand and then the other while performing the exercises. If you're really in a pinch, go through the motions without a weight just to get some movement in your joints. Some movement is better than none.

When you start this routine, you may feel stiff. Your movements will be slow and deliberate. After a few weeks, your body will loosen up and you'll see improvements in range of motion. On days you exercise later in the afternoon or evening, you'll notice your mobility at those sessions is better when you've completed the morning mobility routine.

Tight Muscle Quick Fix

It's often not a traumatic injury that keeps people from exercising but tight spots in muscles or tweaks that feel uncomfortable. Here is a tight muscle quick fix you can use to help loosen a stiff body part.

This series only takes a few minutes to complete. Use it in between sets at the gym, as part of your warm-up, or before participating in an activity that you know will aggravate an already tense muscle. Manual therapy and isometric exercise will help relax the tense muscle. The antagonist activation exercise will relax the opposing tight muscle group. And the dynamic stretch will bring blood flow to the area and establish pain-free ranges of motion.

1. **Manual therapy:** Use massage or another manual therapy technique to loosen up the tight muscle. Spend one to two minutes massaging or rolling over the area. This reduces hypertonicity in the target muscle. *Example:* Use a foam roller or lacrosse ball to massage tight, sore hamstring muscles.

2. **Isometric contraction:** Hold an isometric contraction, either with the assistance of weights or not, for 10 seconds. Use moderate intensity—around a 6 or 7 on the scale of intensity, with 10 being your max effort. The use of isometric muscle contractions triggers autogenic inhibition in tight muscles—a phenomenon known as *postisometric relaxation*.[215] *Example:* Using a leg curl machine or Swiss ball, perform an isometric contraction near the end range of motion (with your knees mostly straight, slightly bent).

3. **Antagonist activation:** Use a light resistance exercise to activate the opposing muscle group. Perform 10–20 repetitions. This technique leverages *reciprocal inhibition*—a neuromuscular reflex that inhibits (relaxes) opposing muscle groups during the movement.[214] *Example:* For tight hamstrings, perform several repetitions of machine leg extensions or narrow stance body-weight squats to target the quadriceps.

4. **Dynamic stretch:** Move in and out of a stretched position targeting the tight muscle for 10 repetitions. ***Example:*** From a standing position, hinge at the hips and reach toward your toes until you feel a stretch in in your hamstrings. Pause momentarily, then stand back up, repeating the motion several times.

Preventing the Big Three

It isn't the mountain ahead that wears you out—it's the grain of sand in your shoe.

— Anonymous

So far, we've covered the basics of pain, movement, mobility, and corrective exercise. While previous chapters aimed to provide an in-depth understanding of why things go wrong in your body and what to do about it, this chapter provides a templated approach to addressing the three most common pain points. There's no way to provide an action plan for all injuries and pain problems. To get safe and proper treatment, you need to see a qualified medical professional such as your physician or physical therapist. There is no singular approach to preventing pain or injury that works for everyone. This is why working with a professional who can assess you and screen your movements for problems is so important. While we can't diagnose and treat anything through a book, we can create principle-based templates that allow you to prevent most pains and imbalances.

Good information technology systems are set up to allow for small, isolated errors that benefit the system's future performance. This is as true in fitness as it is in business and computer programming. When you recognize movement errors and pain responses early, you can fix the small errors before they turn into big ones. Unlike taking time off from exercise every time you feel discomfort, this approach will build your body's resilience and your mental capacities to navigate around physical obstacles. This chapter shows you how to isolate the small errors, keep them small, and keep the system (your body) from crashing. And building on this systems thinking approach, you'll reap the greatest benefits by focusing on the three primary joints that produce the vast majority of pain and misery: the low back, shoulders, and knees—what I call the "Big Three."

In this chapter, I introduce several concepts that can help you prevent the Big Three. You may start feeling overwhelmed at the sheer amount of exercise options and goals. But don't worry, the training program chapter gives you a road map for layering these concepts into your workouts over time for the best results. If, down the road, you are having problems with your back, shoulders, or knees, refer back to these sections and double-down on the suggestions for the body part you're having trouble with—even if it means forgoing your normal training routine temporarily.

Also, I can't stress enough the importance of getting another pair of eyes on you, whether it's a professional or a friend who can review these techniques with you and keep you honest. At least until you become familiar with the exercises. Consider enlisting a friend to work through the program with you.

JOINT-BY-JOINT: STABILITY VS. MOBILITY

All joints have a stability component and a mobility component, but each joint tends to favor one or the other preferably. This is known as the *joint by joint* concept.[216] Here's how the kinetic chain of joints in your body is set up from your feet to your shoulders. Notice how the primary function alternates between stability and mobility as you move up the chain:

- Feet: stability
- Ankles: mobility
- Knees: stability
- Hips: mobility
- Lumbar spine (low back): stability
- Thoracic spine (upper back): mobility
- Scapulothoracic (scapula): stability
- Glenohumeral (shoulder): mobility

Knowing the primary function of each joint helps provide context for establishing preventative goals. For example, your hips are primarily designed for mobility, indicating that maintaining range of motion is paramount. Conversely, your low back is designed mainly for stability, indicating that building stabilizing strength should be the focus—along with mobilizing the joints above and below it to prevent unnecessary movement compensations.

Now, let's get into the common pain points, starting with the mother of all joint pain.

LOW BACK PAIN

When I measured search data for various body parts and pain-related words using Google Trends, "back pain" had more search volume than all the other body parts combined. It's safe to say it is the mother of all joint pain. Not only is it arguably the most painful, it's also severely crippling. Especially low back pain. If you've ever experienced low back pain, you know that your

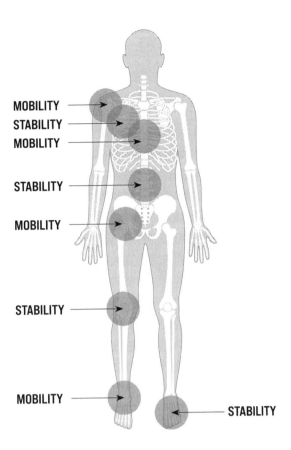

MOBILITY

STABILITY

MOBILITY

STABILITY

MOBILITY

STABILITY

MOBILITY

STABILITY

FIGURE 8.1

Joint-by-joint anatomy depiction.

back is involved in virtually every movement. Sitting up, bending, walking, and even sneezing become painful when your low back is out of sorts. It is the linchpin of your body—which means that a healthy low back prevents many other downstream problems (remember our conversation about how *proximal stability leads to distal mobility*). For these reasons, we'll spend more time addressing low back pain than any other joint pain.

Your back is made of five regions:

- Cervical (neck)
- Thoracic (upper back)
- Lumbar (low back)
- Sacral (bottom of the spine)
- Coccygeal (tailbone)

Our focus will be the lumbar spine. The main function of the lumbar spine (low back) is to hold up the weight of your upper body. It's primarily a stability joint. Your low back stabilizes your trunk while you stand upright, bend over, and twist, all while protecting your spinal cord from injury. Having strong postural muscles, flexible joints above and below, and good movement mechanics all contribute to a healthy, pain-free low back. Here are the most practical and effective ways to prevent low back pain. (Please refer to chapter 11, "Mastering the Movements," for detailed instructions on the exercises listed below.)

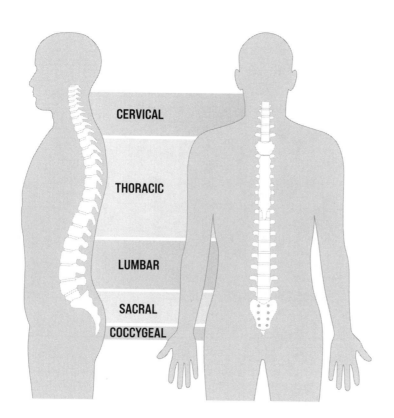

FIGURE 8.2

Five regions of the spine.

1. Activate your glutes.

For as much attention as the glutes get from an aesthetic perspective, they are underrated for their muscular power and role in virtually every lower body movement. Bret Contreras, Ph.D, is the author of *Glute Lab: The Art and Science of Strength and Physique Training*.[217] He's known as the "Glute Guy." Powerlifters and bikini competitors alike turn to Bret when they want to improve the size, shape, and function of their glutes and posterior chain muscles. But as outlined in *Glute Lab*, the glutes do far more for your body than just fill out jeans.

The glutes are (or should be) the prime moving muscles for hip-dominant movements like bending and squatting. They provide joint stability not just for your low back but also your knees and lower legs. Prolonged sitting, imbalanced exercise habits, and a sedentary lifestyle can cause your glute muscles to atrophy and lose their ability to contract properly. This condition is called *gluteal amnesia*. When this happens, synergistic dominance ensues as your low back has to step up. Instead of filling its role as a stabilizing joint, the low back becomes a mobilizing joint. This puts you at risk of acute low back injuries and chronic pain from overuse. Even walking can put unnecessary stress on your joints if you aren't using your glutes properly. It's a common problem. And luckily it can be remedied quickly. Your glutes will remember what they are supposed to do with a little nudging.

If you have a history of low back pain, you should always warm up your glutes with activation exercises before working out. If nothing else, this will

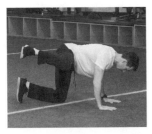

Fire Hydrant

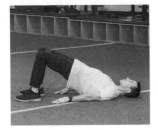

Glute Bridge with Hip Band

remind your body that your glutes are the primary movers during lower body squatting and hinging and that the small muscles of your low back should only act as synergistic supporters. Even if you don't have low back pain, performing glute activation exercises is a great way to improve motor control and muscular power during lower body movements. Activate your glutes, and your low back will thank you.

There are dozens of glute exercises worth exploring and adding to your routine. But these two work for virtually any fitness level and activate all the muscles that make up your butt.

Key exercises

- Fire Hydrant (page 214)
- Glute Bridge with Hip Band (page 213)

2. Mobilize the joints surrounding your low back.

As we've discussed, the low back is primarily designed to be stable—not mobile. Stretching your low back muscles when they're in pain is the last thing you should do.

Instead, focus on mobilizing the joints above and below your low back: the upper back (thoracic spine) and hips. When these joints are flexible, your back has permission to stand strong and stable. When these joints are tight, your low back is forced to flex and carry loads that it's not designed for.

If you have tight hips and upper back muscles, try the dynamic stretch featured below, which targets both simultaneously. It's known affectionately within fitness circles as the "World's Greatest Stretch."

If your low back is too stiff and sore to perform the World's Greatest Stretch, try performing the Cat-Cow exercise first to loosen up muscles in your low back and reduce the overprotective guarding that is preventing you from moving freely. Unlike folding your low back to touch your toes or pulling your knees to your chest, the amount of compression is minimized during the Cat-Cow, making it a safe and gentle option for mobilizing your spine.

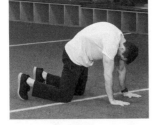

Cat-Cow

Key exercises

- Cat-Cow (page 217)
- World's Greatest Stretch (page 220)

3. Teach your body to hip hinge properly.

One of my favorite diagnostic movement screens is the *bend and lift*. It consists of squatting down from a standing position while holding weights at each side of the body. It's the perfect exercise for examining postural faults

World's Greatest Stretch

and muscle imbalances in the low back and legs. Common faults include shooting the knees too far forward (which indicates a quad dominant squatting motion) and excessively flexing the low back and thoracic spine. The latter is more common, indicating inactive glutes and inability to hinge at the hips properly. This is a dangerous movement fault because it puts your back in a precarious position.

If you've ever watched someone deadlift weight that is far too heavy for them, cringing at the sight of their back curving forward, it's because you intuitively know their spine is at risk. Though your spine is designed to flex, extend, and twist, it is not designed to do so under heavy loads. If you've ever tweaked your low back when moving furniture, it's probably because you didn't stabilize your low back with a proper hip hinge. And like most movement faults, there is also a risk of overuse injury in addition to acute injury when performed repetitively over time.

During a proper hip hinge, the low back remains relatively fixed as you bend toward the ground and back up. So does the upper back. The motion should take place at the hips, allowing the glutes and hamstrings to do most of the work. Because the hip hinge is one of the most fundamental and commonly used movements in daily life, it's important to perfect it. Hip-hinging practice also helps you maintain neutral spine alignment when at rest. That's because maintenance of neutral alignment depends on the quality of your pelvic *force-couples*—the muscle groups that control movement stabilization around your hips. Your hamstrings and hip flexors exert downward forces on the pelvis, while the low back and abdomen muscles exert upward balancing forces. This opposing tension is what allows for quality rotational movement. Train your body to move, and your body will be better equipped to stand still, too.

While deadlift variations reinforce the hip hinge effectively, you can use the cable pull through exercise to train the proper movement patterns. Use this move to improve your hip hinge ability. Add it to your weekly exercise routine and do it prior to heavy lower body movements to reinforce good form. It won't just make you stronger in the gym, it also protects your back in daily life when bending over and standing up.

Key exercise

- Cable Pull Through (page 264)

4. Build your transverse abdominis muscle.

The transverse abdominis (TVA) muscle has come up a few times so far. Because studies show a direct correlation between transverse abdominis development and low back pain, it's worth exploring in more detail. The

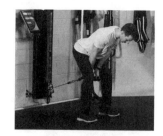

Cable Pull Through

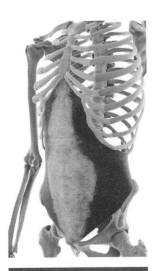

FIGURE 8.3

Transverse abdominis (TVA).

TVA muscle is one of the primary deep-layer core muscles, located in your lower abdomen. Its primary purpose is to stabilize your pelvis during movement. Not only is it the muscle that allows you to suck your "gut" inward, it literally holds your guts in place, earning it the nickname "the Spanxs of the Abdomen." Your TVA performs the same function on your midsection as a weightlifting belt—it tightens, stabilizes, and protects. This is why overusing a weightlifting belt leads to deactivation of the TVA, opening you up to low back pain and injury risk.

A 2013 study published in *The Journal of Physical Therapy Science* compared the development of the transverse abdominis in patients with chronic low back pain (LBP) versus healthy subjects. Researchers found that LBP patients exhibited atrophy of the TVA muscle, whereas healthy subjects were more likely to have well-developed TVA muscles.[218] They went on to suggest that core strengthening exercises designed to increase neuromuscular (mind-muscle) activation of the TVA could prevent muscular atrophy and reduce low back pain risk. Strong TVA and anterior core muscles help stabilize your pelvis and low back during hinging, squatting, and rotational movements.

A 2019 article published in Rehabilitation and Musculoskeletal Health (with the self-explanatory title "The Critical Role of Development of the Transverse Abdominis in the Prevention and Treatment of Low Back Pain") dove deeper into exactly what to do for TVA muscular development. In addition to pointing out that 80% of us will experience low back pain at some point in our lives, researchers provided a few actionable tips: [219]

1. Practice and perfect the "suck it in" maneuver to develop your TVA.

2. Focus on correct posture.

3. Use core stabilization exercises to protect your spine and incorporate those movement habits into daily activities.

The most straightforward way to develop your TVA is to first establish a better mind-muscle connection with it. This can be accomplished with the supine drawing in exercise. Despite the exercise appearing simple, it provides a big bang for your buck. You'll notice a difference in your ability to activate and brace your core after just two or three sessions of performing this exercise. Many people also report improved urinary control, which makes sense; TVA exercises have been shown in studies to improve urinary incontinence and improve urinary output in addition to improving core stability.[220]

Key exercise

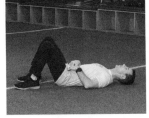

Supine Drawing In

- Supine Drawing In (page 208)

5. Brace your core before heavy movements.

Bracing your core is different from establishing good standing posture. In the posture checklist, the focus is on maintaining the natural S curve of your back—especially if you exhibit the typical slouched, shoulders-forward posture that many people do. But when performing heavy lifts, the goals are different. It's about maximizing intra-abdominal pressure and stability in the muscles surrounding your spine. Not only does this protect your spine, it also helps prevent low back pain and increases your muscular force potential.

Follow this three-step bracing sequence before heavy lifting, picking up furniture, or any other exertion event.

1. Take a deep inhale and hold it, focusing on expanding your belly outward and preventing your chest from rising. This method creates more intra-abdominal pressure and spinal stability than allowing your chest to rise and expand as you breathe in.[221]

2. Tighten your stomach while continuing to hold in the breath, like you are preparing to be punched in the stomach. This cue creates more tension in your core than the popular "suck in your belly" cue (try both now and you'll see what I mean). Bracing for a punch activates your TVA and surrounding core muscles such as the obliques, further reinforcing core stability.

3. Squeeze your butt muscles. This should create a sense of horizontal pressure between your butt and lower abdomen.

Summary: take a big breath into your belly, suck your belly inward, clench your butt muscles. After practicing this a few times, you can shorten your mental cue list to "big belly breath, tighten, butt squeeze."

Then, maintain this positioning as you perform exercises. You'll notice this bracing sequence pulls your thoracic spine downward. That's OK. Again, the goal here is maximum core stability.

With practice, you'll be able to perform this sequence quickly and repeat it between repetitions of heavy lifts. For single lifts or set of only 2–3 repetitions, you can likely get through it with only one breath. For higher repetition sets, or if you feel the need for more air, get your body into a safe position before exhaling and taking another big belly breath.

If you want to see what this looks like at the expert level, watch a powerlifter's stomach just before they perform a squat. You'll see their belly expand outward as they draw in a big breath and their core muscles cinch up around their spine.

6. Build muscular endurance in your low back.

It's #6 on this list, mostly because the previous steps have to do with higher-order goals like mobility and muscle activation, but don't discount the importance of building muscular endurance in your low back. It just may be the most crucial step you take to prevent and resolve low back pain.

Back muscle *endurance* is more important than strength or mobility when it comes to preventing pain. That's because back pain is almost always caused by cumulative stress—such as repetitive use injuries or poor movement mechanics. Without sufficient endurance, your low back cannot maintain good posture throughout the day, let alone maintain optimal spinal alignment during exercises that cause fatigue.

A 2016 study of 55 collegiate athletes from a variety of sports measured the relationship between core muscle endurance and low back pain. Researchers found significant deficits in muscular endurance in subjects with low back pain. The authors of the study recommended that back management programs for athletes should prioritize "strategies to emphasize endurance of core muscles (especially the extensors and flexors)." [222]

A 2006 study of industrial workers published in *Manual Therapy* showed that workers with poor back muscle endurance were more likely to suffer from flexion-related (e.g. bending over) pain than their peers.[223] Even studies of adolescents show a strong relationship between back muscle endurance and low back pain.[224]

Despite dozens of studies demonstrating this concept, most people don't take this message to heart. And most low back pain advice centers around stretching, massage, and strengthening—not muscular endurance. As Dr. Stuart McGill points out, "[back] strength may, or may not, help a particular individual as strength without control and endurance to repeatedly execute perfect form increases risk."[225] After establishing proper movement patterns, your first objective when trying to solve low back pain is to increase muscular endurance. There are dozens of muscles involved in low back muscle endurance, but one muscle in particular is vital for developing endurance along the entire length of your back.

Running vertically along each side of your spinal column is a thin yet powerful muscle called the *multifidus*. This underrated muscle group runs from your tailbone all the way to the top of your upper back. A well-developed multifidus bolsters the stability of your entire back, helping to reduce joint degeneration and prevent low back pain.[226] But it's not just about mechanical support. The multifidus, along with the TVA, is chiefly responsible for sending messages through your spine to your brain about your core's current stability status.[227] These two are the dynamic duo of core stability. This is a perfect example of proximal stability leading to distal mobility. When your

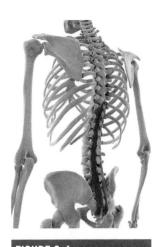

FIGURE 8.4

Multifidus.

multifidus and TVA are well developed and activated, your brain interprets this as a safe environment for movement of your core, hips, upper back, and extremities. Function improves and muscle tension decreases.

While you could build endurance with high-repetition sets of squats and deadlifts, the Bird Dog exercise targets the multifidus. Building on what you know about the roles of both the multifidus and TVA (i.e. coactivation improves spinal stability), you can use the Bird Dog to injury-proof and pain-proof your back.

Key exercise

- Bird Dog (page 209)

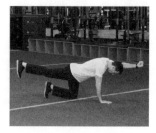

Bird Dog

7. Avoid excessive compression.

If you are prone to low back pain or are recovering from one of those annoying low back tweaks, avoid excessive spinal compression. Let's look at the anatomy of the barbell box squat to illustrate why this matters.

The barbell box squat consists of holding a loaded barbell across your upper back, squatting down until your butt touches a box (usually at a height a few inches higher than your knees), then standing back up. It's a favorite of many powerlifters and strength coaches because it effectively teaches a hip-dominant squat pattern for maximum muscular force production. But it has a dark side. It puts immense strain on the low back from high compression forces. Though our spines have evolved to handle spinal compression without injury, the box squat smashes your spine from both ends. Gravity, your body weight, and the barbell are all compressing your spine from the top down. And if you offload your body weight to the box, even to a small degree, you also have compression forces coming from the bottom.

This is one reason why many coaches (outside of powerlifting especially) are moving away from the box squat. If you suffer from back pain or have instability in your spine from an injury or muscle imbalance, high compression forces could cause further pain and injury. If you have a self-described "bad back," then you may be compression intolerant—at least for the time being. This means that compression forces that normally would not cause problems (like barbell squats and military presses) are pain triggers for you. You can avoid excess compression forces by keeping the load below your low back—or at least below your level of pain. For example, instead of holding a barbell across your upper back, opt for holding dumbbells in each hand by your sides.

Now, am I against squatting with a barbell? Absolutely not. The barbell squat is the king of all exercises. Not just lower body exercises, but *all* exercises. And the box squat is a great tool for teaching proper hip drive and is an effective way to reintroduce barbell squats after recovering from knee tendinopathy. But if you have back pain or want to avoid it, choose exercises that put less compression forces on your low back. At least until you have built up adequate core strength, mobility, and movement mechanics to avoid a pain response.

Tempo matters as well. During squatting and hinging movements, if you bounce out of the bottom of the repetition, you are putting additional compression on your spine. Instead, use slow, controlled movements during the eccentric (lowering) phase, pausing for one to two seconds at the bottom of the repetition. This will reduce compression and have the added benefit of forcing you to stabilize and activate your core, making the exercise more difficult and arguably more effective.

8. Don't sit still.

If you have back pain, your sitting posture is likely an underlying cause and a short-term pain trigger. As Stuart McGill outlines in his book *Back Mechanic*, the best way to desensitize a painful back is to avoid pain triggers—and sitting is at the top of the list.[22] While improving posture can reduce and prevent low back pain, you're better off avoiding the trigger in the first place. Or, more realistically, reducing the power of the trigger.

You can accomplish this by making sitting a more dynamic task. Here are some effective ways to *not* sit still:

- Take regular breaks from sitting to stand, walk, and stretch.
- Exercise, move, and stretch before sitting down for long periods.
- Actively plan to break up long periods of sitting into chunks.
- Get a standing desk.
- Change your posture regularly to prevent muscle shortening.
- Alternate between using a lumbar support pillow or rolled up towel and using your own musculature to maintain low back posture.
- Set alarm reminders throughout the day to adjust your posture, stand up, and stretch.

9. Walk every day.

You already know how I feel about walking. Even 10–20 minutes per day improves lumbar function, decreases dependence on pain killers, increases spinal muscle blood flow, and reduces low back pain (by up to 27%). [174,178,183] Find a time slot you can commit to each day and establish a walking habit.

Best Exercises for Low Back Pain

- 10–20 minute walk
- Cat-Cow
- World's Greatest Stretch
- Supine Drawing In
- Core Bracing Sequence
- Bird Dog
- Fire Hydrant
- Glute Bridge
- Cable Pull Through

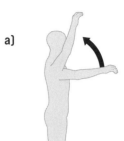

a)

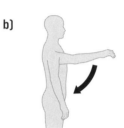

b)

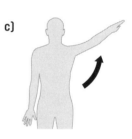

c)

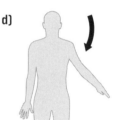

d)

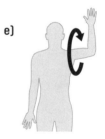

e)

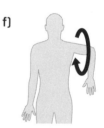

f)

SHOULDER PAIN

Shoulders are the most mobile joints in the human body. But with great mobility come great opportunities for dysfunction. Unlike the hips, which rely on a bony anatomy structure for stability, shoulders rely on muscles and connective tissue.[228] By definition, shoulders are among the least stable of human joints because of their hypermobility. This is the perfect storm for pain and injury. While entire books have been written on shoulder health, I want to focus on three fundamental concepts that will help you understand your shoulder pain and how to prevent it:

1. **Shoulders have extreme ranges of motion through multiple planes:**[228]

   a. *Flexion:* Raising arms up

   b. *Extension:* Lowering arms from a raised position

   c. *Abduction:* Movement away from the midline of the body

   d. *Adduction:* Movement toward the midline of the body

   e. *External rotation:* Rotation away from the midline of the body (primary external rotation muscles are the infraspinatus and teres minor)

   f. *Internal rotation:* Rotation toward the midline of the body (primary internal rotation muscles are the subscapularis, pectoralis major, latissimus dorsi, teres major, and the anterior deltoid)

2. **Shoulder anatomy and pain:**

   - Shoulder function largely depends on the stability and position of the scapula.[229]

   - Shoulder function is heavily influenced by the activity of the larger and more powerful pectoralis major (chest) and latissimus dorsi (lats).

FIGURE 8.5

Shoulder range of motion.

- The rotator cuff is comprised of four muscles that stabilize the shoulder by exerting compressive and downward forces to counteract the actions of the larger shoulder muscles. These four muscles are the subscapularis, supraspinatus, infraspinatus, and teres minor. An imbalance of these muscles is one of the primary causes of shoulder pain.[199]

3. **Shoulder impingement:**

Up to 65% of doctor's visits for shoulder pain are caused by shoulder impingement.[230] This occurs when soft tissues are pinched between bony structures of the shoulder. The primary symptoms are pain during specific movements and reduced pain-free ranges of motion. There are a few different classifications of shoulder impingement, but the most common and preventable type is *subacromial impingement* (a.k.a. swimmer's shoulder). This happens when the supraspinatus tendon and other soft tissues become pinched in the subacromial space—the small gap between your acromion bone (on the top) and the head of your humerus bone (on the bottom).

This is common in overhead athletes and manual laborers who spend time working with extended arms.[231] While the exact cause is difficult to determine, it's typically a combination of poor rotator cuff strength, overactive anterior shoulder muscles, and faulty movement patterns.

Shoulder impingement is annoying but rarely debilitating at first. You can exercise and continue your normal routine despite the discomfort. But like a rope that slowly frays over time from rubbing against metal, your rotator cuff will gradually degenerate, which increases the risk of traumatic injury.

With a basic understanding of common shoulder imbalances, you can use the following concepts to keep your shoulders strong, stable, and pain-free. (Please refer to chapter 11, "Mastering the Movements," for detailed instructions on the exercises listed below.)

1. Mobilize your lats.

The latissimus dorsi (lat) is the biggest muscle in your upper body. It lies just underneath your armpit on each side of your body, extending down to the middle of your low back. With arms at your sides, your lats are in their shortest position. With arms overhead, your lats are fully extended. And that's precisely the problem relating lats to shoulder pain. When you sit at your desk, lie in bed, drive your car—or do virtually any routine task—your arms are at your sides. And your lats are in their shortest position. The amount of time your lats spend elongated is infinitesimally small compared to how often they sit in a shortened position. Naturally, this causes muscle shortening and tightness. Here's the kicker: your lats are responsible for internal rotation of the shoulder. So not only are they the most powerful

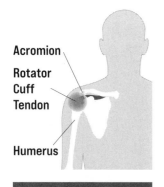

Acromion

Rotator Cuff Tendon

Humerus

FIGURE 8.6

Subacromial impingement.

muscles in your upper body, they are also chronically tight (which prevents overhead flexion) and one of the chief reasons why your shoulders want to pull forward into a hunched position.

You might think of lats as rear-pulling muscles, especially in vertical rowing exercises like the pull-up and lat pull down. Which is true. But your lats are also responsible for internal rotation. Novice weightlifters think they are balancing out their tight chest muscles from twice weekly bench press sessions by adding more lat exercises. In reality, they are creating more tension in their anterior shoulders, not less. From my experience, it's incredibly rare for someone to have adequate lat range of motion without doing it on purpose. It requires direct mobility training.

Here's a quick test you can do: stand in front of a mirror facing sideways. Slowly raise one straightened arm from your side, in front of your body, all the way up over your head. Keep your eyes locked on your back as you do this. As soon as you see your thoracic spine start to tilt or extend at all, stop the movement and hold your arm in place. Wherever your arm stopped, that's the true limit of your shoulder flexion. Meaning you can't get into full overhead arm position without cranking your back into overextension or impinging the front of your shoulder. It's no wonder people experience shoulder pain during pressing movements (e.g. bench press, military press). The lats are preventing proper shoulder motion.

From this, you should take away three main points:

1. You have to prioritize lat mobility to keep your shoulders healthy.

2. Stretching your lats a few times per week isn't enough to balance out all the shortened positions we live in. They need daily work to prevent range of motion restrictions.

3. Before doing any pressing exercises, especially overhead pressing, mobilize your lats. You'll see immediate improvements in shoulder flexion and overhead mobility.

Key exercise

- Anchored Lat Stretch (page 222)

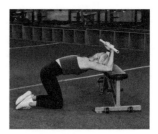

Anchored Lat Stretch

2. Practice ideal shoulder positioning.

Ideal shoulder positioning roughly means your shoulders are "back and down" with the upper arm bones firmly resting in the back of the socket. More importantly, it means your shoulders are in an alignment that allows your skeletal system to work efficiently and without pain. Two main physiological problems prevent ideal shoulder position: kyphosis and anterior shoulder glide. Kyphosis (upper back rounding) is often the result of poor sitting posture. You can quickly improve shoulder positioning through postural training, mobilizing the anterior chest/shoulder complex, and strengthening the upper back. But anterior shoulder glide—where the humerus sits too far forward in the socket—is a bit trickier. This condition alters rotational movements, further causing impingement.

I have a chronically tight left shoulder from capsular plication surgery. (Plication surgery is supposed to improve shoulder stability by tightening up the connective tissue surrounding the shoulder capsule. While it used to be a popular technique for shoulder injuries, it's typically only recommended for chronically unstable shoulders due to the long-term mobility limitations it causes.) Because of the way my connective tissue is structured now, my left shoulder wants to glide forward. This requires more mobility work and posterior shoulder strengthening exercises on my left side. Even if you don't have a sewn-up shoulder, tight anterior and latent posterior shoulder muscles will exert the same dislocating forces on your shoulders.

Addressing the common agonist-antagonist imbalance of tight chest muscles and weak upper back muscles will go a long way toward preventing anterior glide.

Two exercises that train scapula positioning from opposing angles are the Scapular Pull-up and Band Push-up Plus:

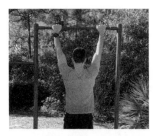

Scapular Pull-up

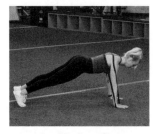

Band Push-up Plus

Key exercises

- Scapular Pull-up (page 223)
- Band Push-up Plus (page 238)

A note on rowing and shoulder position. Rowing motions become a major problem if you have anterior shoulder glide. Even though you may only experience shoulder pain when performing pressing movements, letting your shoulder dump forward while performing rowing motions reinforces bad positioning. Instead, focus on keeping your shoulders back throughout the entire rowing motion: squeeze and hold the contraction in the end position, and only extend your arms as far as you can without letting your shoulders glide forward. This will ingrain the movement pattern and target the muscles that need strengthening most.

3. Improve external rotation.

For weightlifters, shoulder problems caused by poor posture are compounded when internal rotators become even more developed from weight lifting. This is largely due to the power and activity of the lat muscles. Your lats are involved in all pressing movements and rowing exercises, but they are still primarily internal rotation muscles. This creates a synergistic dominance imbalance as the lats take over during horizontal rowing motions that should be controlled by the muscles of the upper back.

If you're curious how internal rotation-dominant you are, perform this test: stand in front a mirror and raise your arms out to each side. Then, relax your arms and let your hands drop down to your hips. Where are the palms of your hands facing? If your palms are facing your body, you have good external rotation function. If your palms are facing backward, you likely lack both external rotation strength and mobility.

There are several reasons this is problematic. Without shoulder external rotation mobility, overhead movements require either excessive extension of your upper back or an impinged anterior shoulder capsule to complete the movement. Neither of these are good options.

It's not just about the flexibility of your muscles. Strength counts just as much, or more. Athletes are more prone to suffer rotator cuff and labrum tears if they lack strength in the muscles that control external rotation.[232] Studies of nonathletes also show decreased external rotation strength is positively correlated with shoulder pain, impingement syndrome, and chronic shoulder instability.[233]

The solution is to:

- Improve active external rotation range of motion (i.e. range of motion you can control with your own muscles, not by an external stretch).

- Strengthen two of the primary external rotators: the infraspinatus and teres minor.

- Maintain adequate internal rotation mobility. Internal rotation is especially important for throwing athletes and weight lifters who need it to prevent their scapula from destabilizing while getting into arms-extended positions.

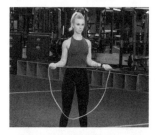

Banded W

Stretching and traditional compound lifts are not enough to achieve these goals. Resistance exercise that targets rotators cuff muscles specifically (versus just doing more pressing and rowing) is the best way to correct muscle imbalances of the shoulder.[234] These muscles need dedicated attention. There's no getting around it.

Key exercises

- Banded W (page 230)
- Band High Pull Apart with External Rotation (page 231)

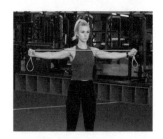

Band High Pull Apart
with External Rotation

4. Build stabilizing strength in your rotator cuff muscles.

The rotator cuff is made up of several muscles and tendons that keep your upper arm bone planted firmly in the shoulder socket. Weakness in these muscles is one of the leading causes of shoulder pain. And it's no wonder—your deltoid muscles want to yank your shoulder out of the socket during abduction and flexion. It's the small muscles of your shoulder, including the supraspinatus, infraspinatus, subscapularis, and teres minor, that prevent it from happening.[197] Luckily, you don't need to memorize shoulder anatomy. You just need to know that the rotator cuff is comprised of several muscles that work together to keep your shoulder strong and stable. And these muscles need a specific type of stimulus to get stronger.

In addition to improving external rotation and posterior shoulder muscle activation, you also need supportive muscle mass and strength in the muscles that surround your shoulder joint on all sides. And those muscles need to be effectively coordinated to carry out all the complex movements shoulders are capable of without injury.

The best way to accomplish this is with a variety of resistance movements that challenge your upper body stability and coordination.[234] Here are two exercises that challenge shoulder stability in novel ways. These movements should be staples in your upper body training.

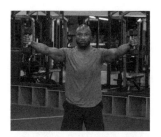

Scapular Plane Dumbbell Raises

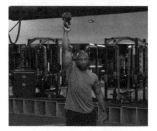

Bottoms-Up Kettlebell Press

Key exercises

- Scapular Plane Dumbbell Raises (page 234)
- Bottoms-Up Kettlebell Press (page 235)

5. Improve thoracic mobility.

Limited upper back mobility is the most overlooked cause of shoulder pain. Shoulder, elbow, and even wrist pain can all be downstream effects that originate from your upper back. The thoracic spine is designed for movement. It's one of the mobility joints in the joint-by-joint model. It can move in all directions: flexion (forward), extension (backward), lateral flexion (sideways), and rotation. You might get away with limited thoracic mobility while performing simple weight training exercises, but not in the real world where twisting, bending, and stabilizing are necessary for pain-free movement.

If you have a stiff upper back, focus on these two exercises. They'll help relieve that annoying upper back muscle tension and free up your shoulders during overhead movements.

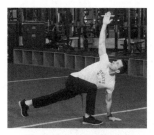

World's Greatest Stretch

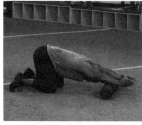

Thoracic Extension
on Foam Roller

Key exercises

- World's Greatest Stretch (page 220)
- Thoracic Extension on Foam Roller (page 229)

6. Get your scapula moving.

Scapulohumeral rhythm is a physiology concept that describes the relationship between your scapula and humerus (upper arm) bone, and how that affects movement mechanics.[235] Any change in scapula position relative to the humerus can disrupt scapulohumeral rhythm (a condition called *scapular dyskinesia*), leading to movement faults and injury. This is why you need the ability to stabilize your scapula and control its movement through various motions.

Closed-kinetic chain (CKC) exercises are movements that involve a more stable distal segment—like your hands and feet. Upper body CKC exercises include push-ups (hands fixed to floor) and pull-ups (hands gripped over bar). Open-Kinetic Chain (OKC) exercises involve a more free-floating distal segment. An example is a standing dumbbell shoulder raise, where your hands are suspended in the air throughout the movement. While both types of movements should be incorporated into training, CKC exercises are generally considered more functional because they shift the primary roles of muscles throughout your body to stabilization. In the case of the Scapular Pull-up exercise, the muscles of your thoracic spine must work hard to keep your scapula in a fixed position. While effective use of CKC exercises will improve your scapular stability, you also need to have a baseline of scapula mobility.

At the risk of talking out of both sides of my mouth, your scapula needs to be fairly mobile. For overhead motions, your scapula contributes around 60 degrees of movement by tilting backward.[235] See **Figure 8.8**. Without enough posterior tilt capability, your shoulder will bear the excess stress. In cases of shoulder impingement, the scapula has failed to rotate upward enough to prevent compression of the subacromial space.[236] Basically, your scapula must be a utility player. The best exercise I've found that accomplishes all three goals of improving stability, strength, and mobility is the Swimmer's Stretch. This exercise will make your parascapular muscles stand up and scream (in a good way).

Another commonly weak movement pattern is scapula protraction—which means moving your shoulder blades forward, away from the spine. It activates the serratus anterior, a fan-shaped muscle that runs parallel along your ribs, just under your armpit.[229] Most people are fairly competent at moving into protraction because their shoulders are accustomed to rounding forward. But the ability to activate the serratus muscle and stabilize in a protracted position is another story. The Band Push-up Plus exercise builds your mind-muscle connection to the serratus anterior. Because much of your shoulder ROM comes from scapula movement, getting this movement pattern right is an effective way to prevent shoulder impingement and build overall pressing strength.

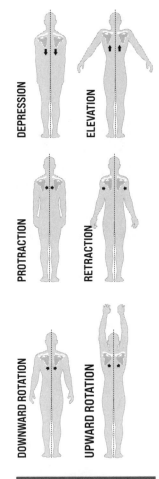

FIGURE 8.7

Movements of the scapula. (Adapted from Paine, R., & Voight, M. L., 2013. The role of the scapula. *International Journal of Sports Physical Therapy, 8,* 617–629.)

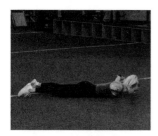

Swimmer's Stretch

Key exercises

- Swimmer's Stretch (page 227)
- Scapular Pull-up (page 223)
- Band Push-up Plus (page 238)

7. Build upper back strength and endurance.

The most common upper body muscle imbalance I see is the agonist/antagonist imbalance of overactive chest and lat muscles, and latent muscles of the upper back—chiefly, the posterior rotator cuff muscles, lower trapezius, and rhomboids. You can stretch tight chest muscles all day long, but if your upper back muscles are lacking, you're still going to experience shoulder pain. You need posterior shoulder strength to balance out the powerful anterior muscles and endurance to keep your shoulder posture in check throughout the day. Without upper back endurance, you'll revert to slumped, impinged shoulders as soon as you get tired. Just as low back muscular endurance is one of the best ways to resolve back pain, the same is true for shoulders. The Band Facepull exercise is unmatched for building upper back endurance.

If you take away nothing else from this section, I want you to remember this: the Band Facepull is the closest thing there is to a magic bullet for shoulder pain—especially if you train it hard, with high reps and high frequency. The exercise doesn't create much joint stress, so you can do it every day. And you should. The key is to maintain good shoulder position while you do to reinforce good movement habits and break bad ones.

If you have tight, overactive lats, you'll want to pull your arms down and forward as you finish the movement. If you have tight or overactive upper traps, you'll shrug your shoulders up toward your ears. Both of these compensations are faulty movement patterns and do not activate the target muscles in your upper back effectively.[199] You want your shoulder blades pinned back and down throughout the exercise. This forces the muscles of your upper back and rotator cuff to do the work. So fight the urge to let your shoulders take the path of least resistance. (Tip: If you're having trouble keeping your shoulders back and down, opt for a neutral or palms-up grip. Exercises that use a pronated grip [palms down] encourage more usage of your internal rotator muscles, which you want to avoid.[229] Also, anchor the band slightly above eye level to reinforce the back and down scapula position.)

The Bent Over Dumbbell Row is another great exercise for overall back development. It forces you to stabilize your low back and thoracic spine while providing a greater opportunity to use heavier loads for more upper back muscle growth.

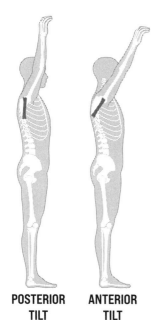

POSTERIOR TILT   **ANTERIOR TILT**

FIGURE 8.8

Scapula tilt refers to the angle of the scapula in relation to the body. Exaggerated anterior tilt leads to shoulder pain. Some posterior tilt is necessary to achieve pain-free overhead motions.

Key exercises

- Band Facepull (page 233)
- Bent Over Dumbbell Row (page 243)

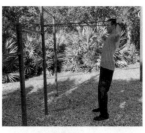

Band Facepull

Best Exercises for Shoulder Pain

- Anchored Lat Stretch
- Scapular Pull-up
- Band Push-up Plus
- Band W
- Band High Pull Apart with External Rotation
- Scapular Plane Dumbbell Raises
- Bottoms-Up Kettlebell Press
- World's Greatest Stretch
- Thoracic Extensions
- Swimmer's Stretch
- Band Facepull
- Bent Over Dumbbell Row

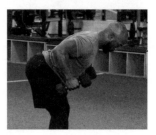

Bent Over Dumbbell Row

KNEE PAIN

Your knees take a beating. Virtually every movement requires your knees to stabilize or move your legs. Adding more repetitive exercise and high-volume training isn't the answer to knee pain, nor is taking a complete break from activity. The only way to bulletproof your knees is to increase their load capacity. That is not accomplished by stretching or mobility work but with slow, controlled repetitions of exercises that progressively challenge the load-bearing capabilities of connective tissue structures around your knees.

The knee is a hinge joint, meaning it's primarily designed to bend back and forth. It is comprised of four primary bones, two shock-absorbing cartilage structures, several fluid-filled sacs called bursae, and numerous surrounding tendons and ligaments.[237] Its main structural purpose is to connect the thigh bone to the shin bone. The four primary bones are:

- Femur (thigh bone)
- Tibia (shin bone)
- Fibula (smaller shin bone)
- Patella (kneecap)

Due to its load-bearing role and limited range of motion (flexion and extension), the knee is prone to dozens of different injuries, making it one of the most common joint pain complaints. You have probably heard of athletes

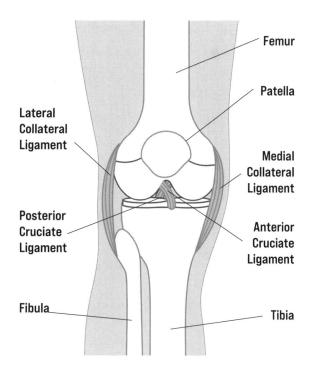

Femur

Patella

Lateral
Collateral
Ligament

Medial
Collateral
Ligament

Posterior
Cruciate
Ligament

Anterior
Cruciate
Ligament

Fibula

Tibia

FIGURE 8.9

Knee anatomy (right knee, frontal view).

suffering from ACL (anterior cruciate ligament) or MCL (medial collateral ligament) injuries that can be career ending. These are common traumatic injuries in athletes whose sport requires sudden changes of direction, like tennis and soccer. Other common minor injuries and sources of pain include:[238]

- **Patellar tendinopathy:** inflammation or degeneration of the patellar tendon, characterized by pain just below the kneecap on the front side of the lower leg.

- **Patellofemoral (compression) syndrome:** irritation of cartilage under the kneecap, characterized by pain inside the middle of the knee joint.

- **Iliotibial band syndrome:** pain that stems from rubbing of the iliotibial band (ligament) against the thigh bone, characterized by pain on the outside of the leg that that spans from hip to knee.

- **Knee effusion:** synovial fluid buildup around the knee joint, characterized by swelling of the knee and difficulty bending and straightening the knee.

- **Knee arthritis:** degenerative condition in which cartilage in the kneecap wears away, characterized (but not always) by the gradual onset of pain over time, general stiffness, and grating sensations within the knee joint.

Osteoarthritis is more pronounced in knees than most other joints because of their weight-bearing role and high activity load. It's not uncommon for older athletes who have experienced severe knee injuries to report to us that an MRI (magnetic resonance imaging) scan showed virtually zero cartilage in their knees. Or their doctor told them that their knees lacked enough cartilage mass to support heavy lower body weight training. This is a difficult problem to work around because it means a critical piece of connective tissue that absorbs and dissipates forces has worn away. If this describes you, consider these two points: (1) you need to be under the guidance of a physical therapist who can lead you through exercise progressions, and (2) you need to double down on functional movement and form while reducing stress on the knee joint. The tips that follow, such as cleaning up your knee track and perfecting a hip-dominant squat pattern, are even more important for you to prevent future knee pain.

If you have mild knee pain that has not substantially limited range of motion, and you're still able to put weight on it, you can likely reduce or eliminate the pain with a few simple tweaks to how you use your knees during movement:

1. Clean up your knee track.

Knee pain is often the result of poor joint positioning during movement. During squatting and lunge movements, it's common for weight lifters to move their knees too far forward, too far inside the midline of their body, or even bend excessively outward. If this is the case for your movement-related knee pain, you can fix it almost instantly by cleaning up your knee track. In a normally functioning knee, the patella sits nicely in a V-shaped groove in your femur.[239] During movement, your patella should slide easily back and forth within this groove. If your knee is not tracking properly, your kneecap could be rubbing against cartilage or putting excessive pulling forces on tendons. Typically, but not always, knee tracking issues are caused by movement faults. While many activities will require your knees to move outside the optimal knee track, maintaining proper knee alignment during load-bearing exercises will reinforce better kinetic chain control and allow you to train without causing tendon or ligament irritation.

The most common movement fault of the lower leg is knee valgus (a.k.a. knock knees), which means your knees collapse inward. Excessive knee valgus during movements like running, squatting, jumping, and landing cause patellofemoral pain syndrome (PFPS)—often referred to as runner's knee. PFPS is characterized by pain and inflammation just behind the front of the kneecap, where the patella intersects with interior cartilage.[240]

The opposite of knee valgus is knee varus (a.k.a. bowlegged knees). This happens when your shin bone turns inward instead of aligning with your thigh, causing the knee to push outward. Knee varus can be simply the result of poor ankle stability or bad movements habits but is often caused by osteoarthritis.[241]

The third common knee fault is excessive forward glide during squatting motions. This indicates overreliance on quadriceps (front thigh muscles) and inactive glutes. The shearing forces created against the knee as it glides forward over the shin bone can cause PFPS, stress the ACL, or—most commonly—lead to patellar tendinopathy.

When you clean up your knee track, you remove the faulty movement patterns that caused pain in the first place. There are even knee tracking devices that use lasers to guide your movements during lunges and squats. You can accomplish the same goal by using a mirror and the Bulgarian Split Squat. First, practice lunging forward with one leg in front of a mirror. Focus on keeping your knee pointed straight ahead, located directly over your foot or just slightly in front of it. Then, move on to the Bulgarian Split Squat to further challenge the movement.

Key exercise

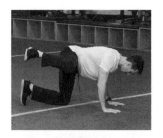

Bulgarian Split Squat

- Bulgarian Split Squat (page 262)

2. Activate your glutes and hip abductors.

If you have inactive glutes or deficits in hip abduction (moving leg away from body), you're more likely to suffer from knee pain. Luckily for you, knee pain caused by hip abductor dysfunction is easy to fix. A 2011 study in the *Journal of Athletic Training* showed that just three weeks of targeted hip abductor strength training reduced knee pain and improved knee function when walking.[242]

Just as activating your glutes takes a load off your low back, so does it with your knees. Mild knee pain can often be resolved simply by activating your glutes and building more of a hip hinge into squatting patterns. This shifts much of the work to your posterior chain (glutes and hamstrings), while taking pressure off your knees. If squatting, lunging, or other lower body movements give your knees trouble, try using the Fire Hydrant and Glute Bridge with Hip Band as glute primers before lower body training. Then, perform a few sets of the Box Stepdown to further reinforce glute and hip abductor engagement.

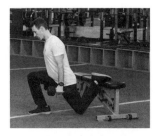

Fire Hydrant

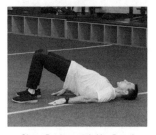

Glute Bridge with Hip Band

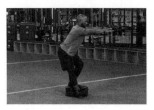

Box Stepdown

Key exercises

- Fire Hydrant (page 214)
- Glute Bridge with Hip Band (page 213)
- Box Stepdown (page 257)

3. Build end-range hamstring strength.

One of the most common agonist-antagonist muscle imbalances is strong quadriceps and weak hamstrings. The larger and more powerful quadriceps force the weaker hamstring muscles to stretch faster than they can contract to counter the force produced, causing hamstring muscle tears and knee injuries. Studies show that hamstring weakness is a dependable indicator of poor knee function and increased risk of knee ligament ruptures.[201]

Unless you target your hamstrings specifically with exercise, you likely have relatively weak hamstrings compared to the rest of your lower body. It's true that most people lack hamstring flexibility. But hamstring weakness, especially the ability to control the eccentric portion of movements, is a bigger problem. This explains why using eccentric-focused hamstring exercises provides a "cumulative protective effect" against muscle damage and injury. With training, you can shift your hamstring muscles' length-tension curve so that peak muscle force is generated at progressively longer muscle lengths.[243] Because many injuries result from movement faults near end ranges of motion, optimizing the angle of peak force production reduces your risk of injury and knee pain.[244]

The most functional exercise for targeting end-range hamstring strength is the supine Swiss Ball Leg Curl. It doesn't look that difficult at first glance, but it's one of the best multitasking lower body exercises. It allows you to create peak muscle tension at the very end range of motion. It also trains flexibility by forcing you to fully lengthen your hamstrings while actively contracting them. Unlike most machine isolation exercises for hamstrings, it trains your ability to coordinate hip extension with peak hamstring contraction. While hip hinge exercises like deadlifts and glute bridges are more functional for movement training, nothing targets hamstring strength, eccentric control, and mobility like the Swiss Ball Leg Curl.

Key exercise

- Swiss Ball Leg Curl (page 267)

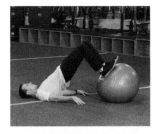

Swiss Ball Leg Curl

4. Improve hip mobility and control.

Your hips control the position of your knees when walking, jumping, and squatting. If your hips are tight or unstable, your knees will suffer the downstream effects. Since the knees are built primarily for stability, not mobility, all this excessive work caused by weak hips leads to pain and injury. Because most people lack both hip stability and mobility, and poor hip control causes low back and knee pain, improving hip function should be a top priority. It may even be more important than strengthening your knees. A 2015 study published in the *Journal of Athletic Training* demonstrated that knee rehabilitation programs focused on hip function reduced knee pain levels faster than those focused on knee function alone.[245]

When it comes to hip strength and control through full ranges of motion, the Cossack Squat hits on all cylinders. It challenges both the hip adductors (muscles that move your thighs closer to your body) and hip abductors (muscles that move your thigh bone away from the midline). It's also great for mobilizing the hamstrings and groin muscles. It's a challenging one, so start slow. Make sure you can control the motion all the way up and down. Stop the movement if you feel excessive tension building in your groin or hips to avoid strains.

No conversation about hip mobility would be complete without discussing the World's Greatest Stretch. It mobilizes and challenges the muscles surrounding your hips on all sides. In my opinion, there is no greater movement for opening up your hips.

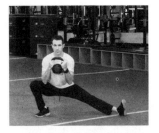

Cossack Squat

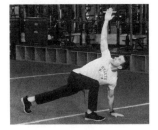

World's Greatest Stretch

Key exercises

- Cossack Squat (page 210)
- World's Greatest Stretch (page 220)

5. Build knee load capacity.

Fixing painful knees is tricky. They already do so much work that you can easily overstress them by adding more exercises and repetitions. This is why using isometric holds and slow resistance training is so effective. It builds tendon load capacity with lower risk of a pain response.[133] If you cannot perform leg exercises without knee pain, take a break from lower body resistance training and work on this progression every other day. You'll feel the burn in your muscles, but you should not feel tendon pain beyond a 3 out of 10 on the pain scale.

- **Wall Sit**: Sit with your back against a wall, feet planted firmly on the ground, and your knees bent at a 90-degree angle. If this causes knee pain, move your feet away from you, increasing the knee angle, until you can sit against the wall without knee pain. Progress to the Single Leg Wall Sit when you can perform a 45-second hold with pain at 3 or less for three consecutive exercise sessions.

- **Single Leg Wall Sit**: The single leg version is performed in the same way as the traditional wall sit but requires you to lift one leg off the ground. Progress to the Bulgarian Split Squat Hold when you can perform a 45-second wall sit with pain at 3 or less for three consecutive sessions.

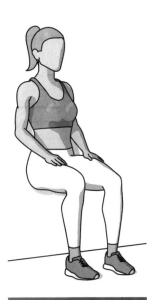

FIGURE 8.10

Wall sit.

- **Bulgarian Split Squat with Isometric Hold:** Get in the Bulgarian Split Squat starting position without any added weight (page 262). Lower your body slowly until you reach the bottom of the repetition, then hold for 10 to 30 seconds. Once you can hold a 30-second contraction on each leg for three consecutive sessions without pain, you're ready to introduce other knee-loading exercises to further build muscle, strength, and joint integrity.

6. Improve ankle mobility.

Ankles are easily my weakest link. Years of repeated sprains left my ankles stiff and full of scar tissue. In order to perform my favorite exercises and activities without pain, I have to stay on top of ankle mobility work. Stiff ankles, especially if you lack dorsiflexion (pulling your toes up toward your body), can lead to both Achilles tendon injuries and knee pain. A certain amount of ankle mobility is necessary to squat and even walk without creating shearing forces that overload the knee.[246] When lacking ankle mobility, your body has two choices to perform squatting motions: (1) lean the upper body forward to allow the hips to descend, which strains the low back, or (2) keep the upper body upright, which strains the tendons and ligaments in the front your knee. Freeing up ankle ranges of motion will allow you to develop stabilizing ankle strength, which provides a better foundation for your knees.

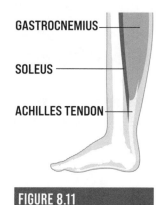

FIGURE 8.11

Lower leg anatomy.

Often, the limiting factor in ankle mobility isn't the actual ankle joint but your calf muscles—specifically, the gastrocnemius. The gastrocnemius is a two-headed muscle that makes up the bulk of your lower leg mass. It attaches the bottom of your thigh bone to the Achilles tendon and heel bone of the foot. Not only do tight calf muscles limit range of motion and put additional stress on your knees, they pull mercilessly on your Achilles tendon, increasing your risk of a rupture and tendinopathy.

The gastrocnemius is a notoriously stiff, stubborn muscle with dense fascia surrounding it, making it difficult to elongate. But you can outsmart it. By leveraging nerve gliding techniques with manual therapy, you can loosen up the gastrocnemius while also improving nerve flow and working out kinks in the fascia surrounding your calves. To do this, perform the Ankle Glide exercise with a foam roll anchor. You should feel this one right away. Studies have shown that only one session of ankle joint mobilization along with manual therapy significantly improves range of motion.[247]

After loosening up your calves with the Ankle Glide exercise, perform a few sets of straight-leg calf raises while standing on a block. Focus on expanding your range of motion at the bottom of the movement. Avoid using momentum. Instead, hold the stretched position for a few seconds during each repetition before raising up on your toes.

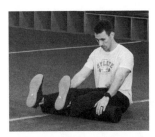

Ankle Glides

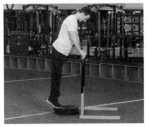

Standing Calf Raise from Block

Key exercises
- Ankle Glides (page 272)
- Standing Calf Raise from Block (page 275)

7. Activate your feet.

The natural arch of your foot is designed to act as a spring during movements, absorb forces, stabilize and align the joints of your lower body, and allow your foot to adapt to surfaces. If you have a healthy arch, there will be space between the floor and the inside sole of your foot when standing. When your arch collapses and the entire sole of your foot touches the ground, whether from genetics, age, or movement mechanics, it's referred to as *flat feet* or *fallen arches*. While some people do not experience any symptoms from flat feet, it puts you at risk of more frequent knee pain and advanced knee cartilage degeneration.[248]

You can test your arch health by standing on both feet (barefoot), then bending over and sliding a finger under the inside of your foot, halfway between your heel and toe. There should be enough space for you to slide your finger a few centimeters under before touching the bottom of your foot.

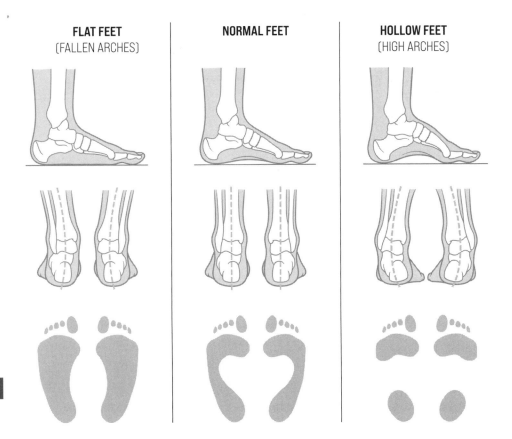

FLAT FEET (FALLEN ARCHES)   **NORMAL FEET**   **HOLLOW FEET** (HIGH ARCHES)

FIGURE 8.12

Foot deformations.

If you can slide your finger under your foot up to the crease of your first finger joint, you have a healthy arch. If there is no space between your sole and the floor, and your finger slams into the inside edge of your foot when you try to slide it under, your arches are collapsed. This is either from having genetically flat feet or from what I call *lazy feet*—when your foot muscles simply haven't been trained to maintain proper position.

While you can't change the foot anatomy you were born with, you can activate your foot muscles and build your arch with targeted exercise. First, let's look at what happens when the arch of your foot collapses and your feet muscles become latent:

1. **Movement faults during exercise are more likely.** A healthy foot arch will keep your heel in line with your knee joint, and your knee joint in line with your hip joint. When your foot collapses, it causes a chain reaction that pulls your entire lower body out of alignment. First, the sole of your foot collapses, causing your heel to kick outward and your ankle to roll inward (ankle eversion). This causes knee valgus, where your knee rolls to the midline of your body, pulling your lower leg and upper leg out of alignment. Not only does this hurt performance, it puts your connective tissue at risk of tearing.

2. **Ligaments in your lower leg and knee are forced to absorb forces.** When your arches fall, you don't just lose anatomical position; you also lose the springlike function of the arch. Instead of the muscles and tendons in your feet and ankles absorbing forces, ligaments and joint capsules do. This causes overuse injuries when you lift weights, run, or jump. Common injuries caused by flat feet include plantar fasciitis (foot pain from stressed ligaments), patellar tendinopathy, and patellofemoral syndrome.

3. **Your feet lose their ability to adjust to the surface environment.** Feet with fallen arches cannot effectively conform to their surface environment when walking, running, or landing from a jump. Instead of your feet bending and flexing naturally, they slam into the ground and send shockwaves from your heel bone up through your low back.

4. **Your butt turns off.** As flat feet force your knees and hips to internally rotate during movements like walking or squatting, your butt gets left out in the cold (gluteal amnesia).[249] That's because when the internal rotation muscles of your hip are activated (adductors), the activity of external rotation muscles (abductors) decreases through the law of reciprocal inhibition. As we've already covered, weak and inactive glutes cause a whole host of problems, including knee pain and low back pain.

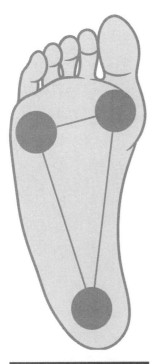

FIGURE 8.13

Three points of contact for ideal foot position.

Foot health doesn't get near the attention it should for preventing knee and low back pain. Whether you have true flat feet or just lazy foot muscles that haven't been adequately trained, activating your feet will improve performance and reduce your risk of knee pain.

Here are two things you can do right now to get your feet in shape:

1. **Master the three points of contact rule.** There are three points of contact that your foot should always maintain with the ground, whether you're going for a walk or squatting 500 pounds. The three points are the heel, ball behind your big toe, and ball behind your pinky toe. Follow this sequence to find your ideal foot positioning:

   Stand barefoot on a flat surface and shift your body weight to your right leg. Next, raise your right heel off the ground and push into the balls of your feet (the area between your toes and arch). Raise the toes of your right foot off the ground and spread them out. You should feel all the weight of your leg on the balls of your feet, balanced between the padded area behind your big toe and padded area behind your pinky toe. Finally, slowly lower your heel to the ground. You'll notice your foot performs an instinctual gripping action against the ground—not unlike a bird or monkey gripping a tree branch with their feet. Repeat this sequence a few times then switch to the left foot.

   Practice walking around barefoot while maintaining this semi-rigid position. With each step, it should feel like you are grabbing the ground with your feet and pressing through your pads. You'll realize how little thought you give to the tone of your feet as you move around.

   Finally, take this new mind-muscle connection into the gym. Practice squatting, lunging, and doing other exercises with active feet. You can perform one-leg balance exercises to further train this position, but I believe establishing a mind-muscle connection with your feet and carrying that into every movement is even more useful. It's not necessary to follow each step of this sequence each time you establish foot position. Just performing it a few times will give you a good feel for how to push through the balls of your feet and balance the three points of contact.

   When you first start doing this, you may find that your feet wobble back and forth, searching for optimal positioning. While this feels like a failure, you're actually training the most important muscle for building your arch: the posterior tibialis. This neglected muscle resides deep in the interior compartment of your lower leg, wrapping around the inside of your foot and attaching near the sole. It is responsible for inversion (rolling onto the outside blade of your foot) and is a crucial muscle for foot stabilization. So, when you see your foot wobbling, it means the posterior tibialis is getting a workout. Over time, as it strengthens and your balance improves, your foot will wobble less and your knees will be more stable. Remember: strong feet, healthy knees.

2. **Don't cramp your feet.** The biggest mistake people make regarding shoes is wearing a size too small. You are better off with a size too large so your toes have room to spread out. Only when your toes are spread can your feet maintain optimal alignment and a solid three points of contact with the ground. Many companies make shoes with wider toe boxes to accommodate toe spreading, which I recommend. Search for "shoes with wide toebox" online or ask a shoe expert at a local store about which shoes provide the most cargo space for toes.

Best Exercises for Knee Pain

- Bulgarian Split Squat
- Fire Hydrant
- Glute Bridge with Hip Band
- Box Stepdown
- Swiss Ball Leg Curl
- Cossack Squat
- World's Greatest Stretch
- Ankle Glides
- Standing Calf Raise from Block
- Active Feet Training

Injury Recovery: Strategy and Tactics

Things are antifragile up to a certain level of stress. Your body benefits from some amount of mishandling. But up to a point. It would not benefit too much from being thrown down from the top of the Tower of Babel.

— Nassim Taleb, author of *Antifragile*

When to seek medical attention

This chapter is not a replacement for medical attention and guidance from a doctor or physical therapist. This is not a complete list of indications for which you should seek immediate medical attention—it only serves to give you a few of the common indications to look out for:

- Abnormal bone, joint, or muscle positioning (e.g. it looks crooked or is misshapen)

- Excessive swelling, bruising, or bleeding

- Sharp pain when performing previously pain-free movements

- Inability to bear weight on the limb or joint without it giving way

- A feeling of abnormal "looseness" in the joint

The medical system is not equipped to help you fully recover from and prevent injuries. Doctors, therapists, and natural health practitioners are limited by their legal scope of practice, time available to spend with you, and specialized knowledge that limits their input to only one or two pieces of the injury management puzzle. If you've been down the conventional medicine path, you already know that treatment revolves around symptoms—not causes. Pills, injections, braces, and suggestions to "stop doing that" are all designed to alleviate pain. What's missing is an understanding of what caused the injury. Without this, you can't confidently move in any direction. It's also rare to find health care providers who are as motivated as you to get you back to full function. "Good enough" becomes the standard. But that's not good enough. Let's replace "stop doing that" and "good enough" with an understanding of why injuries occur, how to heal them, and how to prevent them from happening in the first place.

This chapter isn't a replacement or rebuke of traditional medicine or physical therapy practices. When I'm injured, the first thing I do is see a physical therapist. You should do the same. But the journey from injured to full function and beyond doesn't stop at physical therapy. It's up to you to understand why your injury occurred and how to navigate through the variables specific to you. A good place to start is with the concept of *rest*. Despite seeming harmless and obvious, this topic is one of serious contention in the therapeutic world.

THE PROBLEM WITH REST

Rest. The concept seems simple enough, but it's tricky to nail down. Rest too little, and you aggravate the injury, increasing the time required for full rehabilitation. Rest too much, and you risk losing connective tissue strength, muscle mass, and aerobic capacity. Given this tradeoff, it seems logical to err on the side of too much rest, but there are other factors at play.

First, a couple of definitions.

Passive rest is what people are typically referring to when they use the word *rest* after an injury or repetitive use strain. It means stillness, or complete inactivity. An extreme example is bed rest.

Active rest (a.k.a. active recovery) includes low-intensity movement designed to facilitate healing without aggravating the injury. Examples include massage, low-impact endurance training like walking, body-weight exercises, and light stretching.

When all goes as planned, these two opposing methods don't require much consideration. Here's an example: you sprain your wrist and see a doctor, who suggests wearing a splint for a few weeks to let it heal. Then, after a few weeks, you gradually eliminate the use of the splint while slowly introducing stretches and normal activities. With luck, you're back to normal within a month or two.

Problems arise when a strain becomes a nagging injury that won't heal, or when you are dealing with a repetitive use strain that continues to hurt. In these situations, there is an underlying cause that hasn't been addressed. Rest, ice, and popping ibuprofen only serve to keep symptoms at bay for a while. Here lies the fundamental problem with rest: it doesn't solve underlying mechanical issues or causes. As a physical therapist friend of mine succinctly put it: "The storm that damaged your house is gone, but you haven't fixed the damage."

You can take six weeks off from typing on the computer to prevent wrist pain, but the minute you slouch over your laptop with hands cranked awkwardly to the side, the stressor is back—and the wrist injury will be as well. If you hurt your low back, you can lay off heavy lifting for weeks and find relief, but the first time you lift weights or that massive arm chair in your living room, your atrophied low back muscles will strain from poor dynamic posture.

In the old days, popular opinion was that injuries needed complete rest to fully heal. Now, therapists lean more toward active recovery for a handful of reasons:

1. Passive rest robs athletes of their fitness level, making re-entry into competition difficult. For nonathletes, using passive rest means taking large chunks of time, maybe even months, off from exercise each year. This makes maintaining any kind of fitness level difficult.

2. Long periods of passive rest cause muscle atrophy, shortening of connective tissue (Davis's law), changes in neuromuscular coordination, and weakened bones and joints—leading to a cycle of injury, rest, and reinjury.

3. Studies show active recovery methods such as massage, stretching, and aerobic exercise help ease pain and soreness, reduce inflammation, improve circulation, increase delivery of oxygen and regenerative nutrients, and clear damaged tissue from injury sites to facilitate healing.[250]

4. Active recovery provides the mental and emotional benefits of exercise, warding off stress and keeping mood elevated.

5. Passive rest after an injury completely neglects the law of *mechanotransduction*.[88] Without movement, your tissues do not heal optimally. You're left with weak scar-tissue-like formations that are easily torn and irritated. Movement drives healing.

Unfortunately, it's not as simple as going for a breezy walk or getting a massage a few times per week to expedite injury recovery and relieve pain. There are dozens of individual factors at play. The scientific answer to "What is the optimal amount of passive and active rest?" is: *It depends.* We'll go through injury recovery timelines shortly, but here is a quick guide on how to handle rest when it comes to pain from strains, irritated joints, or other minor flare-ups:

1. **First, do no harm.** Even if you haven't identified the source of the pain yet, make sure you don't do anything to exacerbate it. This involves passive rest during the first 24–48 hours, depending on injury severity.

2. **Don't do anything that hurts.** Don't try to pop your back into place, yank on a painful injured shoulder with a forced stretch, or do anything that causes more pain.

3. **Get professional help.** Determine the extent of the injury and where it's located. Then, seek the appropriate level of medical care as soon as possible.

4. **Stay as active as possible without aggravating the injury.** Focus on low-intensity exercise. If possible, keep your current schedule and exercise frequency. This provides a much-needed mental boost. Make a list of the activities you can do without pain and those that clearly increase pain. In most cases of minor strains and sprains, you can find ways to exercise.

5. **Find the underlying cause.** Steps 1–4 come first because you can implement them immediately, but you should start the detective work as soon as you experience pain. Examine your posture, muscle weaknesses, and inflexible joints. Takes notes on your symptoms and what activities you participated in recently.

6. **Rest early, not later.** The more recent the injury, the more you will benefit from rest. The older the injury, the less you will benefit from rest. In later stages of the injury repair process, you are most likely not suffering from an inflammation problem but from suboptimal connective tissue patterns that need to be realigned and strengthened through movement and exercise.

PRINCIPLES OF MOVEMENT AFTER INJURY

We've established that early movement after an injury aids healing processes (unless of course it puts you at risk of further severe injury). After the initial pain and inflammation has died down, use these principles to get moving safely:

1. Understand the two categories of postinjury training.

There are two main categories of training after an injury: training around the injury and rehabilitating the injury. It's helpful to mentally separate these because each has its own set of goals. Depending on the severity and location of an injury, attempts at exercise can feel fruitless, like it's impossible to complete a training session without aggravating the injury. For back and neck injuries, this can prove true. But in most cases, you can still move and train other body parts. And you should. Finding ways to exercise around an injury allows you to maintain the mental benefits of training and keep the rest of your body strong. You may even find a silver lining, with an injury forcing you to focus on lagging body parts or weak movements. Remember that you are not your injury, and there are still plenty of healthy joints, muscles, and tissues that want your attention.

A common mistake people make is stopping their exercise habits after an injury. They believe that if an injury prevents them from doing what they used to do, exercise is pointless. Don't fall into this trap. Keep moving. Adapt. Find ways to train around the injury. When that nagging injury finally heals, you'll find yourself much more focused and fit.

2. Use pain as your guide.

If a movement does not cause pain and you can complete it with adequate form and control, it's generally safe to do. You'll be surprised by how many movements you can complete with a shoulder strain or busted-up knee. You may have to get creative, but it's worth it. Pain also shows you if you are making progress or regressing. Keep an eye on pain levels during the following one or two days after your postinjury training sessions to see what movements cause lasting discomfort. Avoid these altogether or add them to your rehabilitative exercise routine using light resistance that does not cause you pain.

3. Establish pain-free ranges of motion ASAP.

As soon as you can, figure out what your pain-free ranges of motion are around the injured body part and fight to maintain them. Your muscles don't just shrink from disuse, they also shorten. Braces, splints, and other therapeutic devices will set you back if you overuse them. If your injury requires the use of one of these, make it a priority to work through your full, pain-free ranges of motion a few times per day without use of the device (after getting medical approval).

4. Be clear about your movement priorities.

In the days, weeks, and months following an injury, make sure you are progressing through these stages sequentially:

- **Stability:** Establish a baseline of stability before trying to increase flexibility or build strength. Choose exercises that challenge the affected joint's ability to maintain proper positioning during movement.

- **Movement mechanics:** Before adding greater loads or attempting to increase range of motion, master the movements. Start slow, light, and attentive. You aren't just building strength and endurance, you are establishing motor patterns that will last for a lifetime. Get the movements right early and you'll be able to continue progressing later. Depending on your injury, you may have to relearn proper form as your body fights against what it perceives as a threat. Patience and deliberate practice are key here.

- **Mobility:** Build upon your pain-free ranges of motion, aiming to expand them gradually. Place particular emphasis on getting mobility back to where it was preinjury (or better) in the basic human movements: squat, hip hinge, upper body push, upper body pull, and trunk rotation. Mastering the basics, like the body weight squat, will do more for your full recovery than all the fancy rehab equipment at your gym combined.

- **Strength:** After establishing sufficient stability, form, and mobility, you need to build strength around your injured body part. This not only builds up the load tolerance of tissues around the injury, it also spurs the healing process forward. Most strength gains early after an injury are the result of more efficient motor unit recruitment by the nervous system. Not of building more muscle. Keep that in mind and don't feel like you have to load up the bar or increase resistance every session. Focus on perfecting the form and executing the movement as perfectly as you can. Strength will come.

- **Endurance:** Don't forget endurance training. It's not just for marathon runners. Without muscular endurance, you're just one fatigued movement fault away from reinjury.

5. Be safe in your progressions of intensity and frequency.

Before increasing resistance, develop motor control mastery of the movement. Then, increase load incrementally. Not more than 10%–20% per session. As with strength, increase the intensity of your endurance training only incrementally. And be mindful of adding more frequency, or exercise sessions, into your routine. More frequent exercise is a great way to shield yourself against overuse injuries, but only if you get there gradually. A good rule of thumb is to add only one extra day of training into your weekly routine every four weeks.

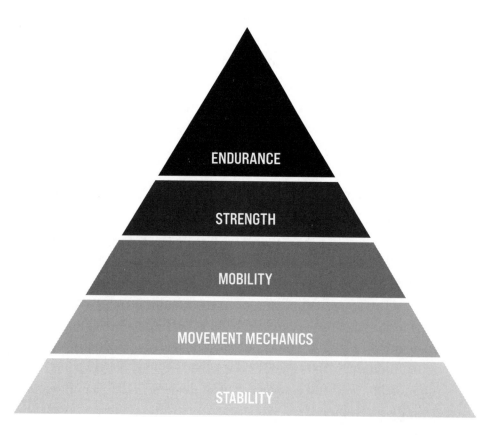

FIGURE 9.1

Injury recovery movement priorities.

Now that you have a long-term strategy for postinjury movement, what should you do immediately following an injury to improve your chances of a full, speedy recovery? If you've been around organized sports or fitness, you have probably heard the acronym RICE, which stands for rest, ice, compression, and elevation. For the last 50 years, this was the gold standard of acute injury care. But new research casts doubt on this technique, and forward-thinking therapists and doctors are using a new method for postinjury care.

THE EVOLUTION OF INJURY RECOVERY ADVICE

In 1978, Dr. Gabe Mirkin coined the term *RICE* in his best seller *The Sportsmedicine Book* to describe a simple method of caring for acute injuries. The concept was straightforward and intuitive and gained immediate widespread acceptance:[251]

- **Rest:** Because you just hurt yourself. No further explanation needed.
- **Ice:** To reduce swelling, inflammation, and pain.
- **Compression:** Wrap or brace the injury to help with all the same stuff as ice.
- **Elevation:** Raise the injured body part above the level of your heart to reduce excess swelling and blood flow.

I can remember several instances where I sprained an ankle or knee and used the RICE protocol. Within seconds, I got some relief. Within minutes, I felt like I was on the mend. That's the thing about the RICE method: you get immediate positive feedback. Swelling goes down and pain vanishes. But as you now know, what works for immediate pain relief doesn't always translate to improved healing outcomes. After decades of unquestioning loyalty to the RICE method, therapists and coaches are wising up to a new way of thinking about injury care.

Studies continue to stack up that show each element of RICE has fatal flaws:

- **Rest:** Movement triggers the mechanotransduction process, where chemical growth factors are released from cells in response to loading. This improves muscle and collagen formations, laying a strong foundation for healing. You don't get that with rest.[252]
- **Ice:** Healing requires inflammation, and any protocols that block inflammation are counterproductive. The acute inflammatory response (immediately following an injury) dilates capillaries and blood vessels, increasing delivery of oxygen and nutrient-rich blood to the injury site. Inflammation also helps mobilize macrophages, a type of cell that speeds up healing and prevents infection by cleaning

up damaged tissue. Macrophages release a hormone called IGF-1 into the damaged tissues, which kick-starts the healing process. Icing an injury blocks inflammation, interrupting the very processes responsible for healing.[253]

- **Compression:** A metastudy covering 20+ scientific articles found no significant evidence that compression aids the healing process.[254]

- **Elevation:** It may help with immediate pain and swelling symptoms but has limited scientific backing for improving outcomes.

If all that's not enough to convince you otherwise, Dr. Mirkin—the creator of the RICE method—has publicly updated his opinion, stating that "both ice and complete rest may delay healing, instead of helping."[251] Which, by the way, is exactly what a good scientist should do, and we should all thank him for that. He even went so far as to cowrite a book with author Gary Reinl and Dr. Kelly Starret titled *ICED! The Illusionary Treatment Option.*

The book *ICED!* lays out an air-tight case against icing and other traditional injury treatment methods, quoting respected journals from all over the world:[255]

"Topical cooling (icing) delays recovery."

—*Journal of Strength and Conditioning Research* (2013)

"Ice is commonly used after acute muscle strains but there are no clinical studies of its effectiveness."

—*British Journal of Sports Medicine* (2012)

"There is insufficient evidence to suggest that cryotherapy [icing] improves clinical outcome."

—*Journal of Emergency Medicine* (2008)

"Ice may not be the best treatment for aching muscles—in fact, it could even be detrimental to recovery."

—University of Pittsburgh Medical Center (2011)

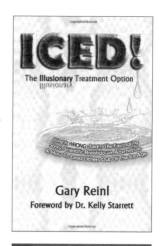

FIGURE 9.2

ICED! The Illusionary Treatment Option (book cover).

END OF THE ICE AGE

RICE has fallen out of favor in the world of injury care. Some clever therapists even started referring to the RICE method as the MICE method (movement, ice, compression, elevation). But as we discussed, ice, compression, and elevation are not always the best methods for supporting the healing process either. We need a completely new paradigm. (And naturally, a completely new acronym.)

A 2020 article published in the *British Journal of Sports Medicine* by researcher Blaise Dubois and colleagues claims that soft-tissue injuries simply need PEACE and LOVE. I'm not kidding. The title of the article is "Soft-Tissue Injuries Simply Need PEACE and LOVE."[256]

The acronym is a bit excessive. But it covers all the bases. And it's grounded in good science:

- **P for PROTECTION**: Protect the injury during the first few days by avoiding movements that cause pain or stress the injured area.

- **E for ELEVATION**: Raise the injured limb (if applicable) higher than the level of your heart to minimize swelling and allow fluid to drain from the area. Follow this for the first day or two postinjury as needed.

- **A for AVOID ANTI-INFLAMMATORIES**: Avoid NSAIDs, ice, and other anti-inflammatories during the first few days postinjury.

- **C for COMPRESSION**: Use elastic bandages, tape, or wraps to reduce swelling so you can continue pain-free movements (but don't become dependent on compression devices that provide stability to your joints—you need to keep those stabilizer muscles strong).

- **E for EDUCATION**: Understand the injury recovery process, let your body do its job, and avoid unnecessary medical interventions that may limit long-term healing outcomes.

- **L for LOAD**: Use pain as your guide for returning to activities. Pain (or lack thereof) will also tell you when it's OK to start adding more resistance and intensity to your movements.

- **O for OPTIMISM**: Injuries take a toll psychologically. Expect it and know that it's normal. Then, work on maintaining a positive, long-term mindset for getting back to full function.

- **V for VASCULARIZATION**: Keep moving. Get creative. Find pain-free exercises you can do that increase circulation and nutrient delivery for optimal healing.

- **E for EXERCISE**: Use targeted corrective exercise to strengthen weak points that may have led to the injury.

You can decide for yourself the best way to remember these fundamental concepts. But one thing is clear: letting your body's natural recovery processes run uninhibited is the real hack for optimizing injury repair.

THE REAL CAUSE OF INJURY

Too often, people injure themselves and never take the time to understand why it happened. They'll follow all the right steps for postinjury care, complete six weeks of intensive physical therapy, then slowly limp back toward their normal way of life. Without an understanding of the real causes of injury, they are prone to reinjury and will likely be plagued by pain and dysfunction for the rest of their days. When I say *cause* of injury, I don't mean the actual traumatic event, like a fall. I mean the series of events that led up to the moment of injury.

Generally, injuries are preceded by two things: (1) underlying muscle imbalances and (2) long periods of slow tissue degeneration. Even traumatic injuries like a broken leg, torn ACL in the knee, or dislocated shoulder follow this rule. I can speak from personal experience on this one.

In 2006, I tore the labrum in my left shoulder while diving for a baseball. I had surgery, completed physical therapy, and returned to play, but my shoulder was never the same. I was in and out of commission with shoulder pain and movement limitations that were made worse every time I stretched the injured shoulder beyond its comfortable range of motion. This caused me to miss the last half of one season and first half of another, and eventually led to the end of my collegiate baseball career. Looking back, I realize that my shoulder injury was years in the making. It was inevitable.

I didn't have the first clue about building strong, stable shoulders. My workouts consisted of the meathead staples: bench press, pull-ups, curls, etc. I lacked upper-back strength, creating a massive agonist-antagonist imbalance around my shoulder joints. Shoulder mobility was a complete joke. I spent no time working on range of motion and could barely get my arms extended above my head without arching to compensate. Now, think about what it takes to dive on the ground with outstretched arms. You need adequate shoulder stability and enough shoulder extension mobility to absorb the impact without straining any tendons, ligaments, or cartilage. I had neither. When I dove for the ball, impact with the ground jammed the head of my humerus upward, ripping the cartilage that connected it to the shoulder socket.

That's not all. I had been experiencing pain in both shoulders all season long. My natural hunched posture and mobility deficits were causing chronic shoulder impingement. Like a rope that frays over time from rubbing against sharp metal, the tendon insertions of my shoulder slowly unraveled as I bench pressed, ran, and swung baseball bats over the months preceding the injury. By the time the actual acute injury occurred, there was likely substantial connective tissue degeneration that predisposed me to a tear.

Ah, if I knew then what I know now. Luckily, you and I don't have to suffer this same fate again. Think about these questions after an injury to make sure you understand and address the underlying causes:

- Is it an acute injury (from a traumatic event) or overuse injury (symptoms increased gradually over time)? Could it be a combination of the two?

- Were you experiencing any ongoing pain, tightness, or discomfort in the weeks leading up to the injury? If so, that indicates a chronic injury and connective tissue degeneration that will need to be rebuilt.

- Are there movement patterns involving the injured body part that you were not able to correctly perform before the injury? This indicates a movement fault that led to repetitive tissue stress.

- Do you have a history of injury at or around the injury site? If so, that indicates you may have scar tissue buildup and mobility deficits that make you prone to future injuries.

- Can you think of any repetitive motions involving the injured body part that you performed regularly leading up to the injury? If so, seek to understand what kind of muscle imbalances that repetitive motion creates, what tissues it could degenerate, and what you can do to reverse the effects of the repetitive motion. Finally, find ways to reduce chronic stress from repetitive motions in the future.

- What postural faults do you have that deviate from optimal static posture? This gives you insight into which muscle imbalances you are at risk of developing that could lead to injury.

THE FINAL STEP: TURNING OFF THE CCTV CAMERAS

In the textbook *Sports Injury Prevention and Rehabilitation*, David Joyce and colleagues lay out a perfect metaphor for the final step of injury healing: turning off the CCTV cameras.[257] CCTV (closed-circuit television) is the common name for private video surveillance technology that allows you to watch recorded events in real time. When you see a TV monitor mounted behind the clerk's desk at a gas station with a view of the pumps, that's CCTV.

Just like a gas station owner who's been burned too many times by thieves, your brain ramps up surveillance of all your movements after an injury. It wants to know what is going on at all times—especially with the injured body part. This leads to *pain sensitization*. While this is helpful in the beginning phases of healing, it becomes a problem as you graduate to the final stages of recovery. At worst, it can lead to an obsessive focus on any uncomfortable sensation. At best, it becomes a distraction that alters movement patterns. Completing the final step—turning off the CCTV cameras—requires understanding three things:

1. Even after the injury site is 99% healed, undesirable neuromuscular changes are likely still present.

2. Foreign sensations, movement alterations, and other changes to your nervous system caused by injury can take months, or longer, to resolve.

3. Your body needs a confident, calm, restorative environment for your central nervous system to back off the surveillance.

This is one of the most unnerving aspects of injury recovery because you can't simply grit your teeth through it. Understanding that injuries have lasting psychological and neurological effects is important so you know what to expect and maintain faith that you'll eventually get past it.

Are you injury-prone?

The term *injury-prone* brings up images of a clumsy kid tripping on his shoestrings. While movement mechanics and coordination variations certainly lead to variances in injury rates, there's more to it than that. Genetics and anatomy affect injury-proneness, as do individual lifestyle variables like movement variation and nutrition. In my experience, there are two common, actionable variables that injury-prone people can influence:

1. **Chronic inflammation:** If your joints are easily inflamed from overuse, you likely have higher levels of total body inflammation or you are simply prone to immune overactions in response to tissue stress. Either way, you'll benefit from more proactive measures to keep inflammation levels in the healthy range.

2. **Failed healing response:** Some people simply recover more slowly than others from injuries (me again)—especially when it comes to connective tissue. A failed healing response describes prolonged periods of immune activity combined with suboptimal tissue healing outcomes.[258] If this describes you, you'll benefit from a more aggressive approach to tissue remodeling—including early ROM training postinjury, slow resistance training, and manual therapy such as deep tissue massage.

KEY TAKEAWAY

There's a lot to talk about when it comes to injury prevention. To avoid getting lost in the weeds, focus on these two concepts:

- **Reduce chronic stressors:** Adjust your lifestyle, posture, and movement habits to avoid repetitive stress. Even for acute injuries, there is usually an element of chronic stress that accumulated over time.

- **Increase load tolerance:** Gradually build your body's ability to handle heavy loads (strength training) through full ranges of motion (mobility training), even in states of extreme fatigue (endurance training).

PART 2

The Training Program

By this point in the book, you have some new tools in your toolbox for resolving joint pain, correcting muscle imbalances, and building a body that lasts. My hope is that you can put this book down right now and apply the concepts covered into your current lifestyle and training program. But I want to take it a step further. In Part 2 of this book, I lay out a periodized training program for rebuilding your body from the ground up.

CHAPTER 10

Exercise Programming and Periodization: Why It's Smart to Be Disciplined

I think the physical therapy profession could learn a lot from strength and conditioning coaches. And vice versa.

— Dr. Aaron Horschig, founder of Squat University
and author of *The Squat Bible*

In this chapter, you'll learn how to layer all the concepts we've covered so far into a coherent, sequential system. Without this chapter, this book is nothing more than a good reference text. If you don't effectively leverage periodization, fitness progress and improved joint health will come only in fleeting moments. Continued, sustainable progress won't happen. Look around you and you'll see evidence of this everywhere you go. Age is a factor, absolutely. But look around your local gym. Even the most committed daily exercise goers are usually stuck right where they're at. Poor movement habits, old injuries, mobility limitations, and lack of smart exercise programming keep them locked firmly in place. They fight just to maintain instead of advancing forward. This doesn't have to happen.

Periodization—the systematic, cyclical planning of training—provides a clear path forward. It's what enables you to assemble all the parts into a working machine. A system. And like any good system, it doesn't depend on willpower, motivation, or memory to work. It thrives on strategic planning, habit formation, templates, and execution. And here's the secret: when you're disciplined with planning, execution—the actual doing—becomes simple. Maybe not easy, but simple. It gives you confidence to focus exclusively and intensely on the task at hand. People who don't exercise think it takes tremendous discipline to go to the gym every day and eat healthy foods. But for people who have established these things as habits, it's as natural as brushing your teeth. The right exercise program frees up your mental energy in the same way.

I'm guessing you aren't in your early 20s, nor does your body work the same way it did all those years ago (if you are in your 20s, then you are ahead of the game). Now is the time to put on your thinking cap. To plan. And to outsmart your younger self. When you think about it, being disciplined with your fitness goals isn't about being tough. It's about being *planful*. That's it. The rest takes care of itself.

CORE CONCEPTS TO PROGRAM

Let's look at some of the core concepts that need to be layered into an effective periodization program for sustainable fitness progress.

- **The dynamic warm-up:** The dynamic warm-up is a fundamental component of any sustainable fitness program. The traditional warm-up of steady-state cardio exercise and stretching has gone the way of the dodo bird, replaced by a new way of thinking about mobility training and movement preparation. You already know about many of the concepts we can leverage to prepare your body for exercise, including pumping more synovial fluid into joints and using dynamic stretching to loosen up joints and muscles. Now it's time to put them into a coordinated system.

- **Corrective exercise:** Without layering corrective exercise into your regular training program, you're building a house of cards, destined to fall when muscle imbalances inevitably lead to movement faults. This includes addressing motor control and mobility, training force couples around key joint systems, and shoring up weak points like your shoulder's rotator cuff. This concept is known as prehab: you're effectively implementing rehabilitative (rehab) movements designed for injury recovery and prevention into daily movement practices. This beats the old model of training as hard as you can, getting injured, completing physical therapy, then starting the whole process over.

- **Traditional training goals:** Training isn't only about preventing injury, it's also about building the capabilities of your body. This is the fun part. It includes neuromuscular coordination, strength, endurance, and agility.

- **Connective tissue training:** We can't forget about connective tissue training. Most people assume joint health is something that they gradually lose over time and there is nothing they can do about it. While age is a factor, your joints can be strengthened and fortified just like muscles. Connective tissue training involves building load tolerance, improving joint stability, and expanding and reinforcing joint mobility.

Sounds like a lot of work, doesn't it? It is. Progressing in all these categories is only possible if you do two things:

1. **Manage time effectively:** Choose only the most effective bang-for-buck exercise, warm up efficiently, and move through your workouts with a deliberate pace.

2. **Create a strategic plan:** Making progress in all these categories isn't simultaneous. It's sequential. By planning out what you want to accomplish over the course of the week, the month, and the next three months, you can cover all your bases in a way that builds upon previous improvements in strength and conditioning.

EXERCISE PROGRAMMING TO PREVENT CONNECTIVE TISSUE INJURY

Prevention of connective tissue injury is not something that is accomplished only by using safe exercise technique and smart applications of movement tempo. It takes planning. The most important principle to get right when constructing your exercise plan is to prevent *accumulated joint stress*. Because tendons and ligaments heal more slowly than muscles, you must balance muscle and strength gains with joint recovery.

Along with utilizing rest days and low-intensity training days, and adding more movement variety, scheduling a *deload* week every four to eight weeks will go a long way toward letting your joints repair. *Deload* simply means backing off the intensity and/or volume to allow muscles, the central nervous system, and connective tissues to heal optimally. Despite fears of losing progress in the gym, an occasional deload week will not cause you to become weak and puny.[259]

I used to implement a deload week every four weeks, then take every eighth week off entirely from weight lifting. I would start each training block by assaulting my body with as much damaging exercise as possible, then lick my wounds during the deload week before starting the cycle all over again. For many people, this logically reinforces the need for deloads. But I don't look at it that way anymore. If your training plan causes such fatigue and joint pain that you need to take time off from exercise every month, then there is a more fundamental problem. The deload is simply a Band-Aid. As researcher Chris Beardsley points out, "If we are doing a strength training program that requires a deload for our connective tissues, then it probably wasn't a particularly well-designed program."[260]

I no longer recommend taking full weeks off from exercise every other month, nor do I advocate for extreme deload weeks where you are essentially going through the motions of exercises without any sort of meaningful stimulus. Deloads are effective tools when appropriately implemented. But your daily and weekly routines should be arranged to prevent the accumulation of joint stress without the need for extreme reductions in volume and intensity.

If all the training methods described so far seem contradictory, it's because they are. Strictly speaking in terms of joint health, you need heavy weights to increase tendon stiffness, slow repetitions for optimal collagen formations, and sustained contractions to induce the greatest adaptive responses. You need all of them. But you can't train all of them at once. In the next section, I'll show you how to layer all these concepts into a training program that optimizes performance now without sacrificing your joints later.

HOW TO USE PERIODIZATION FOR CONSISTENT, INJURY-FREE GAINS

Modern exercise periodization stems from Hans Selye's 1950 General Adaptation Syndrome (GAS) theory.[261] This theory gave names to the three phases of response your body undergoes when experiencing a new stimulus: alarm, resistance, and exhaustion. The fundamental ideas that grew out of this theory still form the backbone of periodization strategy today. That is, mitigate your body's alarm response (shock), maximize resistance (adaptation), and prevent exhaustion. Periodization used to be reserved for Olympians and professional athletes under the tutelage of high-paid trainers who planned their training cycles a year in advance. Now, you can leverage these same principles to make consistent progress while staying healthy for the long haul. A young, hormone-riddled 20-something can ignore this type of planning and wreak havoc in the gym without immediate negative consequences. But you have to be smarter. More strategic.

Periodization schedules for athletes are designed around a distant event. All training goals are directed at peaking for that event. For you, the event is to *keep playing the game.* Since the first step in the periodization planning process is determining the event requirements—and since *longevity is your event*—that should be the primary end-goal of the training program. It trumps all else, and all short-term goals should be sacrificed, if necessary, to achieve that goal. With this framework in mind, let's look at the structure of periodization cycles and a few popular approaches that are relevant for you.

TYPES OF PERIODIZATION FOR RESISTANCE TRAINING

There are three primary types of periodization: linear, undulating, and block.[261–263]

Linear Periodization

Linear periodization is the simplest form of planned resistance programming. Two variables control linear periodization: volume and intensity. Generally, programs following this model start out with higher training volumes (usually more total sets and repetitions) and relatively low intensity, or load. Then, each subsequent training week will consist of less volume and greater load. This continues for several cycles until the workouts consist

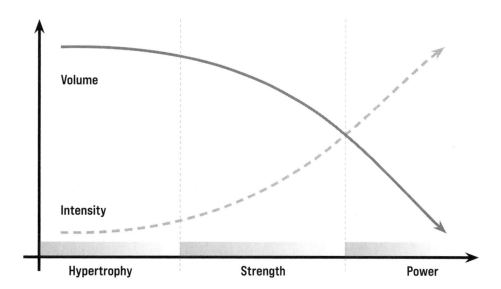

FIGURE 10.1

Linear periodization.

of near maximum effort movements at low work volume. This is usually followed by a deload period, where both volume and intensity are reduced to allow for recovery. Then, the cycle starts over, ideally with newfound strength and conditioning.

Undulating Periodization

Undulating periodization refers to altering the loads and repetition schemes of training sessions throughout the week. The idea is to give your body more frequent recovery periods to prevent neural fatigue while keeping overall training stimulus high enough to trigger a favorable adaptive response. Within each week, you adjust the volume and intensity inversely (as number of repetitions goes up, load goes down, and vice versa). Beyond the neural adaptations, it also more effectively targets the full spectrum of sports performance goals: strength, muscle growth, and endurance.

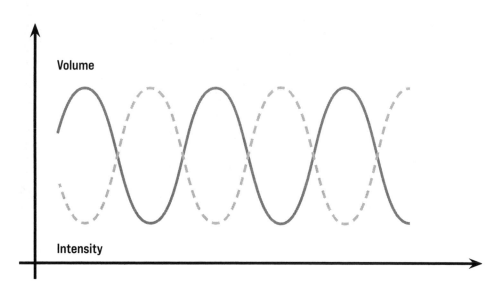

FIGURE 10.2

Undulating periodization.

Block Periodization

Block periodization was born as a solution to the problems created by traditional periodization schedules. Unlike linear and undulating methods, block periodization allows you to focus on one major performance goal for several weeks at a time.[263] This block of time is called a *mesocycle*, and it generally lasts four to eight weeks. After completing one mesocycle, you move on to a subsequent mesocycle that addresses a new goal. Block periodization creates a leapfrog effect where gains from one mesocycle boost the efforts of the next, muscle asymmetries are avoided, and recovery periods balance out more intensive training periods.

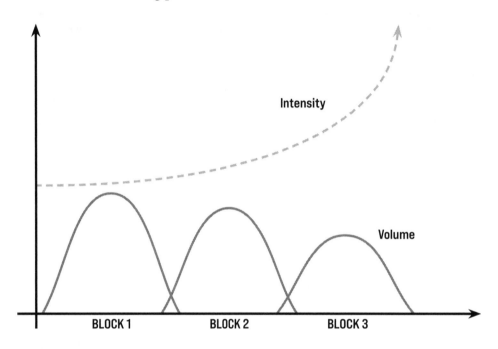

FIGURE 10.3

Block periodization.

Which Is Better?

The strength of linear periodization is its simplicity. It's easy to follow and arguably more effective for gaining strength and muscle than doing the same workouts week after week, at least in novice lifters. But it has two primary weaknesses. First, it's not as effective as periodization techniques that more regularly alter volume and load. A 2009 study published in the *Journal of Strength and Conditioning Research* showed that participants who followed a daily undulating periodization (DUP) program gained more strength than linear periodization participants after 12 weeks of training in the bench press (18.2% increase for LP vs. 25.08% for DUP), leg press (24.71% increase for LP vs. 40.61% for DUP), and arm curl (14.15% LP and 23.53% DUP).[264] In another smaller 12-week study published in the same journal, the undulating periodization group gained almost twice the strength as the linear periodization group.[265]

These differences aren't just *statistically significant*, they're massively significant. Not even close. Researchers believe the vast differences can be explained by linear programming causing neural fatigue and undulating programming resulting in favorable adaptations from more periods of recovery. The concept of progressive neuromuscular fatigue ties into the second weakness of linear periodization: declines in functional movement and increased injury risk.

As I mentioned earlier in the book, being in a state of neuromuscular fatigue puts you at risk of faulty movement patterns that could get you hurt. Therefore, it's important to develop a baseline level of endurance, especially in the muscular systems that you count on most for joint support, like the low back and rear shoulders. But it's not just about preventing fatigue. A 2018 study published in the *Journal of Yoga and Physical Therapy* compared linear and nonlinear periodization for a different reason: to assess changes in postural control, functional movement capabilities, mobility, and injury risk.[266] One of the primary methods of measuring mobility and function is called the Functional Movement Screen (FMS). It consists of analyzing seven basic movement patterns: the squat, hurdle step, in-line lunge, shoulder mobility, straight leg raise, push-up, and trunk rotation. As you might have guessed, the nonlinear periodization groups had higher scores on the FMS and balance tests.

Not only are these improvements directly correlated with strength and performance, they also reduce injury risk. This is an important take-home message: even if you are able to make significant strength, muscle mass, or endurance gains by simply making your workouts harder and heavier over time, you'll be systematically creating muscle asymmetries that will lead to pain and injury. It's just a matter of when.

Undulating periodization also appears to beat block periodization. One study of 17 women aimed at maximizing muscle strength and size showed that weekly undulating periodization (WUD) was more effective than block periodization (BP). In the study, both groups saw significant increases in strength and power, but the WUD group beat the BP group handily in lower-body strength with a 27.7% increase at the end of 10 weeks versus a 15.2% increase in the BP group.[267]

While undulating periodization kicks butt in studies, it has limitations in real life. Unlike the simplistic linear periodization, you can't just count on progressively heavier weights to force you into working harder. When implemented haphazardly, undulating periodization looks like a messy cluster of difficult to follow exercises and repetition schemes. Also, bodybuilding-focused undulating periodization training does not allow for the necessary corrective exercise and joint-supporting work that you need to stay pain-free and injury-free.

PERIODIZATION VARIABLES

Each periodization method has one or two flaws that lead to plateaus and burnout. What we need is a system that pulls the best aspects from all three methods. To do this, let's look deeper into the best ways to manipulate the primary periodization variables: training volume, frequency, and intensity.

Training Volume

To maximize muscle growth and strength gains, more sets and more total work generally leads to better results. For example, a 2015 study from the *Journal of Strength and Conditioning Research* showed that participants who completed 5 sets per exercise built more muscle than those who performed only 1–3 sets after six months of training.[268] It seems that more actually is better. This kind of thinking, supported by the literature that backs it up, causes fitness enthusiasts to ramp up workout volume at the cost of all else. Most people who are motivated to make real progress try to pack in as much work as possible into each training session. They push the limits of their bodies, connective tissue health, and mental health, only leaving the gym when they're completely spent and on the verge of burnout. Every motivational speech about hard work and even scientific literature seems to back up this strategy. But it's shortsighted.

First, high training volume is more important for maximizing muscle growth than it is for increasing strength and endurance. A 2019 study published in *Medicine & Science in Sports & Exercise* demonstrated that while 5 sets per exercise beat out 1–3 sets per exercise for muscle growth, all groups showed significant increases in strength and endurance with "no significant between-group differences."[269] Since the program I recommend focuses on building movement skill and shoring up weaknesses, bodybuilding-level volumes aren't necessary. Secondly, if you ramp up your workout volume too fast, your injury risk skyrockets, especially when you are introducing new exercises and training styles.[169] Third, there is a point of diminishing returns after you reach a certain threshold of training volume. After you have already challenged your body with substantial mechanical load, any additional exercise will only produce marginal improvements at best and may even be counterproductive.

High-volume training doesn't hold up in the real world. I see this play out all the time. A well-intentioned novice performs set after boring set, slogging through the workload they believe is necessary to achieve the body they want. Their focus is lacking during the movements and they subconsciously train with lower intensity to conserve energy, especially toward the end of the training session. This leads to long, grueling workouts and reduced program adherence. I don't know about you, but I'd much rather perform 2–3 intense sets than 5 half-assed sets that produce the same (or worse) results.

Key takeaway

Instead of trying to do maximum damage to your body each session, optimize for consistent incremental gains. Instead of trying to pack in as much training as possible, aim for the minimum effective dose (MED) of training that will allow you to make progress from week to week—at least while you follow the program I've outlined in the next chapter.

Training Frequency

The optimal training frequency for hypertrophy (building muscle) falls somewhere between two and four days per week for most people.[270] For building strength, more frequent sessions with lower volume are better for the necessary neural adaptations. I find it interesting that the more experienced a trainee is, the more they lean toward less frequent, more intensive training sessions. On the surface, the logic seems sound. After developing a base of muscle strength and size, your body requires a greater shock and more training intensity to elicit continued growth. But infrequent muscle training (e.g. training each body part once per week) has drawbacks. Beginners will benefit more from high-frequency training to take advantage of the quick skill-based neural adaptations that occur between sessions. For advanced trainees, more frequent training sessions leads to more time spent in a positive *net protein balance* (i.e. more time in a state of muscle protein synthesis than muscle protein breakdown).[271] Research backs up this logic, illustrating that muscle groups should be trained at least twice per week to maximize growth and strength gains.[272]

Another factor rarely discussed is the impact of training frequency on connective tissue adaptations. We know that collagen synthesis is elevated for around three days after an exercise session, so giving your joints time to recover should be a deciding factor in how you arrange your training schedule.[128] **Figure 10.4** illustrates that both muscle protein synthesis and collagen synthesis rates return to their approximate baselines at around 72 hours (3 days) after intensive training.

Training Intensity

Finally, we can't discuss training frequency without also including training intensity. If you follow a bodybuilding-style program where one or two muscle groups are trained intensely each day, you'll require more rest days between sessions to recuperate fully. If you follow a program that more closely mimics powerlifting training, where heavy loads are used in relatively low volumes, you can train more frequently. In either case, it's important to plan your workouts in a way that enables full central nervous system, muscle, and joint recovery.

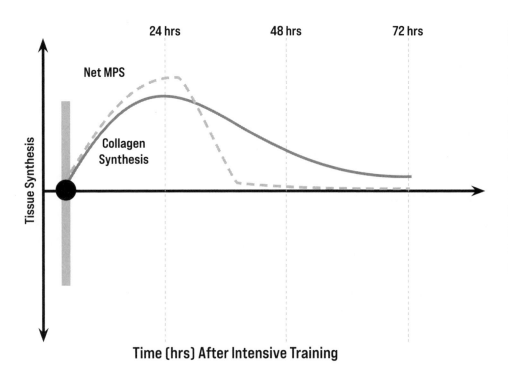

FIGURE 10.4

Muscle protein synthesis (MPS) and collagen synthesis timelines after intensive training. (Tissue synthesis rates are intended to illustrate recovery timelines only, not exact measures.) (Adapted from Magnusson et al., 2010, p. 262–268 and MacDougall et al., 1995, p. 480–486).

There's a great argument to be made for doing full body workouts three times per week—especially for novices who can benefit from "newby gains" and the increased frequency of training the same body parts. But doing full body training each time you hit the gym just doesn't allow enough time to effectively address mobility problems, target weak areas, do corrective exercise work, and perform the big compound movements that drive strength adaptations. I also don't believe that only three training days per week is enough to benefit from the injury prevention paradox (where high-frequency training has a protective effect against injury).[169] Finally, a four-day training split is more likely to create a lasting habit than only two or three sessions per week. The importance of this can't be understated. The more you ingrain your exercise sessions into your weekly schedule, the better your long-term adherence to the program will be.

For these reasons, I recommend a four-day training week consisting of two upper body focused days and two lower body focused days. This schedule is a winning combination of enough mechanical stimulus for muscles to grow and frequency of movement to see positive neural adaptations. It also provides a full three days between targeted exercise sessions so your joints have time to repair.

BUILT FROM BROKEN PERIODIZATION: A WINNING COMBINATION

When you combine proven periodization principles with the science of collagen synthesis, you have a winning formula for consistent, sustainable progress. Weekly undulating periodization will guide the sets and rep schemes of each training day. And weekly "themes" pull the best aspects of block periodization into your training schedule, giving you a singular goal to focus on. Even though linear periodization has serious flaws, the idea of working to progressively increase strength using a gradual tapering of volume with increased loads is not invalid. It just needs to be moderated by sensible adjustments to work volume and intensity—including regular deload periods. Here's how the Built from Broken periodization schedule looks in practice:

Week 1: Connective Tissue Remodeling

Use prolonged repetition speeds (e.g. five seconds down, five seconds up) for maximum connective tissue adaptation. Because each set demands sustained contractions of over a minute, you'll use lighter weights and only complete two sets per exercise. This is your "joint reset" week.

Week 2: Hypertrophy with Heavy Slow Resistance Training

Use slow to moderate repetition speeds (e.g. three seconds down, three seconds up), moderate resistance, and higher volume to maximize muscle growth. Complete three sets of 8–12 repetitions on each exercise.

Week 3: Strength Training

Perform three sets of fewer repetitions, with controlled repetition speeds during the eccentric phase (e.g. three seconds down) and maximum power production during the concentric phase (i.e. lift the weight with as much force as you can). The goal here is to maximize motor unit recruitment and increase strength.

Week 4: Endurance + Energy Loading (Deload Week)

Use light weights that allow you to comfortably perform sets of 15 repetitions or more. While still under control, you will not pause at the start or end of each repetition. Instead, you'll keep the weight in constant motion. This week gives your joints and muscles a reprieve from high intensity but still stimulates neuromuscular endurance adaptations.

• • •

This four-week training block allows for sustainable improvements over time. Unlike many training schedules, you can repeat it indefinitely. I've laid out the exact exercises, sets, and repetition schemes to follow in the next chapters. While you'll get the best results with four training sessions per week, there are also two- and three-day training week options for those of you new to weight training or who are time constrained.

Finding Your Training Schedule

As a trainer and nutrition coach, I've always taken pride in keeping both feet firmly planted on the ground. Not everyone has the time, energy, and resources to train four to five days per week. This has certainly been the case for me in the past, depending on job and personal obligations (and global pandemics that shut down all gyms and schools). But if you can get four training sessions in per week, even if it means getting up earlier or rearranging your schedule, it's worth it. If not, that's OK. You can still make significant progress with three or even two sessions per week. If you're working through a nasty case of tendinopathy or recovering from an injury, starting with fewer sessions per week is advantageous because it gives your connective tissue more time to heal.

If working out fewer or more days per week better suits you, then by all means do what fits your schedule, lifestyle, and interests. I only ask that you give the four-day training split I'm suggesting a shot. Do it for four weeks, then review your progress and decide what you want to do from there. If at that point you decide to back down to only three training days per week, or follow a bodybuilding, powerlifting, endurance, or sport-specific training plan—you'll be doing it with a newly fortified body and a stronger foundation.

Are You Ready for the Advanced Program?

I wrote this book with a certain kind of person in mind: someone who already exercises at least a few days per week but suffers from joint pain and is frustrated by their results. If this describes you, you can jump right into the four days per week training plan. However, if you are not currently doing resistance training at least three days per week, you should spend some time training with weights on two nonconsecutive days per week. If you currently do no weight training, here's how I suggest you ramp up to four days per week:

- **Step 1: Full body weight training: 2 nonconsecutive days per week**—follow for 4 to 8 weeks, then progress to 3 days per week.

- **Step 2: Full body weight training: 3 nonconsecutive days per week**—follow for 4 to 8 weeks, then progress to 4 days per week.

- **Step 3: Weight training 4 days per week** (alternate between upper and lower body strength training days)—follow for 8 weeks, then assess progress, joint health, injury status, etc.

While the exact numbers vary in studies, we know that injury risk skyrockets when your exercise volume jumps up too fast—so be disciplined with how you ramp up exercise frequency.[273]

Keep Moving Between Sessions

Although you will only be doing structured resistance training four days per week, this doesn't mean you are sedentary on the other three days. Like we covered in the chapters on movement and mobility, even your "off" days from working out should be filled with varied movement.

Walking and bicycling are great ways to facilitate circulation and healing in the lower body between resistance training sessions. Swimming is a joint-friendly full-body workout and is especially beneficial for shoulder health. One or two yoga sessions per week between weight training will do wonders for recovery and mobility. Even activities like golf and tennis that you might think of as causing wear and tear can further support your fitness efforts. The opposite is also true—your efforts in the gym will enhance your performance in everyday life. They build on each other, creating a virtuous cycle that allows you to use your body to full potential.

Swimming and Shoulder Health

Swimming is one the most effective full-body active recovery techniques—especially for chronically painful shoulders. It isn't load bearing, so joint stress is minimal. The movements train shoulder stabilization with arms extended and preferentially challenge moving from shoulder protraction to retraction. This provides a nice counter-training effect against all the pressing and slouching you do throughout the week. To prevent repetitive-use injuries from swimming, start with only a couple days per week if you aren't accustomed to it. Keep intensity and volume low—not more than 15–20 minutes at a time. Also, vary your stroke technique to avoid irritating joints. If swimming on consecutive days, focus on the backstroke one day, the breaststroke the next, sidestroke the following day, etc. If you only swim once or twice per week, alternate between these movements every few minutes.

My go-to, joint-friendly stroke for moving through the water effectively without stressing my shoulders is the *sidestroke*. I'm no swimming expert, so I won't pretend to be. But I highly recommend looking up tutorials on the "sidestroke" and "combat sidestroke" (a variation developed by the Navy SEALs). These strokes focus on one side of your body at a time, which allows you to swim continuously while reducing joint stress on each shoulder.

Exercise Selection and Progression

Most fitness authorities recommend performing big, difficult exercises first and accessory work afterward. While this has merit for producing maximum short-term strength gains, it really depends on your goals. If you have weak points that need addressing, you should activate those muscles first. If you need to improve form and control, you should perform exercises that challenge neuromuscular coordination early in the training session. You'll notice that each workout in the next chapter is centered around one or two compound movements per joint system, with accessory work strategically layered in. Perform each exercise in the order listed to optimally mobilize, activate, and strengthen.

As your movement skill and strength increase, you will need to increase the load to continue progressing. If you find an exercise becomes too easy, and you're able to complete all the prescribed repetitions, then increase the weight by 10%–20%. If you cannot complete all the repetitions at a given weight, then drop the weight down until you can at least complete the first set of prescribed repetitions. Here's an example:

If on the Single Arm Dumbbell Row you can complete all three prescribed sets of eight reps with a 70-pound dumbbell, it's time to jump to the 75 or 80 pounders. If you find that you are not able to complete the first set of the prescribed eight repetitions with 80 pounds, then drop back down to 75 pounds. Once you can complete all three sets of eight repetitions, it's time to increase the weight again.

Training with Tendinopathy

I hope the chapters on tendinopathy and collagen synthesis gave you a deep enough understanding of tissue repair processes to modulate your own training schedule as needed. But with so many treatment options and specialized therapies, it's difficult to determine the right course of action. If you work with a physical therapist to heal tendinopathy, they will take you through various isometric exercises, mobility drills, manual therapies, and load management techniques. Highly technical stuff catered to your symptoms and progress. If you have access to a good therapist and your symptoms are severe, I certainly recommend going this route. But there is one training strategy that I've found works better than anything else. It's simple and brutally effective: build tendon strength in your injured body part that far surpasses any reasonable loads you expect to encounter in your life. In practical terms, here's what that means.

Instead of avoiding the exercises that cause tendon pain, face them head-on (after a brief period of unloading that allows inflammation to subside naturally). Pick one or two movements that you can progress in resistance with over time and slowly build your load tolerance. You might have to start with extremely light weights and slow repetitions to avoid aggravating the tendon. Choose the heaviest weight you can lift for several repetitions without triggering a pain response above 3 out of 10 on the pain scale. You might find that you can only lift the bar, or small weights, without increased pain. That's OK. Start there, and slowly, patiently build strength until your tendon can handle much more than it will be tasked with during your normal training sessions and life. You have to be careful, though, because you can't push your tendon to the brink of maladaptation with targeted exercise, then do other stressful movements on top of that. So, it's a combination of focused training to trigger adaptations, removing repetitive motions that cause pain, and avoiding unnecessary aggravation with too much training volume.

The exercise program recommended in the next few sections of this book incorporates movements that challenge every muscle and joint system in your body. You may find that one or two exercises cause a nagging tendon to flare up. In that case, after you have ruled out other injuries or structural problems, back off the weight and slow the repetitions way down. Work on increasing the resistance week after week, as long as your pain scores stay at or below 3 after each session (and you are able to recover fully before the next session). A 3 out of 10 indicates a positive tendon adaptation that should resolve in a few days with rest. Pain level above 3 out of 10 means you are at risk of going back into disrepair and degeneration.

Here are some of the exercises featured in the training program that you can use as therapeutic tendinopathy recovery aids. (Refer to chapter 11, "Mastering the Movements," for detailed instructions on the exercises.) In all cases, focus on building strength through the midrange of motion first. Extreme stretching and end range of motion movements, especially early in the injury recovery process, are more likely to cause flare-ups:

1. Achilles tendinopathy (pain on back of ankle): **Standing Calf Raises**

2. Patellar tendinopathy (pain in patellar tendon, just below kneecap): **Goblet Squat**

3. Medial elbow tendinopathy, a.k.a. golfer's elbow (pain on inside of elbow, just below elbow joint): **Alternating Dumbbell Curls**

4. Lateral elbow tendinopathy, a.k.a. tennis elbow (pain on outside of elbow, just below elbow joint): **Zottman Curl**

5. Bicep tendinopathy (pain near intersection of your upper arm bone and front of shoulder): **Dumbbell Fly Press**

6. Tricep tendinopathy (pain in lower tricep region, near where tendon inserts into elbow): **Bottoms-Up Kettlebell Press**

7. Shoulder tendinopathy (pain in the interior of shoulder): **Cable Facepull**

EXERCISE LIMITATIONS

The program that follows consists of exercises that are either joint friendly or designed to challenge commonly weak areas with light loads. Still, you may find you are simply unable to perform some of the movements if you have a pre-existing condition or injury. If this happens, find a pain-free alternative and move on. If you must modify an exercise initially, you'll more than likely build the necessary stability and mobility by the end of the program to perform that movement pain-free. One step back, two steps forward.

SETS, REPS, AND REST SCHEMES

The optimal rep ranges for hypertrophy range from 8 to 12 per set. For pure strength, it's closer to 5 repetitions per set. For endurance, sets of 15 to 20 are optimal.[4,274] You will be utilizing a mix of rep ranges based on accomplishing these goals, along with building connective tissue resilience.

Some of these repetition progressions resemble intensive physical therapy programs, where you are drilling a movement over and over with high repetition sets to retrain motor patterns, wake up latent muscles, and repair joints. In my opinion, this type of high-repetition training is more difficult than using heavier weights and fewer reps. But it's necessary. Other repetition schemes in the program more closely resemble traditional weightlifting based on increased intensity and decreased volume, with the occasional deload. The literature on training volume, reps, intensity, etc. helpfully points us in the right direction, but it should not be taken as gospel for accomplishing your goals. For example, even though endurance may not be your primary goal, training with higher repetition sets allows you to get more practice perfecting the movement. And when implemented correctly, these workouts will trigger a massive metabolic and muscle growth response. Especially in the early phases, don't get too caught up in how much weight you are moving or what percentage of your one-repetition maximum you're using. Instead, challenge yourself with loads that match the repetition suggestions while still maintaining proper movement form. The last thing you want to do is sacrifice quality for quantity.

Optimal rest periods also vary by training goal. For strength, studies show resting up to three minutes between sets optimizes adaptations. For hypertrophy, resting 60–90 seconds between sets is best. Still, other research shows that even shorter rest periods of 30–60 seconds create a greater hormonal response—increased growth hormone release and metabolic rate changes.[275] For the sake of time management, I'm a big fan of keeping rest periods as short as possible without sacrificing movement quality. It keeps you engaged in the workout and allows you to get more work done in less time. Even though the workouts suggested in the next chapter consist of only five or six exercises, you could easily draw the session out to 1.5 or 2 hours if you drag your feet. Don't let this happen. Throughout this program, rest one to two minutes between sets. This is long enough to catch your breath and let your muscles recharge. If you're like me, you'll find that shorter rest periods keep the workout interesting, keep your mind engaged, and produce better results.

REP SPEED/TEMPO

Recommended tempos will be indicated in this format: 3131. This means a 3-second eccentric phase, 1-second hold at the bottom of the movement, 3-second concentric phase, and 1-second hold at the top of the movement. If you are new to using slower repetition speeds, start out by performing movements in front of a clock and watching the second hand move. Count to yourself along with the clock until you get an accurate sense of counting in your head. It sounds silly, but everyone subconsciously speeds up their count when the exercise gets difficult.

As you get further into the program, you can let up on the micromanagement of rep speed and let intuition take a more active role. Even if you aren't perfect in your repetition timing, you'll still accomplish the exercise's goal if you remember the purpose of the rep speed. For three- to five-second repetition speeds, the most important concept is controlling the weight through each degree of motion. For one-second rep speeds, you don't have to worry about completing the movement in exactly one second. Instead, work on moving the weight deliberately and quickly while still maintaining control. And remember that you're always better off going too slow than too fast.

HOW TO WARM UP

Fitness dogma dictates that you spend 5–10 minutes "warming up" before doing any real exercise. Typically, this involves slogging along on the treadmill, riding an elliptical machine, or half-heartedly yanking on your joints to limber up followed by several lightweight sets of whatever exercise you're doing in the gym that day. There are several problems with this approach. First, it's boring. I avoid machines like the plague because I simply don't like them. And I offer the same courtesy to any clients I work with because I don't want them to hate working out either. Second, there are much more effective ways to warm your body up for exercise and prime your central nervous system for performance. Third, studies show *less is more* when it comes to warming up. According to a study published in the *Journal of Applied Physiology*, the "standard warm-up causes fatigue and less warm-up permits greater…power output" (for cyclists in the case of this study).[276]

Instead of the traditional warm-up, I propose performing a short (~5–10 minutes) series of dynamic stretches, light resistance exercises, and skill-based movements. This is referred to as a *dynamic warm-up*. In addition to utilizing dynamic stretching to improve mobility, it also more effectively primes your central nervous system for exercise. Although an effective dynamic warm-up will raise your core temperature (the primary goal of the old-school warm-up), it's equally valuable for improving movement patterns. The skill-based aspect keeps your mind engaged. It's rewarding to see yourself becoming more proficient at executing body-weight movements from week to week. And you'll quickly see the carryover into your main weight training lifts. One of the most important reasons to use a dynamic warm-up is the least talked about—it serves as a diagnostic ritual to see what is going on with your body that day. What joints are extra stiff, what muscles are tight, and what movement patterns just aren't working. This awareness allows you to address any potential problems early, which can prevent a minor tweak from developing into a full-blown injury.

If you work out early in the morning, or you find your body feels better after a few minutes of steady-state exercise to raise your heart rate, then by all means go for it. Walking, jogging, riding a stationary bike—they're all perfectly acceptable if you have the time and energy. But keep it short. No more than five minutes. Instead, lean on the dynamic warm-up to prepare your mind and body for training. Your heart rate will speed up, your core temperature will increase, and your central nervous system will stand at attention—all without draining your energy and wasting time.

The second component of warming up is preparing your body for specific movements. I cringe when I see someone walk into the gym, crawl under the bench press, and start banging out heavy reps. They are playing Russian roulette with their shoulders. Not to mention, shortchanging themselves on strength. On the opposite end of the spectrum, some people warm up too much, performing set after set of light movements before getting to their working sets. This not only causes fatigue; it causes the workout to drag on much longer than necessary, leading to poor program adherence and half-hearted training intensity. Instead of following either of these common paths, use what Dr. John Rusin calls *ramp-up* sets.

RAMP-UP SETS

John Rusin is a doctor of physical therapy and renowned strength coach. In the fitness industry, he's known as the go-to guy for elite performers suffering from pain. In addition to working with athletes in the NFL, MLB,

CrossFit Games, and IFBB professional bodybuilders, he also founded the Pain-Free Performance Specialist Certification (PPSC). This advanced certification teaches trainers and strength coaches how to help their clients avoid injuries.

In addition to incorporating a dynamic warm-up before each training session, Rusin recommends following a streamlined ramp-up approach. For compound lifts like the barbell squat, deadlift, and bench press he recommends the following:[277]

- **Ramp-Up Set 1**—50% of the working load for the prescribed number of working reps
- **Ramp-Up Set 2**—75% of the working load for half the reps in the working sets
- **Ramp-Up Set 3**—110% of the working load for one single rep (explosively)
- Working Sets (the actual training)—Perform the prescribed sets, reps, and load suggestions.

What's markedly different about this approach is that it relies on fewer reps and explosive, full-intensity movements to prime your body. The final ramp-up set uses a heavier weight than your working set—but only for one repetition—which makes your working sets feel lighter and increases strength. This is a brilliant way to leverage *postactivation potentiation*—where your muscles heighten contraction efficiency after they experience a brief maximum voluntary contraction.[278]

Move through the ramp-up sets at a brisk pace, pausing just long enough to change the weights and catch your breath. After completing all the ramp-up sets, take a short break (1–2 minutes maximum) until you feel fully recovered but still primed for movement. Then, dig straight into the prescribed working sets. The only modification I will occasionally make to the ramp-up scheme is adding an initial set of 20–25 reps with little to no resistance—often just using the bar or 5- to 10-pound dumbbells. For stiff joints or problem areas, this helps increase blood flow and synovial fluid circulation for better joint lubrication. The key is to use a weight that doesn't fatigue your muscles too much. Ramp-up sets are more important for compound movements early in your exercise routine, and less important for accessory work later in the routine when you're already warm. If your muscles are ready to go, keep ramp-up sets to a minimum.

AN EVEN SIMPLER WAY TO WARM UP

If following a ramp-up set scheme seems like too much math and micro-management, do this instead:

- **Ramp-Up Set #1**—Before each working set, grab a weight you think you can lift at least 15 times. Perform 10 smooth, controlled repetitions with this weight. Rest just long enough to catch your breath.

- **Ramp-Up Set #2**—Grab a weight you can lift at least 10 times. Perform 5 repetitions. Catch your breath.

- **Ramp-Up Set #3**—Choose a weight that is 10%–20% heavier than you plan on using for your working sets. Perform 1–2 repetitions just to get a feel for it. This will often show you that you can lift much more (or less) than you thought, allowing you to choose an appropriate weight more effectively.

Most seasoned lifters (besides competitive powerlifters and arithmetic junkies) use an intuitive ramp-up scheme like this one. The more you get comfortable with a specific exercise, the less time and energy you will have to spend figuring out how to choose your weights.

WHAT ABOUT FOAM ROLLING?

As mentioned earlier in the book, studies show self-myofascial release techniques such as foam rolling can help increase flexibility, reduce joint pain, and improve recovery.[212] I often use and recommend foam rolling during the warm-up phase for tight muscles. For muscles surrounding injured joints that you can't safely stretch, manual therapy is a great way to loosen up without aggravating the damaged joint. But in my opinion, it feels good more than it is an effective healing agent. That's why it isn't programmed into the training schedule.

If foam rolling helps, keep doing it. If you want to try it for loosening up sore muscles, go for it! Spend a few minutes (limit yourself to five) targeting stiff, sore muscles either before or after training (and don't hammer on already sore tendons and ligaments). If you have a joint injury you are recovering from, I suggest spending a few minutes targeting the muscles above and below the joint before your rehabilitative routine. Foam rolling can be an effective supplement to a corrective exercise routine, but don't expect it to be a magic bullet. Your primary therapeutic tools will always be load training and dynamic movements that take you through full ranges of motion.

CHAPTER 11

Mastering the Movements

Mastery requires both impatience and patience. The impatience
to have a bias toward action, to not waste time, and to work with
a sense of urgency each day. The patience to delay gratification,
to wait for your actions to accumulate, and to trust the process.

— James Clear, author of *Atomic Habits*

This chapter provides an exercise database with instructions for all movements in the training program. There is an infinite number of exercises you can use to optimize your body. You can and should explore more than those listed here. But for the sake of simplicity, I recommend sticking to these movements exclusively while following the program. These exercises were hand-picked for their overall effectiveness and their ability to address the most common muscle imbalances. For reference purposes, I've categorized each exercise into primary movement sections.

Keep in mind that these are not isolation movements for specific muscles. Virtually all train multiple muscle groups at once. For example, the Facepull is technically an upper body pull exercise, but the intent of the movement is to prime your shoulders for lifting and correct imbalances, so it's listed in the shoulder stability section.

The sections are divided as follows so you can easily find exercises by type:

- Mobility, Core, and Dynamic Warm-up
- Shoulder Stability
- Upper Body Push
- Upper Body Pull
- Upper Body Accessory Work
- Squat/Knee Dominant Movements
- Hinge/Hip Dominant Movements
- Lower Body Accessory Work

EQUIPMENT AND GYM ACCESS

These exercises were hand-picked based on the assumption that you can access exercise equipment available at most gyms. While this program can be completed with minimal equipment when you use modifications, there's no doubt that having access to barbells, cable machines, dumbbells, and various benches gives you an advantage. However, you never know when you'll lose access to your gym, have to work out from home, or need to travel without all the equipment you are used to. So, for each exercise I've included acceptable alternatives and modifications that will allow you to train with minimal equipment if necessary.

This isn't an exhaustive list, but here is what I recommend you have access to:

- Barbell and weights
- Dumbbells
- Kettlebells
- Adjustable workout bench
- Pull-up bar
- Jump box or low, solid stool
- Swiss ball (a.k.a. Physioball)
- Cable pulley machine
- TRX Suspension Trainer system or other strap-based suspension device
- Accessories: Most gyms carry versions of these—but you should have your own:
  - ▶ **Exercise band set:** Get yourself a set of exercise bands that range from light to heavy (a set of four bands ranging from ~15 pounds of resistance to ~125+ pounds will be plenty). I prefer the thick, flat, looped resistance bands instead of the cylindrical ones for heavy-loaded exercises (they don't snap as easily). For light exercises, a set of cylindrical bands with handles will come in handy. You can find band sets by searching for "pull-up assistance bands" and "elastic resistance bands." Some brands with quality sets include Crossover Symmetry, Theraband, Elite FTS, WODFitters, Intey, Power Guidance, and Draper's Strength.
  - ▶ **Hip band (glute band):** The hip band is a thick, high-resistance loop about 14 to 16 inches wide when folded. This little band is worth its weight in gold and is unmatched for activating the often-neglected hip abductors and glutes. Some quality brands of hip bands include Mark Bell's Sling Shot, Crossover Symmetry, ProFitness, Gymshark, Hurdilen, and Untold Performance.

▸ **Stopwatch:** For tracking rest periods and rep speeds. Use one you don't mind roughing up a bit.

And here's a minimalist list of equipment you can use for at-home or travel workouts. While there are some great body-weight programs and exercises you can use for on-the-go workouts, having access to these resistance tools will enable you to challenge your muscles and connective tissues in ways that body-weight moves simply cannot.

With these tools, you can accomplish most of the exercises I recommend with challenging loads:

- **Exercise band set** (set of four resistance levels)
- **Hip band**
- **1–2 light kettlebells:** Light enough that you can press the kettlebell over your head with one arm for 10+ repetitions.
- **1–2 heavy kettlebells:** Heavy enough that pressing over your head with one arm more than 4–5 times is not possible, but light enough that you can get the weight into the goblet position (held with both arms in front of your chest).
- **Set of (2) light dumbbells:** Light enough that you can perform at least 15 repetitions of overhead presses.
- **Sturdy box, chair, or stool**
- **Stopwatch**

With some creativity, you can substitute dumbbells for kettlebells and vice versa. Resistance bands can be substituted for weights with some movements, but this is not ideal. Traditional weights provide load through the entire range of motion while resistance bands only challenge you toward the end of the movement when they are fully stretched. Resistance bands are great for strategically challenging end ranges of motion and joint stabilization but are not the best option for load training.

If your budget and living space allow it, having a portable pull-up bar and suspension straps (like the TRX Suspension Trainer) gives you even more options. Word of caution: Doorway-anchored pull-up bars are dangerous. If you go this route, make sure you properly install the bar and use a sturdy door frame. I've broken enough doorway trim, so I don't use these anymore. You're better off getting an actual steel pipe or bar that can be professionally installed in your home for safety or doing what I do when in a pinch—find a sturdy tree limb.

SUPPORTIVE EQUIPMENT, BRACES, AND WRAPS

Weightlifting belts, braces, wraps, and sleeves should only be used for two reasons: (1) to provide extra joint stability on heavy (near maximum) lifts or (2) to guard a pre-existing injury. One notable exception is wrist wraps used for gripping barbells on movements like the deadlift, where your grip is often the weakest link. But like any supportive device, it can become a crutch. Use sparingly if at all.

Try to use the minimum amount of supportive equipment. This program is about shoring up weak links throughout your body. By wearing a heavyweight belt or wrapping up your knees, you are defeating the purpose of the corrective exercises. I'm not asking you to do anything that hurts. But the truth is, if you can't do an exercise without being wrapped up like a mummy, you shouldn't be doing it. At least not with heavy loads.

Another common piece of equipment worth mentioning is your shoes. For weightlifting and skill-based training that doesn't involve running, your best bet is to wear cross-trainers or minimalist shoes with a low profile and thinner sole. Virtually any exercise-intended shoe will work. Just stay away from high-top basketball shoes with high ankle support (unless you need it to protect a pre-existing injury), and avoid overly cushioned running shoes. The more cushion between your foot and the floor, the more force you lose during movements. Heavily cushioned shoes also destabilize your knees when performing lower body load training. Reebok and Nike are two popular brands that make shoes specifically for exercise without too much cushion. The old Converse "Chuck Taylor" model shoes are still popular among weightlifters because they provide a flat, solid base with minimal cushion.

If you have not worn minimalist shoes without cushy soles before, start slow and easy. Ankles and feet are commonly injured when people start using minimalist shoes without letting their feet acclimate (usually during the first 10–12 weeks after switching from more supportive shoes).[279]

If you have any doubts about shoes, equipment, or other devices and how you might be affected, check with your doctor or physical therapist first. There is no shame in using tools that allow you to exercise pain-free, as long as you aren't using them as crutches to avoid addressing underlying muscle imbalances.

WHAT'S MISSING?

A few exercises are conspicuously missing from my list: the barbell bench press, the barbell squat, and the barbell deadlift. These are arguably the three most productive resistance exercises you can do for building muscle and strength. I have nothing against them and believe they should be fundamental parts of strength training programs for people without pre-existing back, knee, or shoulder issues. But the truth is that these three exercises are responsible for the lion's share of workout-related aches and pains.

Many people lack the core strength, mobility, and training to perform these exercises under heavy loads. Even if you're not one of those people—and these barbell moves are your go-to exercises—I challenge you to step away from them for a few weeks. Challenge your squat, hinge, and pressing capabilities in different ways. Exercises like the Romanian Deadlift, Spanish Squat, and Bulgarian Split Squat will wake up muscles you didn't know were there. If you do return to heavy barbell training after completing this program, I'm confident that your movements will be cleaner and your base stronger than before.

You'll also notice that supersets, giant sets, rest-pause sets, and other variations on exercise timing aren't used often in this program. While these methods can effectively increase intensity, you'll be better served to focus on executing the exercises in order, one at a time, to the best of your ability. This will ultimately lead to more rapid progress as you master the exercises and increase load volumes.

LOWER BODY
Supine Drawing In

The purpose of the Supine Drawing In exercise is to establish a mind-muscle connection with your transverse abdominis muscle (TVA) and other deep layer muscles of the core.

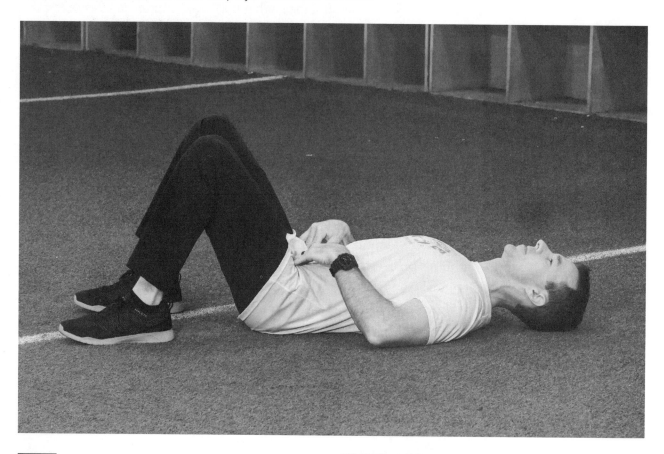

SETUP

Lie on your back with your knees bent and feet comfortably planted on the ground. Place the fingers of both hands on your waistline, just inside the bony protrusions of your hips on each side.

EXECUTION

Take a deep breath and slowly exhale all the air from your lungs. At the end of your breath out, brace your stomach as if you were about to get punched. Then, further activate your TVA by drawing your belly button inward as if you were trying to touch it to your spine. Hold this position for a few moments, then release the contraction and take a breath in. Complete 10 total repetitions before heavy lifting workouts.

COMMON MISTAKES

- Not bracing hard enough to activate all the other muscles of your core besides the TVA.
- Moving through the repetitions too fast without holding the peak contraction.

CUES

Brace your stomach like you're about to get punched, then pull your belly button to your spine.

VARIATIONS

Once you are comfortable with the supine version, you can increase the difficulty and intensity by moving to a kneeling position or standing position with one leg lifted off the ground (the latter being the most difficult).

LOWER BODY
Bird Dog

The Bird Dog is an excellent tool for teaching stability through your entire posterior chain and improving low back endurance. When not performed correctly, it's a waste of time. The key is to keep your core and upper back braced forcefully, nonstop, through the entire movement.

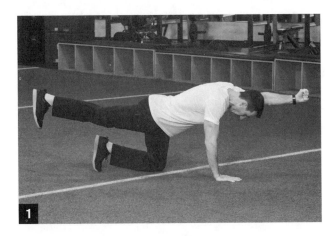

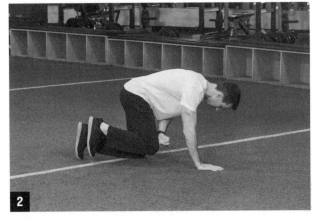

SETUP

Get into the quadruped position (hands and knees on floor—shoulders directly over wrists, knees directly under hips). Activate your TVA by drawing your naval inward. Make sure your lumbar spine is neutral. Next, flex your glutes. You should have tension throughout your entire pelvic region at this point.

EXECUTION

Bring one hand into a tightly clenched fist and extend your arm outward in front you without arching your upper back. Keep the thumb side of your hand facing the ceiling. Keep your gaze on the ground in front of you with your chin tucked. Extend the opposite leg out away from your body. Do NOT raise your leg up—push it straight out as far as you can without causing your hip to drop backward. Activate your glute muscle on that leg hard. Mentally scan your posture to ensure your body is in a straight line. This completes a repetition on one side of your body. Complete all repetitions on one side of your body before moving to the opposite side. TIP: Check your posture periodically through different segments of the movement by positioning yourself sideways next to a mirror.

CUES

Neutral spine, brace hard, arm straight out, leg straight out.

COMMON MISTAKES

- Overarching your lumbar spine during extension and rounding your back during flexion.
- Raising your arm too far up toward the ceiling, creating a compensating arch in the upper back and low back.
- Letting your core muscles relax after each repetition.
- Not bracing your core and upper back strongly enough to create full-body stability.
- Moving too quickly through the motion and losing dynamic posture quality.

LOWER BODY

Cossack Squat

The Cossack Squat is a multitasking mobility exercise for the hips, hamstrings, and ankles. When performed while holding a weight, it becomes an effective strength-building move.

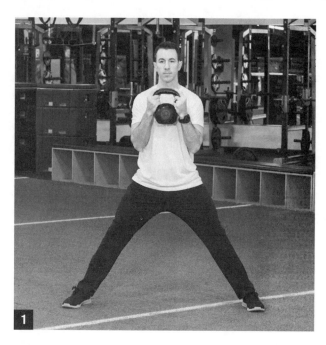

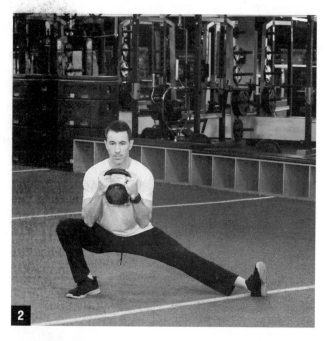

SETUP

Start with only your body weight until you have developed enough range of motion, strength, and comfort to use increased loads safely. To set up the move, stand with your feet spread wide and toes pointed out slightly.

EXECUTION

Shift your body weight onto one leg by bending at the knee, keeping your upper body as upright as you can. Continue moving into the stretched position until your groin and hamstring flexibility limits you or you start to lose posture in your back. Then, reverse the motion and return to the starting position with your body weight balanced on both legs. You can immediately perform another repetition on the opposite leg or complete a set of consecutive reps on one leg before switching.

CUES

Neutral spine, active feet, side lunge, then push with your glutes.

COMMON MISTAKES

- Letting your upper back round during the lowering phase.
- Failing to widen your stance enough in the starting position.
- Moving too fast or progressing too quickly, putting the groin and hamstring at risk.

VARIATIONS

If you have trouble maintaining your balance, or want to focus on safely getting into a fully stretched position, you can start with hands placed on the floor in front of you for balance.

Once you are comfortable with the Cossack Squat, you can further challenge the movement by increasing the width of your stance in the starting position and rotating your extended leg onto the heel of your foot. This increases the mobility demands on the hips, groin, hamstrings, and ankles.

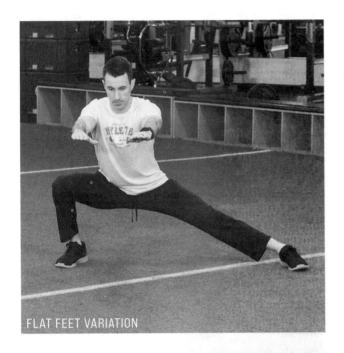

FLAT FEET VARIATION

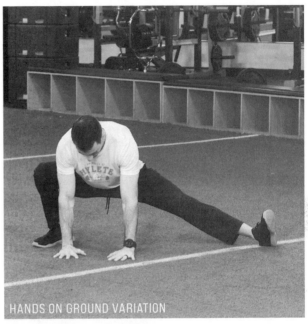

HANDS ON GROUND VARIATION

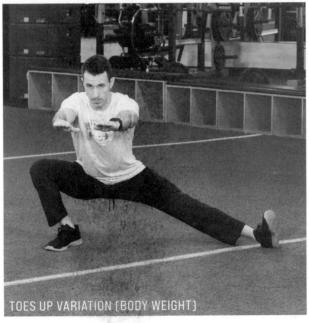

TOES UP VARIATION (BODY WEIGHT)

LOWER BODY
Glute Bridge

The reason your glutes aren't doing their job might be the fault of tight hip flexors, which shut off glute activation and overwork the low back and hamstrings. This exercise both mobilizes the hip flexors and activates the glutes and hamstrings. This should be a staple in your warm-up routine before lower body training. It can also be loaded with resistance to build strength, muscle, and power in your posterior chain.

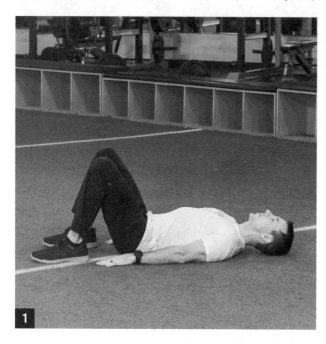

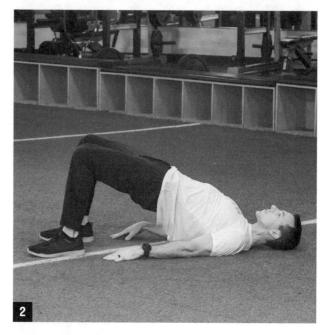

SETUP

Lie on your back with hands at your sides, knees bent, and feet planted firmly on the floor.

EXECUTION

Brace your core, contract your glutes, and push your feet down into the floor to raise your hips off the ground. Continue raising your hips until your upper body and thighs are in a straight line. Hold at the top of the movement and contract the glutes again to ensure peak muscle tension, then slowly lower your hips to the ground.

CUES

Squeeze your glutes and push through your heels.

COMMON MISTAKES

- Unstable footing.
- Craning your neck upward instead of keeping the back of your head on the ground.
- Moving too quickly and not fully contracting your glutes at the top of the movement.
- Arching the low back instead of using your glutes to drive the movement.

VARIATIONS

- **Glute Bridge with Hip Band:** Place a hip band around both legs, just above the knees, to intensify the contraction and activate the hip abductor muscles.
- **Glute Bridge with Groin Squeeze:** Squeeze a medicine ball or other soccer-ball sized tool between your legs during the movement to activate the groin muscles.
- **Single Leg Glute Bridge:** Perform the glute bridge with one leg lifted off the ground and knee extended. This increases the difficulty and adds an element of antirotation training for core stability.

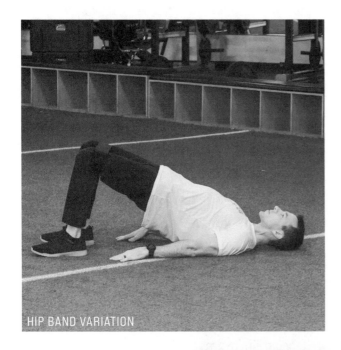

HIP BAND VARIATION

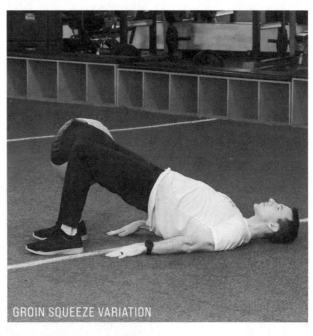

GROIN SQUEEZE VARIATION

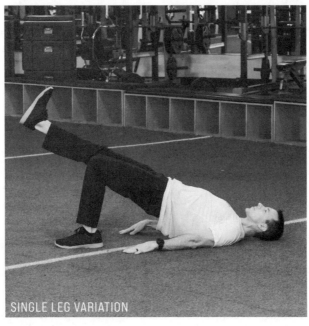

SINGLE LEG VARIATION

LOWER BODY

Fire Hydrant

The Fire Hydrant (a.k.a. hip abduction from quadruped position) is simple and effective for improving hip abduction function and activating the glutes. It's a favorite prehab exercise among powerlifters and is easy enough for any novice to employ successfully.

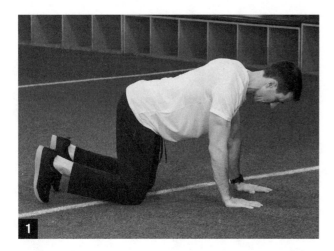

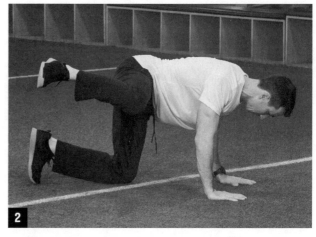

SETUP

Assume the quadruped position (on hands and knees). Brace your core and tuck your chin, looking at the ground.

EXECUTION

While keeping the rest of your body as still and braced as possible, open your hip on one side of your body, raising your thigh as high as you can without falling out of alignment. Maintain a consistent knee angle throughout the movement. Contract your glutes and the muscles on the outside of your hip at the top of the movement, holding briefly before slowly lowering your leg back to the ground. Complete all reps on one side of your body before moving to the opposite.

CUES

Neutral spine, knee bent, hip straight out to the side.

COMMON MISTAKES

- Twisting your low back and core instead of keeping it rigid and braced.
- Using momentum to swing your leg up instead of slowly contracting the hip abductors.
- Overarching or rounding your low back.
- Creating a fault in your cervical spine by looking up (not tucking chin).

VARIATIONS

If you can easily perform 25 repetitions on each leg without feeling fatigue, it's time to increase the difficulty. Here are two options:

- **Standing Fire Hydrant:** Perform the exercise from a single leg standing position, holding on to a bench or wall to assist you in staying balanced.
- **Banded Fire Hydrant** (not pictured): Perform the exercise with a hip band looped around both legs, just above or below the knees. This will shorten the range of motion but intensify the contraction and abductor activation.

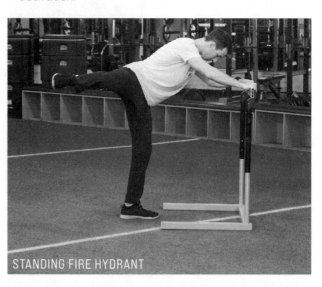

STANDING FIRE HYDRANT

LOWER BODY

Pigeon Stretch

The Pigeon Stretch, an exercise borrowed from yoga, is one of the most effective hip opening static stretches when performed correctly. When performed incorrectly, it places stress on the low back and knees. Make this part of your weekly routine and you'll see improvements in squat and hinge-based movements.

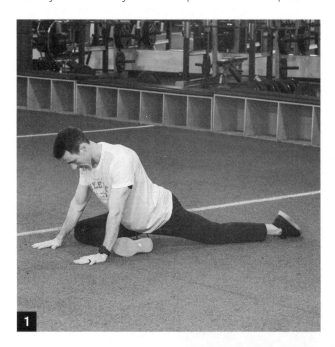

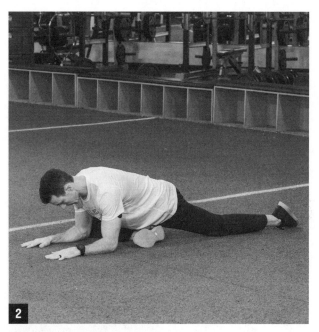

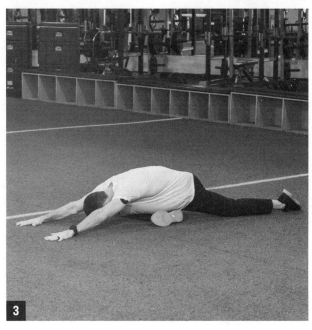

Continued on next page

SETUP

Assume a lunge position with your left leg forward and right leg extended behind you.

EXECUTION

Slide your right leg backward, lowering your body to the ground as far as your hips will comfortably allow you. Lower your hands to the ground for support on each side of your body. From there, slowly allow your left knee to fall away from your body. Ideally, your knee will remain at a 90 degree angle as your leg folds all the way down to the ground. Keeping your low back in alignment, gently lean forward with the assistance of your hands until you feel a stretch in the outside of your left hip. Repeat on the opposite side.

CUES

Lunge, fold open front hip, lean forward.

COMMON MISTAKES

- Rounding the low back and thoracic spine.
- Attempting a more aggressive stretch than your hips and knees are prepared for.

VARIATIONS

To make the exercise easier, use a block or rolled up towel under the bent knee to take pressure off your hip joint.

SUBSTITUTES

Thread the Needle: If you don't feel like you can safely perform the Pigeon Stretch, opt for the Thread the Needle exercise from the supine position. To perform Thread the Needle, lie on your back and cross one leg over the other, forming a 90-degree angle with your knee. Gently pull both legs toward your body, keeping your low back posture in check, until you feel a stretch in the outside hip of your bent leg.

BLOCK UNDER KNEE VARIATION

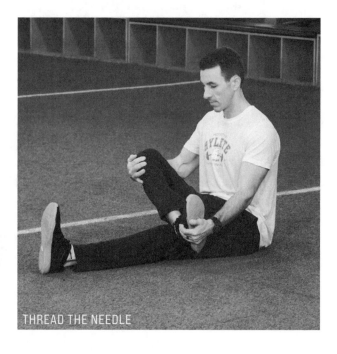

THREAD THE NEEDLE

LOWER BODY
Cat-Cow

Though the low back is primarily designed for stability, the Cat-Cow effectively loosens up tight back muscles. This is a great exercise to perform as a warm-up before training lower body movements or working out with a stiff, sore low back.

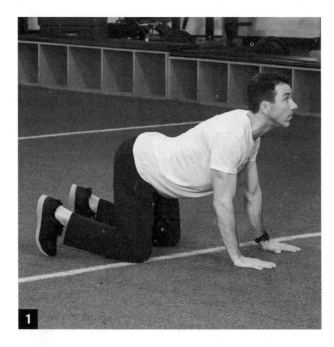

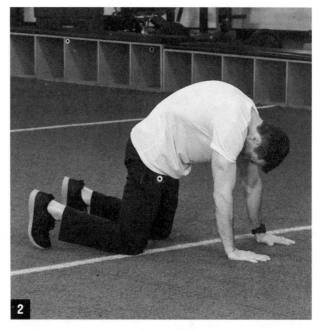

SETUP

Assume the quadruped position with your hands directly below your shoulders.

EXECUTION

(the Cow) Let your belly fall downward as your low back arches. Roll your shoulders back and down and lift your gaze to the ceiling as you gently extend your neck upward. Take a deep breath inward as you move through this phase.

(the Cat) To execute the Cat phase of Cat-Cow, you will reverse the Cow movement described above. Lift your rib cage toward the ceiling, drawing your naval inward to activate your TVA. Push your hands down through the floor, letting your shoulders move into a protracted position with your upper back rounded (this is one time when upper back rounding is OK). Lower your gaze to the ground slowly, gently bending your neck until you are looking at your belly button. During the Cat phase of the exercise, release your breath outward.

As you become more comfortable with the movement, practice synchronizing your breath with each repetition.

CUES

Arch and look up, then round and look down.

COMMON MISTAKES

- Forgetting to roll your shoulders back and down during the Cow phase.
- Forgetting to round your upper back during the Cat phase.
- Moving too quickly through the movement.
- Failing to match breath with movement.

LOWER BODY
Hinge to Squat

The Hinge to Squat is one of my favorite lower body mobility exercises for three reasons: (1) it trains solid foot position in a way that translates well to lower body exercises, (2) it teaches dominant hip squatting, and (3) it illustrates how the squat and hinge are not necessarily separate, but different points on the same spectrum of lower body movement. More hip angle and less knee angle creates a hinge. More knee angle and less hip angle creates a squat. Practicing the transition from hinge to squat will make you better at both, while also mobilizing your posterior chain and hip flexors.

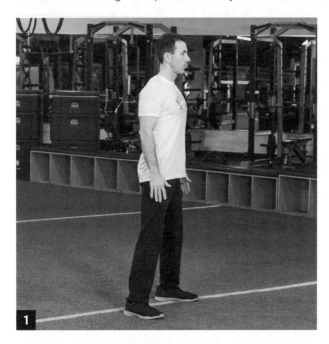

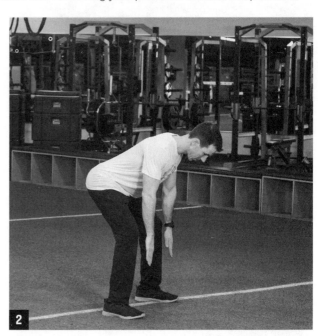

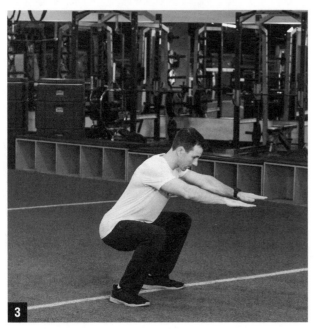

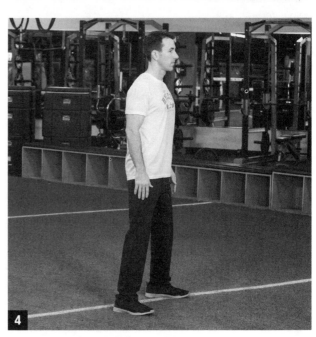

SETUP

Begin in a standing position with feet shoulder-width apart.

EXECUTION

Push your butt backward and hinge toward the ground (while maintaining a neutral spine from your low back to the crown of your head). Stop when you feel tension in your hamstrings. From there, keep your weight back and sink your butt into the bottom position of a squat. Think about pulling yourself into the squat position with your hamstrings. Stand back up to complete one repetition.

CUES

Hinge, pull into squat, stand up.

COMMON MISTAKES

- Rounding your low back.
- Rocking forward onto your toes during the transition from hinge to squat instead of keeping your weight back.
- Pushing your knees forward during the transition and losing tension in your posterior chain.

VARIATIONS

If you have trouble going from hinge to squat, try widening your stance and pointing your toes out slightly.

LOWER BODY

World's Greatest Stretch

If I could only do one mobility exercise for the rest of my life, it would be the World's Greatest Stretch. It's a brilliant move because it mobilizes two of the most common hypertonic body parts (the thoracic spine and hips) and forces cooperation between your upper and lower body.

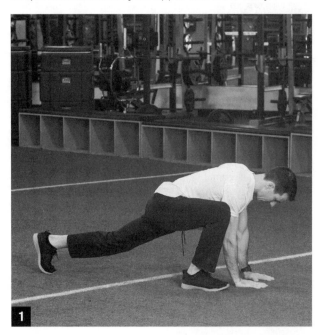

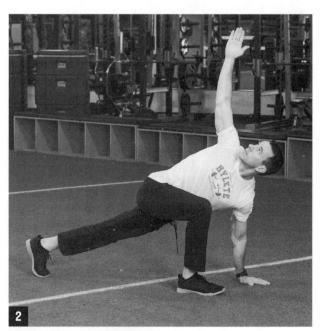

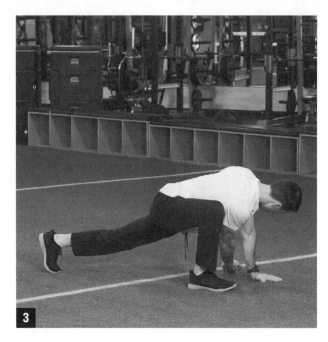

SETUP

From a lunge position with your right leg extended behind you, lower your hands to the ground with extended arms. Straighten your right knee.

EXECUTION

Shift your upper body weight into your right hand and punch through the ground, moving your shoulder into a protracted position. Keeping your left arm fully extended, open your chest and reach toward the sky, letting your gaze follow. You should feel a stretch in your right hip flexor, left hip abductors, and upper back. Reverse the motion and return to the starting position. Without stopping the motion, scoop your left arm underneath your right arm and reach to the right side of your body as far as you can. You should feel a stretch in your left hip, hamstring, and upper back. Complete all repetitions with your right leg extended behind you, then switch sides and complete the same number of repetitions with your left leg extended behind you.

CUES

Lunge, twist and reach to the ceiling, then reverse and reach under your other arm.

COMMON MISTAKES

- Not straightening the back leg.
- Losing foot stability and rocking onto the blades of your feet.
- Losing lower body stability near the top of the movement as the thoracic spine becomes the focus.
- Failing to drop your shoulder toward the ground as you reach under the opposite arm.

VARIATIONS

Yogis will tell you this movement should be performed with the bent knee pointed straight forward. This creates more lower body stability and shifts the stretch emphasis to the thoracic spine. This is difficult to do even for flexible people, which is why most strength athletes who perform this stretch let the hip of their bent leg open up away from their body. Naturally, this creates a better hip-opening response and takes some of the pressure off your midback. As long as you aren't rocking onto the blade of your foot as you twist, this is perfectly acceptable.

If you are not able to feel any upper back stretch during the World's Greatest Stretch due to extremely tight hips, you can try dropping your back knee to the ground. This will reduce the effectiveness of the exercise as a hip opener but will allow you to put more focus on mobilizing your thoracic spine.

Knee on Ground Variation

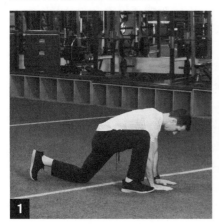
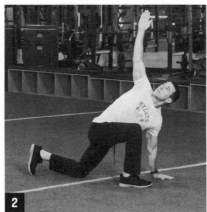
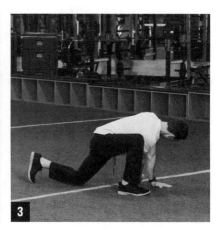

UPPER BODY

Anchored Lat Stretch

Because they are internal rotators, tight lats can cause shoulder pain, movement faults, and other muscle imbalances that lead to injury. The Anchored Lat Stretch mobilizes tight lats and improves overhead range of motion.

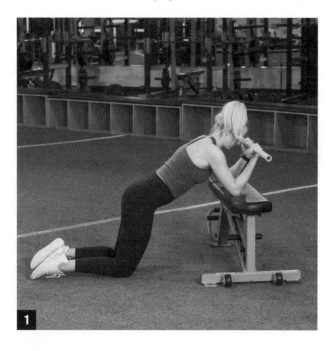

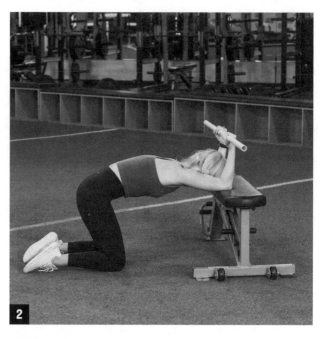

SETUP

From a kneeling position, place your elbows on a bench, foam roller, or box while grasping a PVC pipe or straight bar with a palms-up grip, shoulder-width apart. Round your low back slightly to protect it from overextension during the stretch.

EXECUTION

Bend your elbows to 90 degrees and drive them down into the bench. You should feel a stretch in the lats and muscles just behind your armpits.

CUES

Round your low back and drive downward with your elbows.

COMMON MISTAKES

- Hands too close together (should be about shoulder-width).
- Arching your low back.
- Knees too close to the bench which reduces the amount of force you are able to apply.

VARIATIONS

If you don't have access to a rigid pipe or bar, you can use a resistance band instead. This variation makes it more difficult to keep your shoulders from rotating inward, so pay attention to keeping your palms up and shoulders wide during the movement.

SUBSTITUTES

Suspension Trainer Lat Stretch (not pictured): You can mimic the Anchored Lat Stretch with a suspension trainer: facing away from the suspension straps, bend your arms to 90 degrees with your palms facing behind you and lean into the stretch. Be sure to keep your low back arched so the emphasis stays on the lats. This is a great stretch, but it doesn't allow you to place as much isolated force into the lats as the Anchored Lat Stretch.

UPPER BODY

Scapular Pull-up (Active Bar Hanging)

The Scapular Pull-up (a.k.a. Active Bar Hanging) prepares your scapula and shoulders for vertical pulling movements and mobilizes your lats in a functional way. This move involves static hanging from a pull-up bar with intermittent repetitions of scapula activation. You'll also get the back-relieving benefits of spinal decompression—where your spine is gently stretched by gravity (a nice counter to all the compression forces we encounter in the gym). However, this exercise does require a minimum threshold of low back strength, shoulder stability, and grip strength to perform safely.

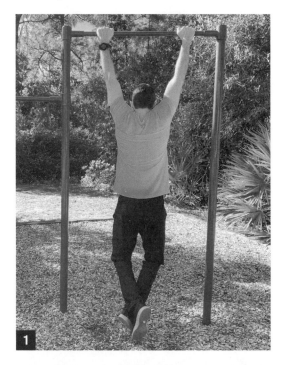

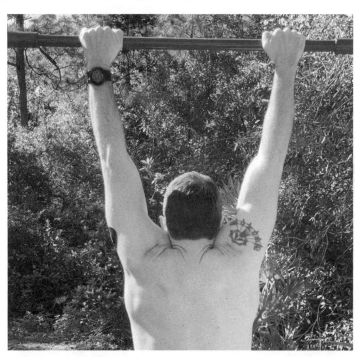

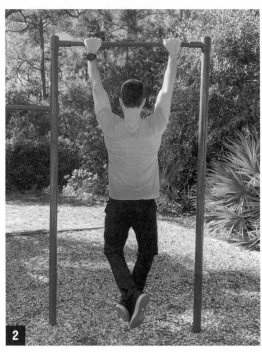

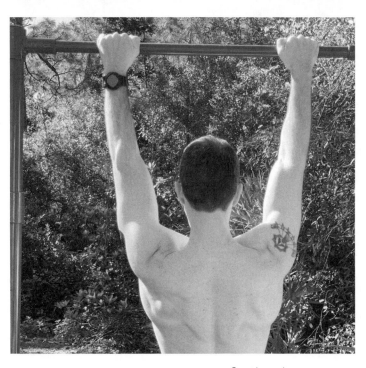

Continued on next page

SETUP

Start by hanging from a pull-up bar with an overhand (pronated) grip.

EXECUTION

With your arms fully extended in the hanging position, pull against bar while keeping your elbows completely straight. Wrap your thumbs over the bar as opposed to gripping it like a baseball bat. You should feel your entire shoulder girdle shift down a few inches as the rest of your body moves upward. Hold the position for a moment, then relax your shoulders and allow them to raise up again. The range of motion is minimal, and this does require practice to get it right. You will notice that your body moves a few inches backward in the contracted position, placing your arms slightly in front of your body. This puts your arms into the scapular plane, where the lats are stretched and shoulders out of impingement danger.

CUES

Pull down on the bar with elbows completely straight.

COMMON MISTAKES

- Bending your elbows.
- Rocking or using momentum to create the movement.

VARIATIONS

If you are unable to support your body weight from the hanging position or shoulder pain is holding you back, you can perform this exercise with your feet on the ground (assuming you can find a bar close enough to the ground).

SUBSTITUTES

- **Anchored Lat Stretch**
- **Suspension Trainer Scapula Activation:** If you do not have access to a pull-up bar or you cannot perform Scapular Pull-ups without pain, perform the same exercise but with your feet planted on the ground while holding onto the handles of a suspension training system. To enhance the exercise, start with a palms down (pronated) grip with your shoulders in the forward, protracted position. Then, externally rotate into a neutral grip with palms facing each other as you pull your scapulas together.

UPPER BODY

Band Pass Through

The Band Pass Through is a dynamic stretch that effectively opens up the chest, improves shoulder flexion, and trains proper scapula movement and thoracic extension during overhead exercises. This movement can be performed with a broom handle or rigid bar, but a resistance band's elasticity reduces shoulder joint stress.

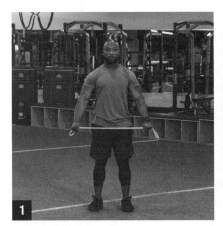
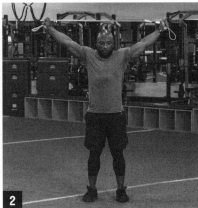
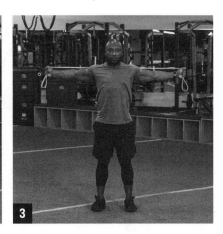

SETUP

Stand with a resistance band gripped in both hands with an overhand grip. Raise the band in front of you to eye level.

EXECUTION

Slowly raise your extended arms up over your head. As your arms reach the overhead position, shrug your shoulders up to upwardly rotate your scapula. Continue pulling the band behind your head, lowering your shoulder blades back to the down and retracted position as the band drops further toward the ground. Stop when you feel a healthy stretch in your anterior shoulder capsule, then slowly reverse the motion. Do not force the stretch to complete a full range of motion.

CUES

Raise arms overhead, shrug shoulders up, then pull the band behind you.

COMMON MISTAKES

- Using momentum instead of controlling each segment of the movement.
- Letting your shoulders dump forward to increase range of motion.
- Failing to move the scapula up and down when necessary during the movement.

VARIATIONS

You can substitute a broom handle, PVC pipe, or any other rigid bar for this exercise.

UPPER BODY

Modified Bully Stretch (Retract and Depress)

The Modified Bully Stretch teaches the proper back-and-down shoulder position without encouraging a forward dumping of the shoulder joints like the traditional Bully Stretch does. It also effectively mobilizes tight muscles near the front of the shoulder capsule. This one of my favorite stretches for taking pressure off chronically impinged shoulders.

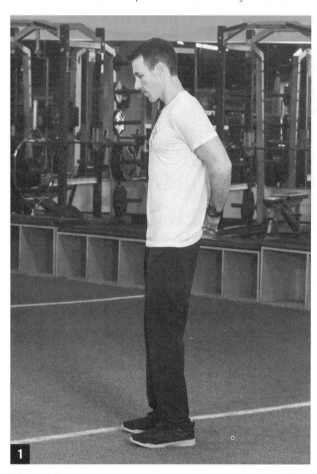

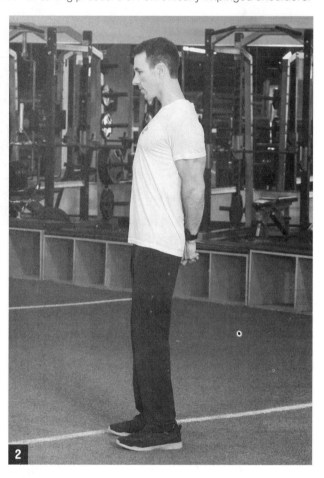

SETUP

Stand with feet shoulder-width apart and clasp both hands behind your back with fingers interlaced.

EXECUTION

Pinch your shoulder blades together, raise your chest, and extend your thoracic spine. Tuck your chin to prevent neck extension during the next phase of the movement. Then, depress your scapula by gently pulling down with both arms. Your shoulders should feel "back and down" in this position, and you should feel a stretch in the front of your shoulder capsule. Hold for a moment, then release the tension and allow your shoulders to relax. This completes one repetition.

CUES

Clasp hands, shoulders back, pull down.

COMMON MISTAKES

- Failing to fully retract the scapula before pulling down.
- Extending the neck upward, which encourages your shoulders to dump forward out of proper position.
- Arching the low back to compensate instead of keeping the focus on the scapula/shoulder complex.

UPPER BODY
Swimmer's Stretch

Few trainees use this underrated shoulder mobility drill. It doesn't just stretch your shoulders; it also reinforces optimal scapula position and activates your upper back muscles. When executed correctly, it's extremely difficult to perform the exercise with good posture for more than a few repetitions. If I only had time for one upper-body mobility drill per day, this would be it. Be patient with this one and use slow movements. After a few sessions, you'll see the difference it makes in upper body posture, mobility, and endurance. If you have never performed this exercise, start with the 45-degree Swiss ball variation described below.

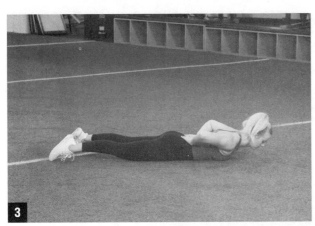

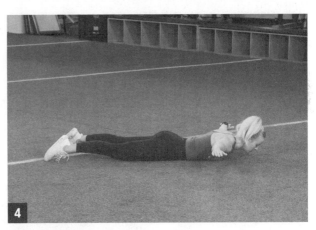

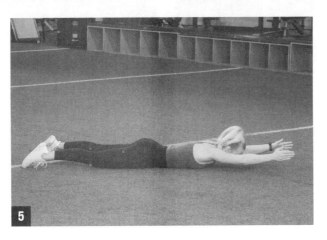

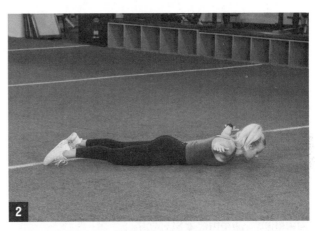

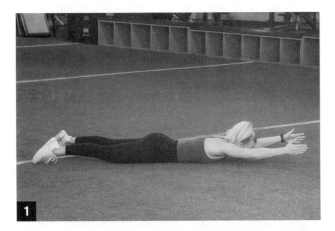

Continued on next page

SETUP

Lie face down on the floor with your feet together.

EXECUTION

Reach both arms overhead, shrugging your shoulders up with your thumbs facing the ceiling to externally rotate your shoulders. Pull your scapula back and down, then bring your arms down until they are straight out to your sides in a T shape. Rotate your thumbs toward the ground, then bend your elbows and tuck your hands behind your back. Press the backs of your hands into your low back, adjusting your scapula back and down again to prevent slouching. Hold this stretched position for a moment before reversing the motion.

CUES

Shoulders overhead and externally rotated, then down to your sides and tucked behind your back.

COMMON MISTAKES

- Moving too fast.
- Failing to start the movement with shoulders externally rotated.
- Letting your shoulders dump forward, which takes the focus off of your scapula and upper back.

VARIATIONS

- **Kneeling Swimmer's Stretch:** The least difficult version is from the kneeling position with your upper body straight up and down.
- **Swiss Ball Swimmer's Stretch:** To increase the difficulty, lie with your chest anchored against a Swiss ball or bench with your upper body at a 45-degree angle to the ground.

Kneeling Swimmer's Stretch

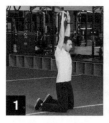 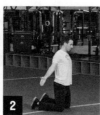 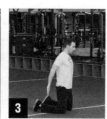 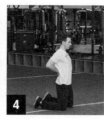 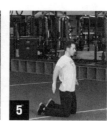 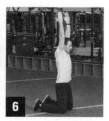

Swiss Ball Swimmer's Stretch

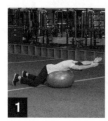 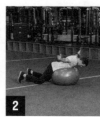 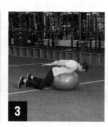 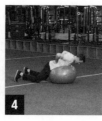 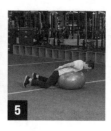 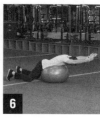

UPPER BODY

Thoracic Extension on Foam Roller

You can mobilize your thoracic spine by lying on your back with a foam roller placed perpendicular to your body, directly under your scapula. Some people even get a little joint crack or pop doing it that way. It's not a bad stretch, but it easily brings the low back into play unnecessarily. Instead, try the opposite. By placing the foam roller under your forearms in the prone position, you can target thoracic spine extension more effectively without stressing your low back. This version adds an element of loaded stretching, helps establish upward scapular rotation, and reinforces shoulder external rotation.

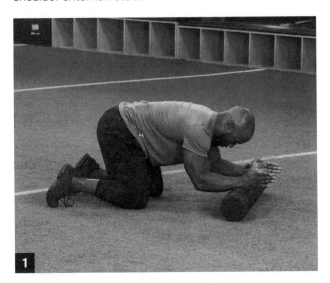

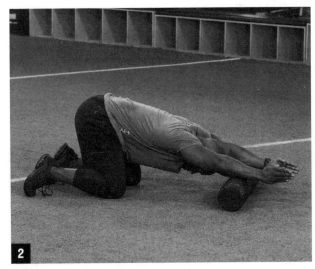

SETUP

From the quadruped position (on hands and knees), place a foam roller in front of you, a few inches forward of your head position. With your elbows bent at 90 degrees, place your wrists on the foam roller. Point your thumbs to the ceiling. Round your low back slightly and brace your core muscles to prevent low back stress.

EXECUTION

Push down with your wrists into the foam roller to engage your lats. Then, slowly straighten your elbows while leaning forward, continuing the downward pressure. Continue moving forward, lowering your torso to the ground (core still braced), until the foam roller slides up to your elbows and your arms are fully extended. Hold for a moment, then slowly reverse the motion by contracting your lats. Keep your shoulders back and down throughout. You should feel an active stretch in your lats and shoulder capsule as the foam roller rolls away from you. Think of this move as trying to touch your armpits to the floor in the fully extended position.

CUES

Round your back slightly, then extend your arms and push the foam roller down through the floor. Push your armpits toward the floor.

COMMON MISTAKES

- Arching your low back.
- Failing to activate your lats while pressing downward.
- Not maintaining constant downward pressure into the foam roller.

VARIATIONS

If you don't have a foam roller handy, you can mimic this movement by getting into the quadruped position and anchoring your forearms against a bench or chair. The key to this exercise is active contraction of the lats downward and engagement of the stabilizing muscles of your upper back.

THE EXERCISES SHOULDER STABILITY

Another category of movement conspicuously missing from the list of exercises is overhead pressing. That's because without sufficient mobility and synergist activation, overhead pressing causes shoulder impingement and pain. Besides, you can build significant shoulder strength, muscle mass, and stability without a traditional overhead press. That's why we are going to focus on improving shoulder function and building shoulder stability with exercises that are less stressful to the shoulder joint. It all starts with bringing up the posterior shoulder muscles.

SHOULDER STABILITY

Banded W

The Banded W isolates the external rotator muscles of the shoulder. Use a light resistance band and focus on getting maximum range of motion. This exercise is more about developing end range of motion control and stability than it is building raw strength. It's also a great warm-up exercise before pressing movements to alleviate cranky shoulders.

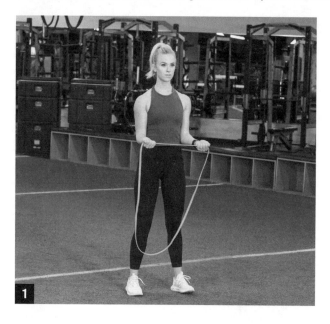

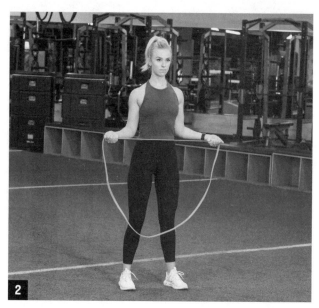

SETUP

Stand with your elbows tucked in by your armpits. Grab a light resistance band with a palms-up grip. Hold in front of your chest with tension in the band in the starting position. Pull your shoulders into the back and down position and tuck your chin.

EXECUTION

Keeping your elbows tucked in, rotate your forearms away from your body until your hands are pointing to each side. Keep your elbows stationary. Hold for a moment, then slowly reverse the motion.

CUES

Elbows in, palms up, externally rotate.

COMMON MISTAKES

- Failing to establish back-and-down shoulder position initially.
- Arching the back at the end range of motion.
- Using a resistance band that is too heavy and limits range of motion.

SUBSTITUTES

You can lie on your side and use a light dumbbell to perform the external rotation exercise instead of a band. However, resistance bands are superior because they provide greater tension at the end range of motion (where we are trying to establish control) and are easier on the shoulder joint.

SHOULDER STABILITY

Band High Pull Apart with External Rotation

The Band High Pull Apart exercise retrains any synergistic dominance caused by overactive deltoids and lats. It activates the neglected middle back muscles (e.g. lower trapezius and rhomboids) and external rotators (e.g. infraspinatus and teres minor).

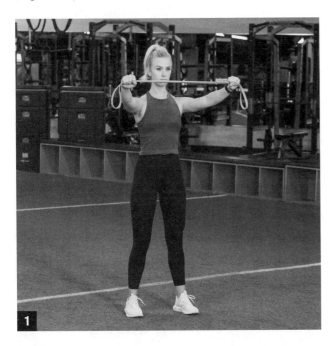

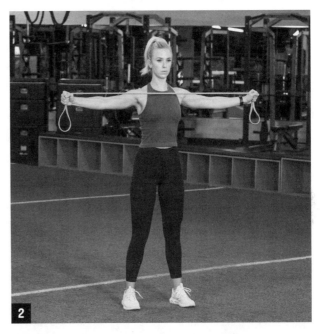

SETUP

Grasp the resistance band on each end with an overhand grip. Straighten your arms in front of you, holding the band at eye level with hands shoulder-width apart. Retract your shoulders and brace your core. There should be a small amount of tension in the band at the starting position.

EXECUTION

With elbows straight, pull your arms backward in a slight arc so they end up straight out to your sides, forming a T shape (this slight downward arc is important for preventing activation of the overused upper traps). As you move through this motion, rotate your elbow pits toward the ceiling. In the end position, your arms will be extended out to your sides in a "T" shape with the middle of the band touching your upper chest.

It's a two-part movement—your shoulders extend straight out to your sides, and your forearms rotate from a pronated (palms down) position to a supinated (palms up) position.

CUES

Pull your arms into a "T" position while rotating your elbow pits up to the ceiling.

COMMON MISTAKES

- Starting the exercise with hands below eye level, which encourages shoulder shrugging.
- External rotating at the wrists instead of at the forearm (think about rotating your elbows, not your hands).
- Protracting your shoulders in the starting position instead of keeping them retracted and depressed (back and down).

VARIATIONS

Anchored Band Pull Apart (not pictured): You can perform this exercise with a band anchored to an object in front of you. This is a good option if you want to increase the resistance of the exercise. To perform this variation, anchor a resistance band to a solid surface at eye level as you stand in front of it.

SHOULDER STABILITY
Seated Cable High Facepull

The Facepull improves external rotation function and targets neglected middle back muscles like the lower trapezius. But it's easy to mess up. A common mistake is performing the exercise with a slight upward angle, where the pulley is anchored below the height of your shoulders. This makes it difficult to keep your scapula down and encourages you to shrug your shoulders upward, using the already overworked upper traps instead of the rear delts and rotator cuff muscles.

Another common problem with the Facepull is internal shoulder rotation. This is the opposite of what you want to accomplish and could lead to shoulder impingement. To prevent this, opt for a neutral grip with palms facing each other instead of an overhand grip.[229] Though there are several variations, I recommend primarily using the seated cable version. From the seated position, you can more effectively stabilize your lower body and eliminate back movement.

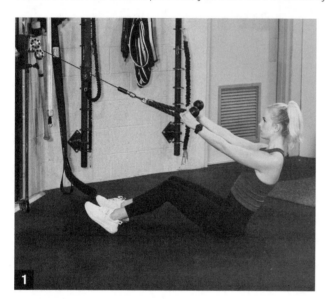
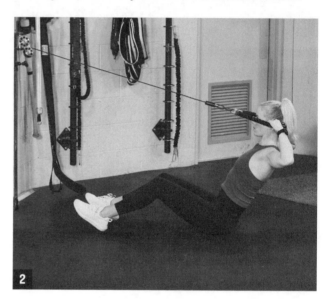

Standing Cable Facepull

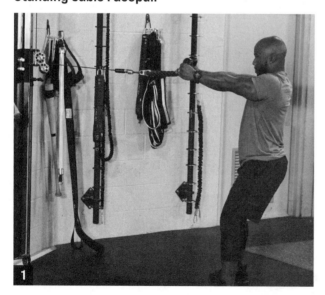
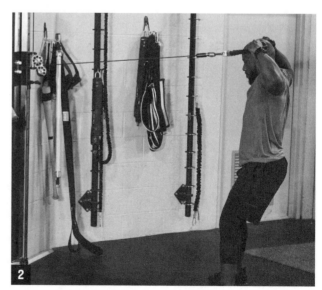

SETUP

Position a cable pulley with the rope attachment at or just above eye level when you are in the seated position. Grasp the rope from underneath the attachment so your palms are facing each other, and your thumbs are pointed backward. Sit down with your knees bent and feet firmly planted on the floor. Make sure your upper body is straight up and down—not leaning forward or backward. You may need to perform a few test reps to ensure the cable height is correct and the exercise path has a slight downward angle. Pull your scapula back and down. Hold it there throughout the exercise.

EXECUTION

Pull the handles toward your ears, spreading your hands apart as you pull. Continue pulling until each side of the rope attachment is outside your ears and your shoulders are in the externally rotated position. Your elbows should be bent to about 80 degrees. Pause briefly, then slowly extend your arms, taking care not to allow your scapula to protract or shoulders to internally rotate. Stop the lowering portion of the exercise when your elbows are straight.

CUES

Neutral grip, shoulders back and down, pull to the ears and externally rotate.

COMMON MISTAKES

- Using an overhand grip instead of a neutral grip.
- Letting your shoulders dump forward and internally rotate during the eccentric (lowering) phase.
- Pulling the cable too high or too low (you should pull the rope straight to your ears).
- Leaning backward or using momentum during the pulling motion—"cheating" the movement.
- Using a weight that is too heavy, causing the delts and lats to come into play.

VARIATIONS

- **Standing Cable Facepull:** Perform the same motion from a standing position, which further challenges balance and core stabilization.
- **Dumbbell Facepull:** Lying on an incline bench or bent over (if no access to bench), perform the same basic motion by rowing the dumbbells toward your ears.
- **Band (High) Facepull:** For warming up or building endurance, anchor a resistance band to a fixed object just above eye level to perform the Band Facepull.

Dumbbell Facepull

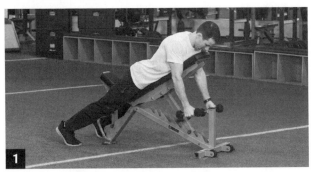

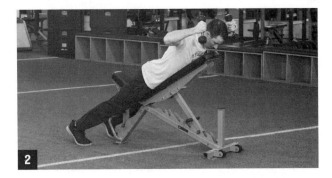

Band (High) Facepull

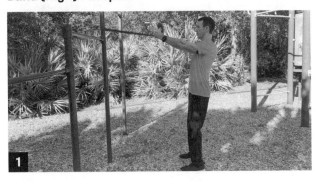

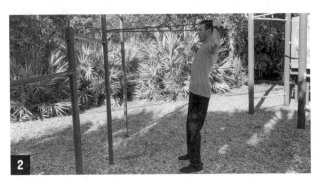

SHOULDER STABILITY

Scapular Plane Dumbbell Raises

Unlike a typical front or side dumbbell raise that isolates the deltoid muscles, the Scapular Plane Dumbbell Raise trains scapula stability and total shoulder joint strength. More importantly, research shows that it more effectively maintains the subacromial space during motion, preventing shoulder impingement.[280]

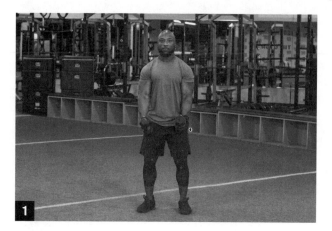

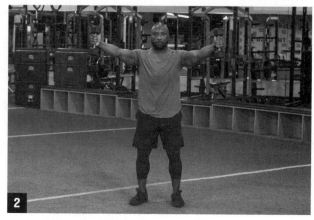

SETUP

Stand with feet shoulder-width apart, holding a pair of dumbbells by your sides, with elbows slightly bent.

EXECUTION

With a thumbs-up, neutral grip, raise your arms out to the sides of your body and just slightly forward—around 30 to 45 degrees forward from the frontal plane. Stop the motion when your arms are parallel with the ground. Control the weight at the top of the movement by pausing briefly before slowly lowering the weights back down.

CUES

Thumbs up, dumbbells to your sides and slightly forward.

COMMON MISTAKES

- Using momentum instead of controlling each segment of the movement.
- Letting shoulders dump forward instead of keeping them back and down.
- Using too heavy of a weight.

VARIATIONS

Scapular Plane Resistance Band Raises: If this movement causes pain even with light weight, substitute a thin resistance band for the dumbbell. This will allow for peak contraction at the top of the movement while minimizing shoulder joint stress.

Scapular Plane Resistance Band Raises

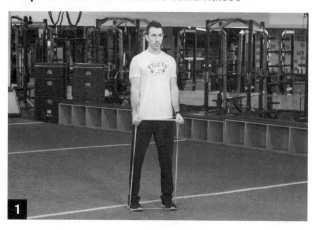

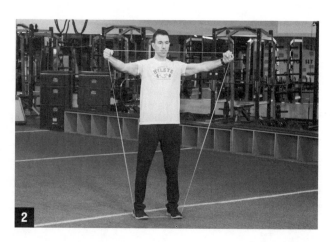

SHOULDER STABILITY

Bottoms-Up Kettlebell Press

The Bottoms-Up Kettlebell Press will put your ego in its place. Instead of the round part of the kettlebell facing downward, you will hold it "bottom up." Because of the challenging stabilization component, you'll have to use a weight that is much lighter than you would normally use for a dumbbell overhead press or standard kettlebell overhead press.

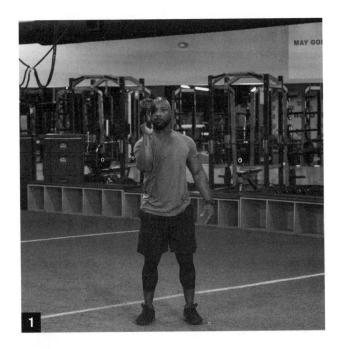

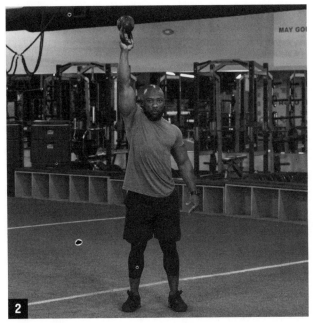

SETUP

Stand with feet shoulder-width apart holding a kettlebell in one hand. Either swing the kettlebell up or use a two-handed grip to safely get it into the starting position. To start the pressing movement, the kettlebell should be balanced just in front of your shoulder at about chin height. Keep a firm grip on the handle to prevent the weight from wobbling.

EXECUTION

Brace your core and extend the weight straight over your head, finishing with your arm pointed straight up in the air and the kettlebell balanced in the bottoms-up position. You will notice that to fully extend your arm, the weight will travel posterior as you press it up. If you have tight lats, getting into the overhead position may be a challenge at first. Hold the weight in the extended position for a moment before slowly reversing the motion.

CUES

Bottom up, front rack position, press straight up to the ceiling.

COMMON MISTAKES

- Starting with the weight either too close to your body or too far away.
- Pressing and lowering the weight too fast.
- Failing to firmly grip the handle to stabilize the weight.
- Failing to fully extend overhead, usually due to tight lat muscles.

SUBSTITUTES

If you don't have access to a kettlebell, you can substitute a dumbbell and perform the same motion. This will not create the same stabilizing stimulus but works as a stand-in if necessary.

UPPER BODY PUSH

Incline Dumbbell Fly Press

The Incline Dumbbell Fly Press is a combination of a traditional fly and chest press. Instead of having your arms fully extended, as dumbbell flys are often performed, you'll have a slight bend in the elbows. This takes pressure off your shoulder joint and allows you to use a heavier weight for a greater mechanical load. It also mobilizes the commonly tight anterior shoulder capsule and chest muscles more effectively than a flat, noninclined movement.

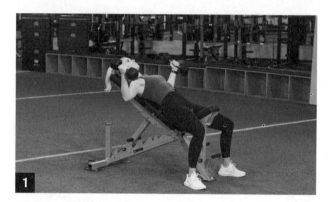

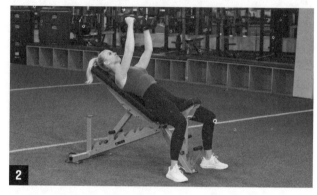

SETUP

Position yourself on an incline bench with a pair of dumbbells resting on your knees. Using a kick-up motion from your knees to assist, press the dumbbells straight up with palms facing each other. Make sure your feet are planted firmly on the ground, your core is tight and neutral, and your shoulders are back and down (not protracted forward). The back of your head should be in contact with the bench.

EXECUTION

With the dumbbells already pressed overhead, begin the first repetition by bending your elbows to about 90 degrees. You'll have to drop the dumbbells down slightly to do this. This will give you an accurate gauge to measure your elbow angle. Then, open up your elbow angle about 20 degrees further (to about 110 degrees).

Keep your elbows fixed at this angle, and slowly lower the weights until you feel a gentle stretch in your upper chest. In this position, your upper arms and shoulders should be even with or just below the plane of your body. You may be able to stretch beyond this range, but doing so increases the risk of shoulder injury.[280] Hold the bottom position for a few moments while keeping a forceful contraction present in your chest and arms, then raise the dumbbells back up to the top, never losing the 110 degree angle of your elbows.

The elbow angle doesn't have to be perfect. And the optimal angle will vary from person to person. Choose an elbow position that allows you to use a fairly heavy weight, does not cause you any shoulder stress, and allows you to feel a stretch at the bottom of the ROM.

CUES

Elbows bent slightly wider than 90 degrees, lower to plane of body, and hold.

COMMON MISTAKES

- Failing to establish proper shoulder position before beginning the movement.
- Losing the consistency of your elbow angle during the movement.
- Arching your back at the bottom of the ROM instead of maintaining a neutral spine.
- Lowering the weights too far (beyond the plane of your body).

SUBSTITUTES

If you don't have access to an incline bench, you can perform the same motion on a flat bench (or the floor). Alternatively, you can use a Swiss ball to re-create the incline bench position.

UPPER BODY PUSH

Incline Dumbbell Press

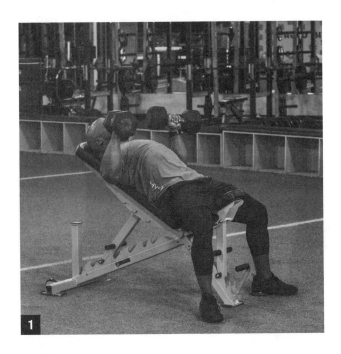

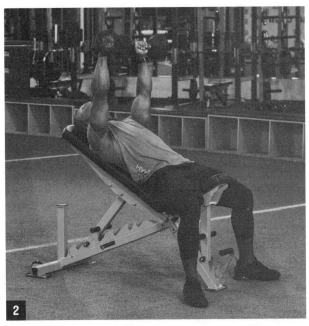

SETUP

Position yourself on an incline bench with a pair of dumbbells resting on your knees. Using a kick-up motion from your knees to assist, press the dumbbells straight up with palms facing down. Then, supinate your forearms to about 45 degrees. This will make it easier to keep your shoulders in position. Make sure your feet are planted firmly on the ground, your core is tight and neutral, and your shoulders are back and down (not protracted forward). The back of your head should be in contact with the bench.

EXECUTION

With the dumbbells already pressed overhead, begin the first repetition by lowering the weights to your sides. Try to keep the angle of your elbow-to-armpit at about 45 degrees. This places less stress on the shoulder capsule than the more common method of flaring the shoulders out wide. Stop the lowering portion of the movement when you feel a stretch in your upper chest. In this

position, your upper arms should be at or just below the plane of your body. Control the weight in the bottom position momentarily, then press back up to the starting position.

CUES

45-degree forearm angle, 45-degree armpit angle.

COMMON MISTAKES

- Failing to establish proper shoulder position before beginning the movement.
- Arching your back at the bottom of the ROM instead of maintaining a neutral spine.
- Lowering the weights too far (beyond the plane of your body).

SUBSTITUTES

If you don't have access to an incline bench, you can perform the same motion on a flat bench (or the floor).

UPPER BODY PUSH

Band Push-up Plus

The Banded Push-up Plus adds an element of scapular stabilization to the traditional push-up. Essentially, you perform a regular push-up, then protract your shoulders forward, further elevating yourself off the ground. I've talked a lot about keeping the shoulders back and down. This exercise has a different goal: improving shoulder stability in extended and protected positions. When you add a heavy band as resistance and use isometric holds, the Band Push-up Plus becomes an effective upper body push exercise for building strength, muscle, endurance, and coordination. Once you get comfortable with the exercise, challenge yourself by using the heaviest resistance band you can while still maintaining proper form.

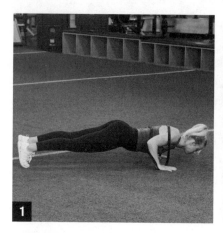

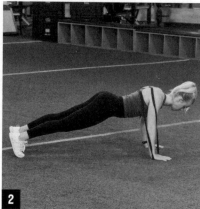

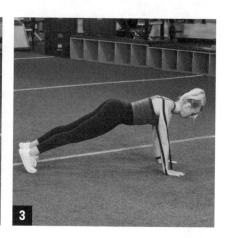

SETUP

From a kneeling position, grab a resistance band in each hand with the length of band wrapped around your upper back. Move into the bottom position of a push-up with your hands parallel with your chest.

EXECUTION

Push your hands down into the floor to keep the band secured in place. Next, brace your core hard to keep your spine in alignment (the band will cause your torso to drop if you don't resist). Complete a push-up. Pause briefly, then protract your shoulders forward as if you are trying to push yourself as far away from the ground as possible. Hold this position, then allow your shoulders to slide back and down again so that you are in the top position of a regular push-up. Slowly lower yourself to the ground.

CUES

Keep your low back neutral, push up, protract.

COMMON MISTAKES

- Allowing your hips to drop toward the ground.
- Failing to fully protract your shoulders at the top of the motion.
- Taking breaks after each repetition instead of keeping constant muscle tension.

VARIATIONS

- **On fists:** If you have bad wrists, or are strong enough to use a heavy pull-up-assistance band during this move, try performing the Push-up Plus on your fists. This will also help you secure the band in your hands when you squeeze your fists together. Use a foam mat, yoga mat, or rolled up towel to create a cushion between the floor and your knuckles.

- **Feet lowered:** If you have trouble performing this exercise on flat ground, use a bench or chair to elevate your upper body. Try to make your body form a 45-degree angle from the floor. If you are struggling with the Band Push-up Plus, I would rather you perform this variation with the band than revert to a traditional push-up with no band resistance.

- **Feet raised:** To increase the resistance, elevate your feet off the ground using a bench or chair.

- **Serratus emphasis** (not pictured): Another way to make this exercise more challenging and effective is to slide your hands a few inches toward your head. This will force the serratus muscles to contract harder and increase the load on your core.[281]

THAT'S IT?

Yes, just three horizontal push exercises is all I recommend during the first phases of the BFB program. Most people do too much pressing anyway, which exacerbates muscle imbalances around the shoulder. And remember, your shoulders are going to be challenged from multiple angles with other exercises.

The loaded stretch element of the Fly Press and shoulder stabilization challenge from the Push-up Plus will boost your pressing power and build your chest muscles. Take a break from the machines and barbells. You'll be surprised by how much you can improve your pressing with these few simple movements.

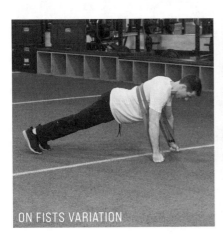

ON FISTS VARIATION

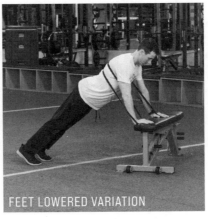

FEET LOWERED VARIATION

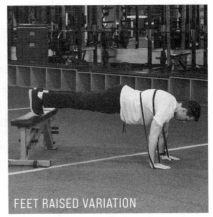

FEET RAISED VARIATION

UPPER BODY PULL

Single Arm Strict Dumbbell Row

Make friends with the Single Arm Strict Dumbbell Row. It's going to be your #1 back builder. This exercise challenges stability and control more effectively than any machine or cable system. Because you only use one side of your body at a time, it helps correct any side-dominant muscle imbalances. Unlike barbells, it allows you to keep your wrists in a neutral position for less elbow and wrist stress. And, it enables you to challenge your back and posterior shoulder muscles with heavy loads safely.

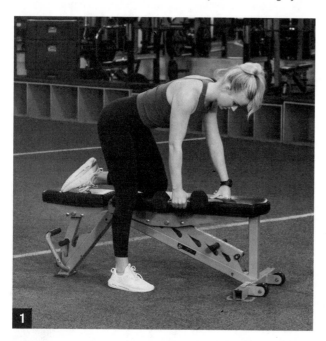

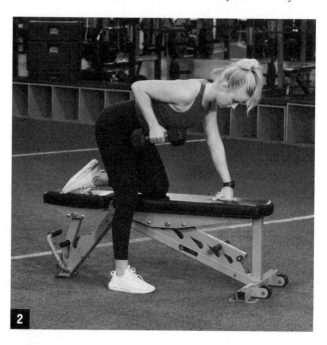

SETUP

For the knee-anchored variation, set one dumbbell next to a flat bench. Place one knee on the bench, with the opposite foot firmly planted on the ground. Use your hand on the knee-anchored side to stabilize your upper body against the bench. Bend down and grasp the dumbbell. Straighten up and pull your weight-loaded shoulder into the back-and-down position.

EXECUTION

Achieve neutral spine and brace your core forcefully. Execute a row by driving your elbow up toward the ceiling, keeping your elbow close to your body throughout the movement. Stop the motion when you can no longer pull the weight further without your shoulder dumping forward or losing scapula position. Squeeze your back muscles at the top, then slowly lower the weight.

CUES

Shoulder back and down, core tight, pull elbow toward your hip.

COMMON MISTAKES

- Using momentum instead of controlling each segment of the movement.
- Letting the shoulder protract forward through the bottom range of motion.
- Rotating the body to "cheat" the movement instead of keeping core tight and neutral.

VARIATIONS

- **Single Arm Strict Dumbbell Row:** The variation I described above is the strict variation—where your scapula is retracted throughout the movement. You'll notice this variation is much harder than haphazardly yanking the dumbbell up like a lawnmower cord. It creates extreme fatigue in your posterior shoulder and forces you to take the momentum out of the exercise. This variation is more therapeutic for the shoulders and arguably a more functional exercise than letting your shoulder stretch down toward the ground at the bottom of the motion.

- **Single Arm Full Range Dumbbell Row:** The full range variation is performed in the same way as described above, except you reach further toward the ground during the eccentric portion of the exercise. This increases the range of motion and stretches the lat muscles further before contracting. It also allows you to use heavier weights. There is nothing inherently wrong with performing the exercise this way, but be careful about not slinging the dumbbell out of the bottom. This will reduce muscular contraction in the middle and top ranges of the motion (where you probably need the most work—especially if you have hunched forward shoulder posture).

- **Single Arm Split Stance Dumbbell Row:** Instead of kneeling against a bench, bend over at the waist and use one hand to anchor your body against a rack or bench. This variation is more challenging for the core and low back muscles to stabilize.

- **Single Arm Staggered Stance Dumbbell Row:** The staggered stance row is performed from a lunge position, which challenges the muscles of the posterior oblique sling (hamstrings, butt, low back).

Single Arm Full Range Dumbbell Row

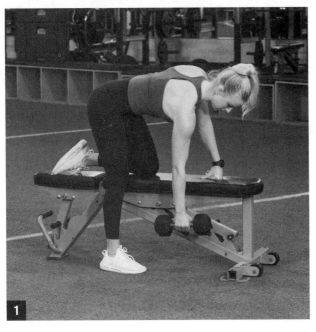

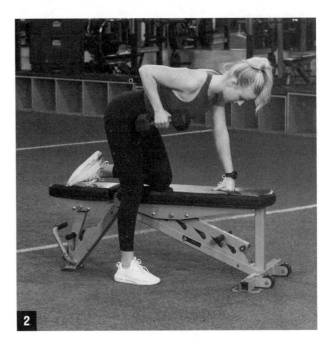

Continued on next page

Single Arm Split Stance Dumbbell Row

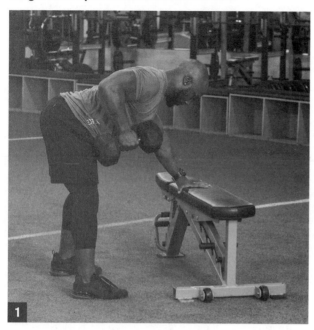
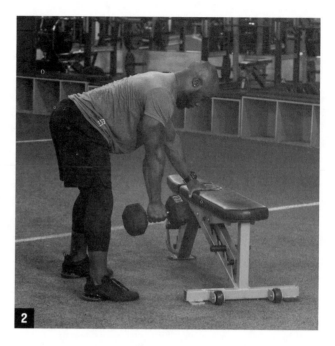

Single Arm Staggered Stance Dumbbell Row

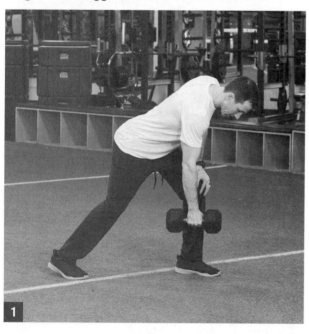
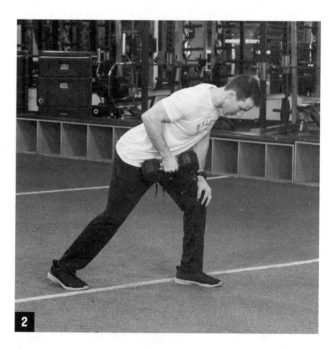

UPPER BODY PULL

Bent Over Dumbbell Row

The dual (two-handed) row develops posterior chain coordination. It places greater emphasis on the muscles surrounding the low back and thoracic spine, making it an effective postural exercise.

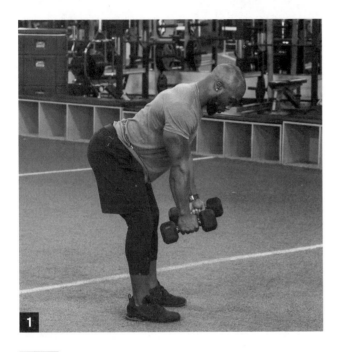

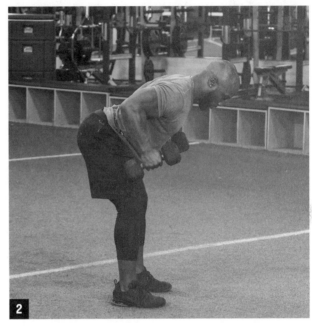

SETUP

For the bent-over variation, start in the standing position with dumbbells held in each hand. Brace your core and push your butt backward to initiate a hip hinge. Let your arms hang straight out in front of you, keeping your shoulders in the backs of their sockets. Aim for a 45-degree angle between your torso and the floor. Use a mirror or partner for guidance.

EXECUTION

With palms facing each other, tuck your chin and pull your elbows up toward the ceiling, keeping your arms close to your body. Squeeze your shoulder blades together at the top of the movement, then slowly lower the weights back down.

CUES

Row straight up and squeeze the shoulder blades.

COMMON MISTAKES

- Rounding the low back (be careful here!).
- Failing to squeeze the shoulder blades at the top (usually because the weight is too heavy).

VARIATIONS

- **Incline Dumbbell Row:** Instead of bending over at the waist, lie face down on an incline bench. This takes your lower body out of the equation, further isolating the upper back and rear deltoids.

- **Incline Dumbbell High Row:** This variation is performed lying face down on an incline bench, but with a different arm angle to the body than the standard dumbbell row. Instead of keeping your elbows close to your body, flare them out to the sides. This is similar to a Facepull with one key difference: you will not externally rotate your shoulders at the top of this movement. Instead, you will use a heavier weight that only allows you to row up toward your face, placing more emphasis on the upper back and rear deltoids.

- **Strict vs. full range:** For the Dual Dumbbell Row, I recommend performing each repetition with strict form—where your scapula stays retracted throughout the movement.

Continued on next page

Incline Dumbbell Row

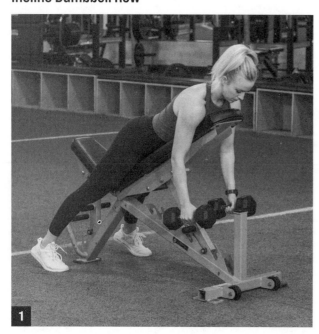

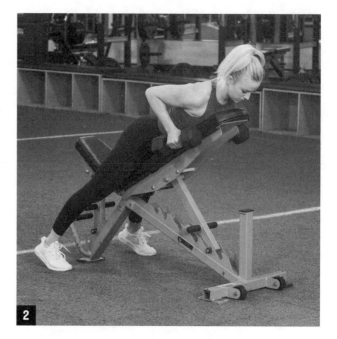

UPPER BODY PULL

Suspension Trainer High Row

Suspension training systems, such as the popular TRX, use your body weight as resistance. While there are hundreds of exercises you can perform with suspension straps, my favorite is the Suspension Trainer High Row. It allows you to adapt your grip, foot position, and body angle to create a joint-friendly pull.

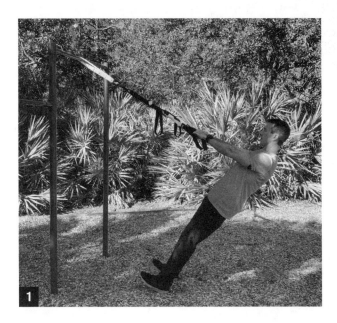

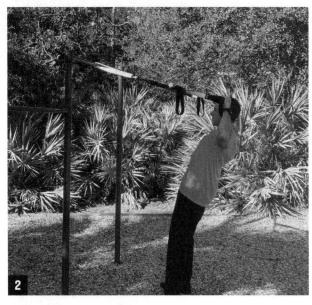

SETUP

Using a suspension trainer with straps anchored above your head to a wall, adjust the straps so you can lean backward to about 45 degrees while keeping your arms straight. Your palms should be facing each other (neutral grip) and your body should be straight from toes to head.

EXECUTION

With a neutral grip, pull your hands toward your head, finishing the movement with your hands just outside your ears and your thumbs pointed backward. Both your arm angle to your body and your elbow angle should end at about 90 degrees. Squeeze your shoulder blades together at the top, then slowly lower your body back down to the starting position.

CUES

Body straight, neutral grip, pull to your ears with arms at 90 degrees.

COMMON MISTAKES

- Extending your hips forward during the pulling phase.

- Incorrect foot positioning: the closer your feet are to the wall where the straps are anchored, the more challenging the exercise will be.
- Using your arms and elbows to drive the movement instead of forcefully contracting your upper back muscles.

VARIATIONS

Suspension Trainer High Row with Straight Arm Lowering: To add an extra element of posterior shoulder strengthening, perform the lowering portion with straight arms instead of bent arms. To use this variation, straighten your arms into a "T" after completing the row, then slowly lean backward, allowing your body to lower under the control of your posterior shoulder muscles.

SUBSTITUTES

If you don't have access to a suspension trainer, you can substitute one of the following exercises: Standing Cable Facepull, Band Facepull, Bent Over Dual Dumbbell High Row.

Continued on next page

Suspension Trainer High Row with Straight Arm Lowering

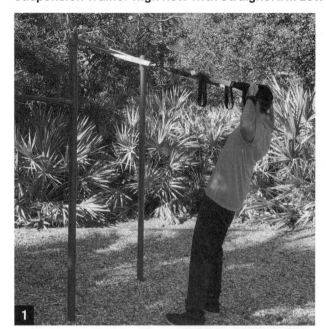

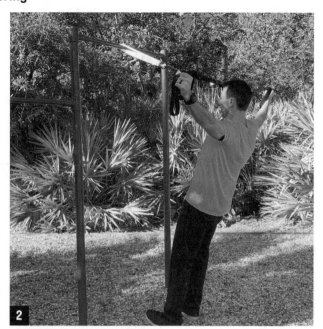

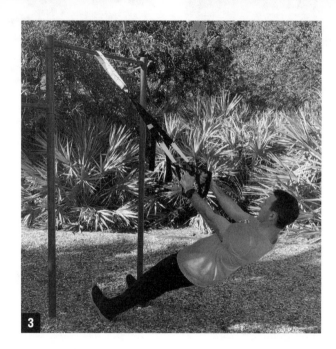

UPPER BODY PULL
Reverse Grip Cable Pulldowns

The Reverse Grip Cable Pulldown creates a muscle-lengthening loaded stretch on the lats in addition to being a great muscle and strength builder.

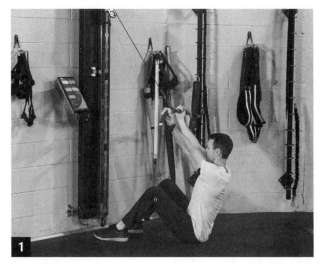

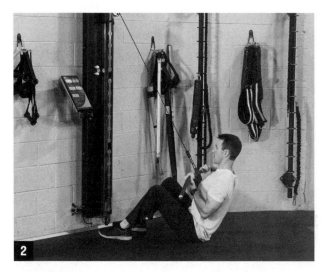

SETUP

Using a lat pulldown machine, grab a straight bar with an underhand grip, hands just inside shoulder-width. Lock your shoulders in the back-and-down position. Lean back slightly, which engages your upper back in addition to your lats and discourages shoulder rounding.

EXECUTION

Pull the bar straight down toward your chest, resisting the urge to let your shoulders dump forward. Squeeze your lats and shoulder blades at the bottom of the movement, then slowly straighten your arms. At the top of the movement, lean forward slightly while still maintaining the back-and-down shoulder position. This should provide a gentle stretch in your lat muscles.

CUES

Shoulders back and down, pull to your chest, lean forward and stretch at the top.

COMMON MISTAKES

- Rounding your shoulders forward during the pulling phase.
- Shrugging your shoulders upward at the top of the movement instead of keeping your shoulders back and down.

VARIATIONS

You can play with the angle of this movement by leaning further backward. This will take some emphasis off your lat stretch at the top of the motion, but it may be necessary depending on your height and the type of machine you are using.

SUBSTITUTES

Chin-up: A pull-up is performed with an overhand grip while a chin-up is performed with an underhand grip. Both are excellent exercises, but in my opinion the chin-up is superior for fully lengthening the lats and keeping the shoulders in a safe, stable position. If you are able to complete an underhand chin-up safely and with good form, use it instead of the Reverse Grip Cable Pulldown.

It is not necessary to literally get your chin over the bar, which usually results in protruding your head forward and hunching your shoulders. Stop the movement when you can no longer pull yourself upward further without hunching your shoulders forward.

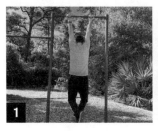

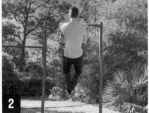

UPPER BODY PULL

Lying Dumbbell Pullover

The Lying Dumbbell Pullover activates the serratus muscles and lengthens the lats. Think of this exercise as a mobility tool rather than a muscle builder. You will want to use a weight that is light enough to control the movement without putting your shoulders at risk.

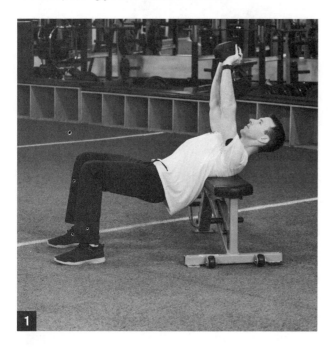

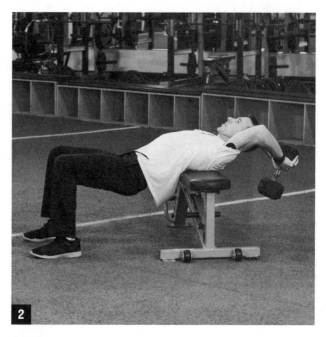

SETUP

Lie perpendicular across a padded flat bench, with your upper back resting on the bench and both feet planted firmly on the floor. Alternatively, you can perform this exercise while lying on a Swiss ball. Grasp a dumbbell with both hands, using a baseball grip or hands interlocked. Press the weight straight up to the ceiling and allow a slight bend in your elbows. (You may find it easier to lay the dumbbell on the bench next to you before getting into position.)

EXECUTION

Brace your core to ensure your low back does not arch during the movement. Slowly lower the dumbbell behind your head. Stop the motion as your upper arms cross the plane of your body, or when you feel a stretch in your lats and upper back. Hold for a moment, then return to the starting position.

CUES

Abs tight, lower until you feel a stretch in your lats.

COMMON MISTAKES

- Failing to prevent lower back movement during the lift (not bracing core).
- Lowering the dumbbell too far behind you.
- Using your triceps to initiate the movement instead of keeping a consistent elbow angle and using your lats, serratus, and upper back muscles.

THE EXERCISES **UPPER BODY ACCESSORY (ELBOWS AND WRISTS)**

UPPER BODY ACCESSORY

Alternating Dumbbell Curl with Supination

Dumbbell curls are ideal for building strong biceps and forearm supination patterns without wrecking your elbows and wrists. Curls aren't just for vanity, either. By training with the dumbbell curl variations below, you will fortify your lower arms against injury and improve one of the most functional categories of strength: *grip strength.*

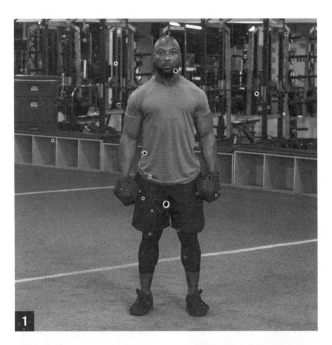

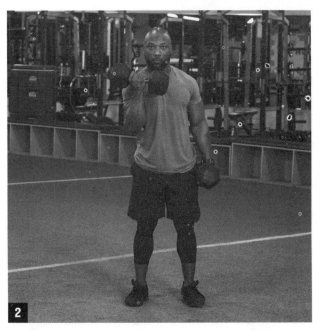

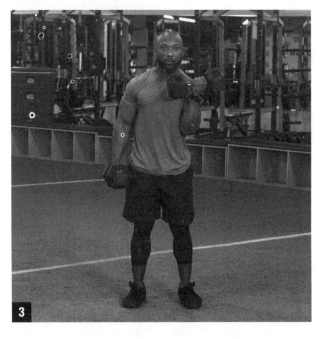

Continued on next page

For the alternating curl variation, start from a standing position with a dumbbell in each hand, palms facing your body (neutral grip). Because we want to emphasize the commonly weak supination movement—rotating your forearm and hand outward—slide your hand up to the thumb side of the dumbbell instead of gripping it in the middle of the handle. This will demand more outward rotating force, making the exercise more effective.

EXECUTION

Lift one of the weights by bending at the elbow and simultaneously rotating the pinky-side of your hand inward and toward the sky (supination). Try to initiate the supination motion at your forearm instead of merely twisting your wrist joint. Finish the curl when the weight is in front of your shoulder and your palm is facing the ceiling. Keep tension on your bicep at the top for a moment, then slowly lower the weight. Alternate sides with each repetition.

CUES

Curl and rotate your forearm outward (supination).

COMMON MISTAKES

- Rotating the wrist joint instead of rotating at the forearm.

- Leaning back, slinging the weight, or otherwise cheating the movement with a weight that is too heavy.
- Failing to control the lowering (eccentric) portion of the exercise.

VARIATIONS

- **Hammer Curl:** The hammer curl is performed with neutral wrists. It targets the muscles that underly the biceps, the brachialis. The brachialis is called the "work horse" of the elbow, producing most of the force during elbow flexion. Strengthening this muscle, especially with slow eccentric-biased movements, helps prevent elbow and wrist injuries. The hammer curl can be performed with both arms simultaneously or alternating.
- **Zottman Curl:** The Zottman Curl is the most multitasking of all curling movements. It trains the commonly weak wrist extensor muscles and trains both pronation (palms down) and supination (palms up). To perform the Zottman Curl, start by performing a traditional dual dumbbell curl and supinating your forearms at the top (as described above). At the top of the motion, turn your palms toward the ground so you are holding the dumbbells with an overhand grip. Slowly lower the dumbbells toward your sides.
- **Band Zottman Curl:** In a pinch, you can also perform the Zottman Curl with a resistance band.

Hammer Curl

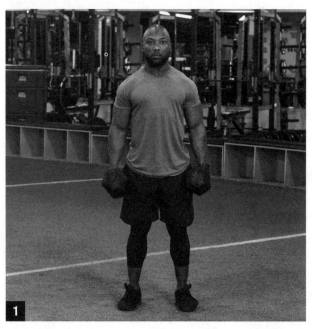

1

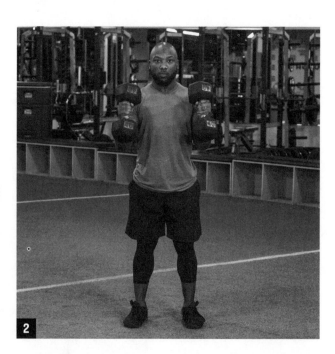

2

Zottman Curl

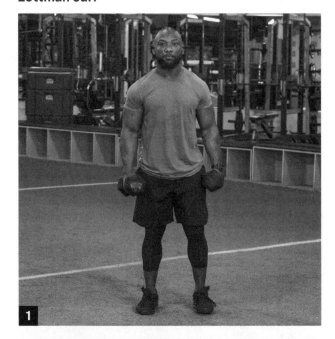

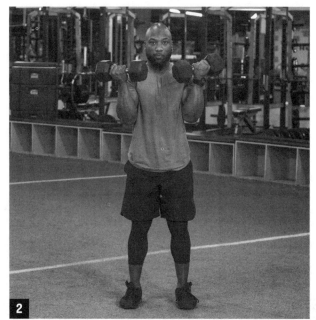

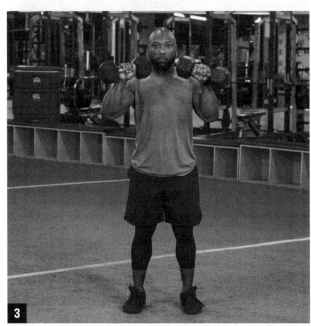

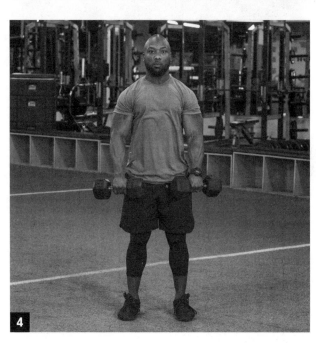

UPPER BODY ACCESSORY

Forearm Tendon Glides

I was introduced to a variation of this exercise by a physical therapist. After years of managing my elbow tendinopathy and months of working through a wrist injury, I had plateaued. I could perform most exercises but still had occasional painful movements. Adding tendon glides to my daily routine has been transformational. This simple exercise improves the tendon's flow through the carpal and cubital tunnels, helping to reduce nerve pain and improve motor unit recruitment of muscles in the hands and forearms. Through the principle of irradiation, training your wrists and hands to contract with full force enables more efficient transfer of force across joints, which translates to greater strength.[282]

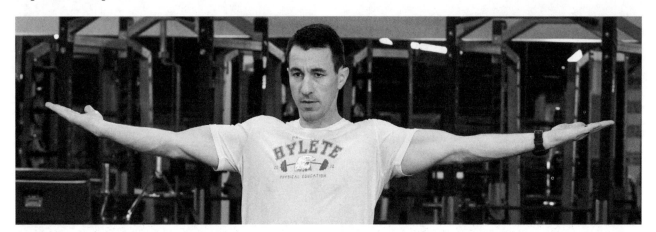

SETUP

From a standing position, extend both arms out to your sides in the shape of a "T." Externally rotate your shoulders, pulling them back and down with your palms facing up. Spread your fingers wide open and extend your wrists toward the ground. This sets up a nice neural stretch before you start the movement.

EXECUTION

Starting from the last digits on your fingers, make a slow fist, rolling up your fingers one joint at a time. Then, flex your wrist and squeeze the muscles of your forearm. Reverse the movement by opening up the fingers and extending the wrist back the other direction. If you are doing this right, the muscles in your lower arms will be fatigued.

CUES

Roll your fingers into a fist, flex your wrist, open your hand, extend your wrist.

COMMON MISTAKES

- Failing to squeeze the fist and extend the wrist with enough contraction force.
- Not holding the end positions long enough.

VARIATIONS

You can perform tendon glides with arms at your sides or in any comfortable arm positon. The arms extended variation above enhances the neural stretch through the elbow joint.

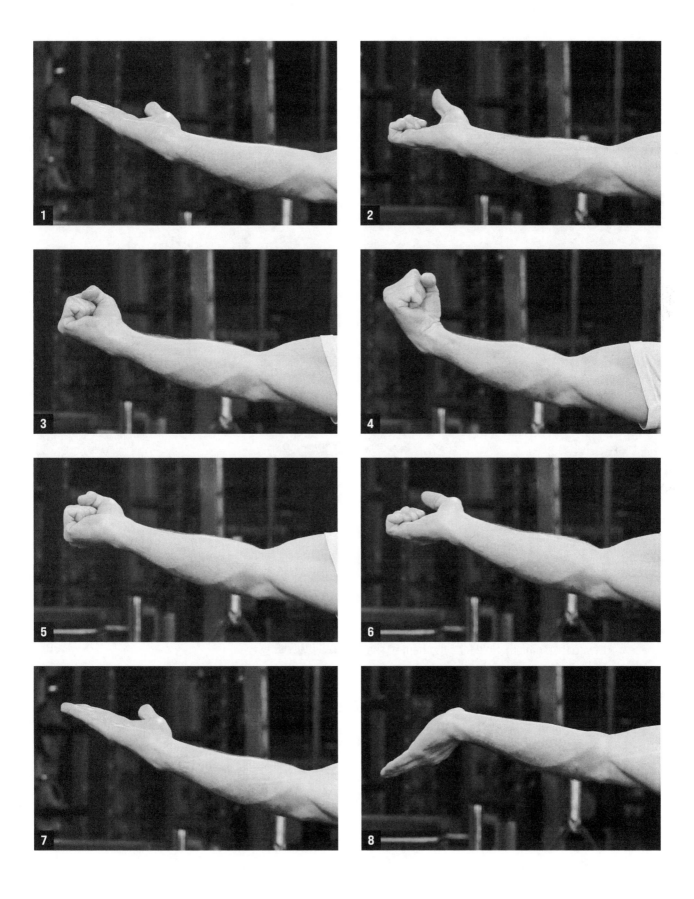

UPPER BODY ACCESSORY

Dumbbell Pronation/Supination

The forearm flexors (curling your wrist inward) and pronators (rotating your thumb down) are the two most overworked muscular systems of the lower arm. Conversely, the extensors (opposite to flexors) and supinators (opposite to pronators) are typically weak. This is largely due to how we use our hands in everyday life and which exercises we choose to perform. The dumbbell pronation/supination combination below will help rebalance any existing asymmetries in your forearms and wrists.

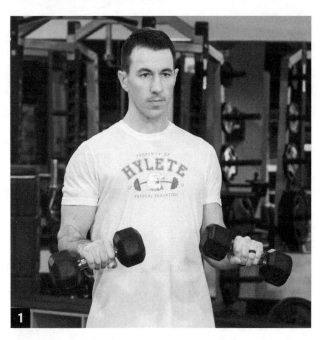

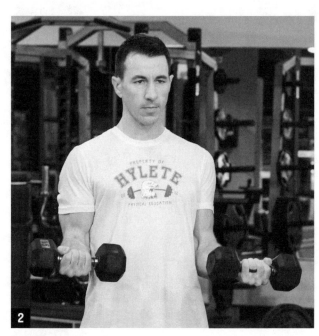

SETUP

Hold a dumbbell in each hand in front of your body with elbows bent at 90 degrees.

EXECUTION

Slowly rotate your palms to the ground (pronation) until you reach the end of your range of motion. Hold for a moment, then reverse the movement by rotating your forearm outward (supination). Hold for a moment at the end range. This completes one repetition.

CUES

Elbows tucked in and bent 90 degrees, rotate at the forearm.

COMMON MISTAKES

- Using momentum instead of controlling each segment of the movement (going too fast could cause injuries to the ligaments in your wrists).
- Cranking your elbows away from your body at the end range (this is usually an unconscious compensation to get more movement out of the exercise).

VARIATIONS

You can make this exercise more challenging by performing the straight arm variation. Instead of using bent elbows, extend your elbows fully in front of you. The weights should be slightly lower than the height of your shoulders. Perform the same motion, taking care to rotate primarily at the elbows (not the shoulder or wrist)

Straight Arm Variation

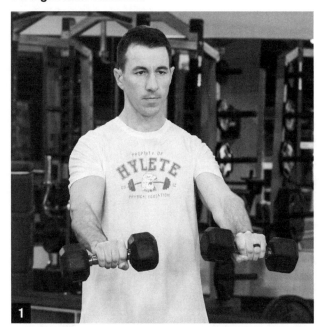

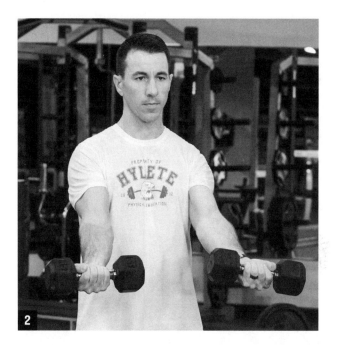

UPPER BODY ACCESSORY

Standing Dumbell Pullover

The Standing Dumbbell Pullover combines two isolation movements (lat pullover and tricep extension) into a compound movement that mobilizes tight muscles of the upper back and improves thoracic extension. It's a great countermovement to all the forward flexing you do throughout the day.

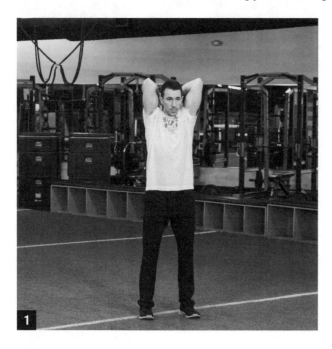

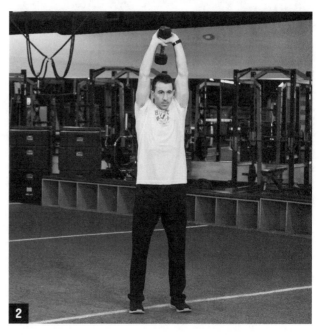

SETUP

From a standing position, grasp a dumbbell with both hands, using a baseball grip or hands interlocked. Press the weight straight up to the ceiling and lock out your elbows. Achieve neutral spine and tighten your abs to protect your low back.

EXECUTION

Bend your elbows and slowly lower the weight behind your head, taking care not to lose your flexed ab position. When you reach the end range of your elbow flexion, push the weight further backward by extending your thoracic spine. You should feel a stretch in your lats and triceps. Hold for a moment before reversing the motion and extending the weight straight over your head.

CUES

Tight abs, thoracic extension, then press the weight overhead.

COMMON MISTAKES

- Arching the low back (protect your back!).
- Using a weight that is too heavy, which could cause shoulder or elbow distress in the bent position.

LOWER BODY PUSH

Box Stepdown

The Box Stepdown teaches hip-dominant squatting, which helps prevent low back and knee pain. It also challenges knee stability and ankle mobility. You will find that performing this exercise prior to other lower body movements improves your balance, movement patterning, and glute activation.

Start with a 4- to 5-inch elevation and work your way up as you develop movement proficiency. You are better off with a 4-inch elevation and perfect form than a 12-inch elevation and sloppy form. This exercise is not about blasting your leg muscles. It's about mastering the right movement patterns.

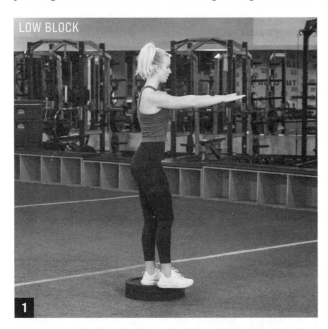

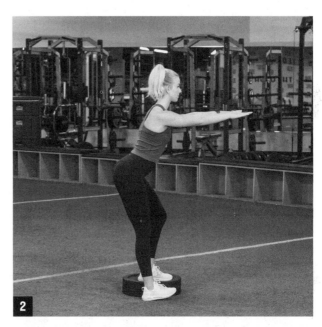

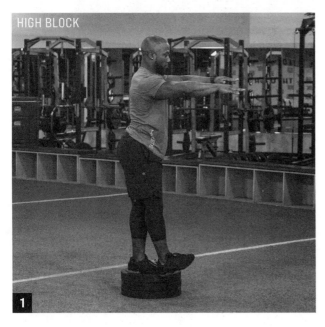

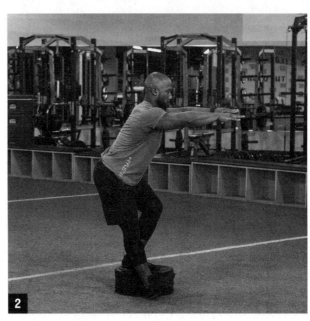

Continued on next page

SETUP

Stand on a sturdy box, bench, or stacked barbell plates—anything that will give you elevation from the ground and a sturdy base. Place one foot near the center of the box and let the other dangle off to the side. To start the movement, balance on one leg while the other is suspended.

EXECUTION

Hinge at the hips and push your butt back to initiate the movement. Straighten your arms in front of you for balance. Focus on maintaining alignment between your knee and foot from left to right. Then, continue lowering your body while lifting the toes of your suspended leg up toward the ceiling. Touch your heel to the ground without taking the weight off of your opposite leg. Pause momentarily, then drive your hips forward and stand back up straight.

CUES

Hip hinge, align knee over foot, touch heel to the ground.

COMMON MISTAKES

- Failing to hinge at the hips to start the movement, which places strain on the knee.
- Not stabilizing the loaded foot by pressing firmly into the main three points of contact (balls of your feet and heel).
- Using a box that is too high for your current skill level.

VARIATIONS

This is a vital movement, so there are no suitable variations. But, if you have trouble balancing, you can hold onto a wall or other anchor for balance. This is a skill-based movement. So even if you start out struggling, stick with it and you will progress quickly.

LOWER BODY PUSH

Spanish Squat

There are two main categories of trainees who use the Spanish Squat: powerlifters looking to get the last bit of force potential out of their knee extension efforts, and physical therapy clients recovering from knee surgery or tendinopathy. Most general population clients and healthy athletes don't utilize this one. But they are missing out. The Spanish Squat maximizes muscle force production at the very end of your knee extension range of motion, where most people are the weakest. It's a great exercise for building knee joint resilience, improving lower leg endurance, and pumping up your quadriceps.

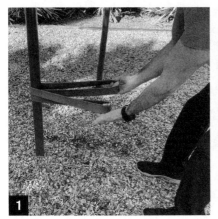
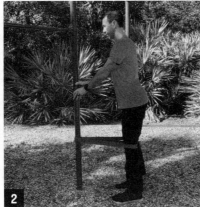
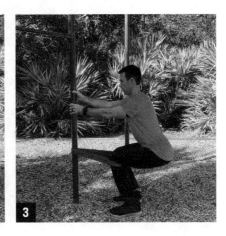

SETUP

To start, anchor a heavy loop band around a stable structure such as a weight rack or pull-up bar fixed to the wall (be careful here—make sure that anything you strap the loop to has no chance of falling on top of you when the band starts pulling). You will need to wrap the loop band around the anchor in front of you, just above knee height. The band should create two loops for you to place your feet through. After stepping through each loop, move the band up to your knee pits. Then, shuffle away from the anchor to create band tension—at least enough so that you have to consciously keep your knees locked out to prevent the band from bending them forward. If necessary, grab onto something in front of you for balance. I prefer a squat rack or pull-up bar that has been bolted to the floor. At home, the base of a tree or a strong (and trusting) partner holding the band for you can work as an anchor.

EXECUTION

Push your butt backward and squat down until your thighs are parallel with the ground, keeping your torso as upright as you can. Maintain a neutral spine (no low back rounding allowed). Pause in the bottom of the squat briefly, then stand back up. In this top position, consciously contract your glutes and quadriceps simultaneously. Your goal is to produce a maximum contraction at the top of the movement. If you do this right, your thighs will be burning after a few repetitions.

CUES

Push your butt back to lower, contract the glutes/quads hard at the top.

COMMON MISTAKES

- Getting lazy at the top of the motion and not forcefully contracting the leg muscles.
- Anchoring the loop band lopsided so that one leg receives more band resistance than the other.
- Letting the band pull your torso forward instead of keeping it upright (a mirror is beneficial here).
- Not shuffling away from your band anchor far enough to create tension against the backs of your knees.

SUBSTITUTES

It's worth purchasing your own set of loop bands if only so you can perform it. However, if you don't have access to quality loop resistance bands, you can substitute a leg extension machine. It does not have the same effect, but you can still build peak end range force potential by holding an isometric contraction with knees extended.

LOWER BODY PUSH

Goblet Squat

The Goblet Squat is easier on your low back than barbell variations, but don't be fooled. It demands forceful stabilization of your core and allows for safe, full-range squats—which all add up to a gut-busting exercise. You can perform the goblet squat with a dumbbell, kettlebell, or even a cable machine or resistance band.

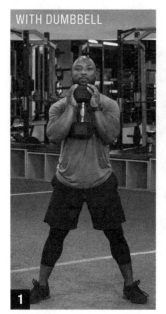
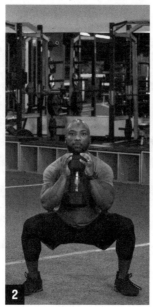
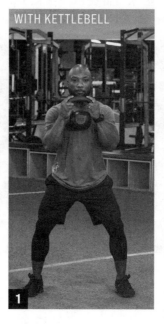
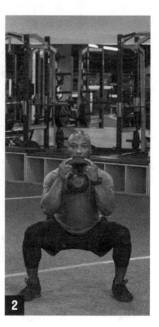

WITH DUMBBELL

WITH KETTLEBELL

SETUP

Stand with feet slightly wider than shoulder-width, toes pointed out a few degrees. Grasp a dumbbell under one of the plated sides and lift it directly in front of your chest.

EXECUTION

Pull your elbows in tight against your body, take a big breath in, and brace your core. Initiate the squat by driving your butt backward, keeping your upper body as vertical as possible. Descend until your thighs are parallel with the ground or you cannot go any lower without falling forward. Pause briefly, then stand back up, continuing to brace your core forcefully to prevent your upper body from leaning forward.

CUES

Elbows in tight, butt back, upper body upright.

COMMON MISTAKES

- Letting the weight drift away from your body, placing additional stress on your low back.
- Rounding your low back or leaning forward to get into the bottom position.
- Using too narrow of a stance, making it difficult to achieve full ROM without stressing your knees.

LOWER BODY PUSH

Dumbbell Front Squat, Heels Elevated

The Dumbbell Front Squat creates an even greater demand for upper body stabilization than the Goblet Squat. Due to the more forward position of the weights in this exercise and your heels being elevated, you should be able to get into deeper squat positions. You will also notice fatigue in your ab muscles as they contract to prevent your body from falling forward. As with all elevated heel squatting, start slow and use a slow tempo. The muscles and connective tissue surrounding your knees will be working harder. This is good for building resilient knees as long as you don't jump into the deep end too quickly.

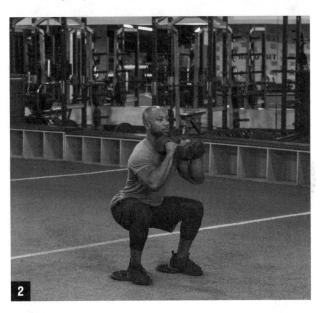

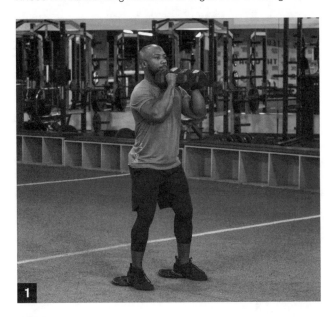

SETUP

Place two 2.5-pound barbell weights on the floor, about shoulder-width apart from one another. In a pinch, you could use a foam mat, folded yoga mat, or folded towel. Aim for heel elevation of around ½ inch. Stand with the back halves of your feet resting on the plates and the front halves on the ground. Point your toes forward unless mobility limitations force you to turn them out slightly to squat with proper form. Lift two dumbbells into the front rack position. Press the plates of each dumbbell against one another hard enough to force your chest muscles to contract.

EXECUTION

Pull your elbows in tight against your body, take a big breath in, and brace your core. Initiate the squat by driving your butt backward, keeping your upper body as vertical as possible. Continue pushing the dumbbells inward against one another. Descend until your thighs are just below parallel with the ground or you cannot go any lower without falling forward. Pause briefly, then stand back up, continuing to brace your core forcefully to prevent your upper body from leaning forward.

CUES

Elbows in tight, butt back, keep your upper body upright.

COMMON MISTAKES

- Using too high of a heel elevation, placing stress on the knees.
- Moving too fast and failing to pause at the bottom of the squat.
- Rounding your low back or leaning forward to get into the bottom position.

VARIATIONS

If you have a history of knee pain, either go very light and slow on this exercise or remove the heel elevation element. If you do not use a heel elevation, widen your stance and point your toes out far enough so that you can get into the bottom position of a squat (thighs parallel to the ground) without your upper body falling forward.

SUBSTITUTES

Goblet Squat

LOWER BODY PUSH

Bulgarian Split Squat

Think of the Bulgarian Split Squat as your new gold standard of lower body strength. To be strong at this exercise, you will need more than muscle power. It takes hip mobility, knee stability, balance, and a coordinated posterior chain.

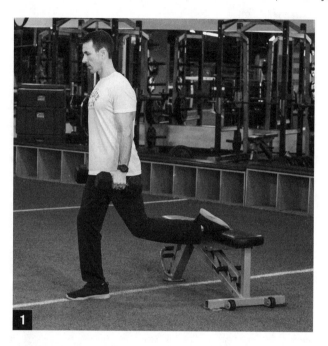

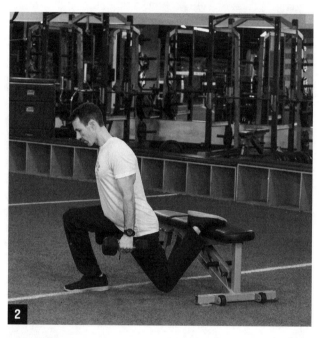

SETUP

Before adding weight to this exercise, practice anchoring one leg behind you on top of a weight bench. In the rear leg elevated position, the knee of your front leg should be directly over the middle of your foot. If your starting knee position is too far forward, it puts a strain on your knees. If your knee position is over your heel or further back, it will also stress your knee and rear hip flexor. Once you start moving, your knee will travel forward over your toes. This is OK. But getting the starting position right is vital.

Stand in front of a weight bench holding a dumbbell in each hand. Lift one leg up and backward, resting the instep of your foot against the bench. Lean forward slightly, placing more weight on your front leg and taking the stress off of your back knee.

EXECUTION

Lower your body until your front thigh is parallel with the ground. Pause briefly, then stand back up until your front knee is straight. Focus on keeping your knee in alignment with your foot—never traveling too far left or right. Perform all repetitions on one leg before switching to the opposite.

CUES

Front knee directly over foot, weight on front leg.

COMMON MISTAKES

- Placing the toes of your rear foot against the bench instead of your instep. This creates an unstable environment and can tweak your rear knee.
- Not taking enough time to get the front foot position correct before beginning.
- Placing too much weight on the back leg.

VARIATIONS

- **Contralateral Variation:** Instead of two dumbbells, hold one heavy dumbbell in the hand opposite to your front leg. This is an excellent option if you are having trouble preventing knee valgus (knee caving inward) using the standard variation. The contralateral force required to counterbalance the weight activates stabilizing muscles that help keep your front knee in proper alignment.

- **Body-Weight Variation:** Most people lack the mobility and knee stability to load up the Bulgarian Split Squat with heavy weights safely. If you are having trouble with the weighted variations, there is no shame in perfecting the body-weight-only variation before adding more load.

SUBSTITUTES

If you lack the balance required to perform even the body-weight variation of the Bulgarian Split Squat, use a standard split squat—where both feet are planted on flat ground. Perform this exercise in the same manner as described above, except you will start the exercise from a lunge position. Be careful not to slam your kneecap into the ground, which could cause a patella injury.

Contralateral Variation

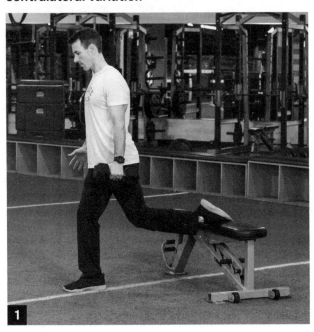

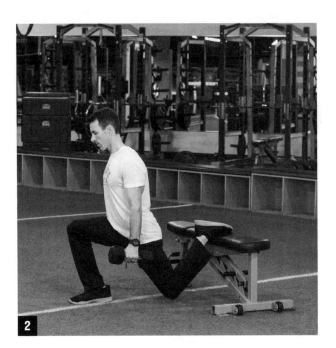

LOWER BODY PULL

Cable Pull Through

The cable pull through teaches hip hinge mechanics and is a great strength primer for lower body resistance training. The key is to make your glutes and hamstrings drive the movement—not your low back.

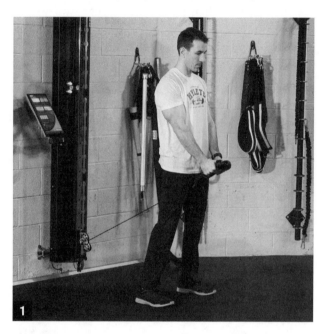

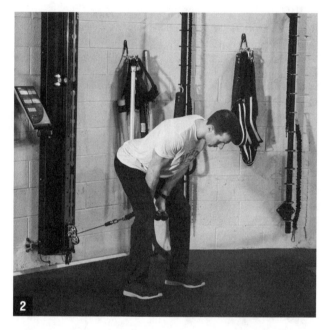

SETUP

Using a cable pulley machine, place a rope handle attachment at the bottom of the cable's anchor position near the floor. With feet shoulder-width apart, face away from the cable pulley. Position your feet close enough to the cable rope attachment that you can bend over and pick it up between your legs.

EXECUTION

Grip the rope attachment and extend your hips into the standing position, finishing with the rope attachment gripped just in front of your legs and hands touching your inner thighs. This is the top of the range of motion, but it will be your official starting point for the exercise. From here, brace your core and keep your low back in neutral position. With knees slightly bent, push your hips backward to initiate the downward movement, keeping your back straight and chin tucked. Stop the range of motion when you can no longer bend further without your low back rounding. Pause long enough to control the movement, then activate your glutes and drive

your hips forward into the standing position. Finish the movement by contracting your glutes forcefully.

CUES

Brace core, knees slightly bent, push hips back.

COMMON MISTAKES

- Overextending hips at the top of the movement and rounding back at bottom of movement.
- Gazing too far up or down, causing poor neck posture.
- Setting up too close or too far away to effectively utilize the cable's load.
- Using the low back muscles to drive the movement instead of the glutes and hamstrings.

SUBSTITUTES

If you don't have access to a cable machine, you can mimic the movement by anchoring a resistance band near the floor and using it in the same way you would a rope handle attached to a pulley.

LOWER BODY PULL

Dumbbell Romanian Deadlift

The Romanian Deadlift (RDL) is a deadlift variation that focuses on glute and hamstring activation. Unlike the traditional deadlift where the bar starts on the floor, the RDL starts from a standing position. It's easier on the low back than the conventional deadlift and effectively expands hip hinge range of motion.

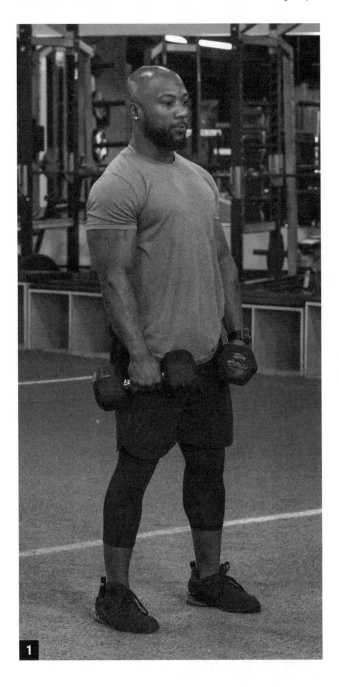

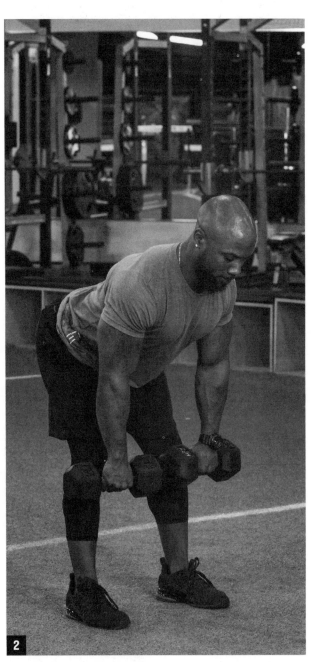

Continued on next page

SETUP

For the dumbbell variation, stand with feet shoulder-width apart, grasping two dumbbells with an overhand grip. Bend your knees slightly. Achieve neutral spine, tuck your chin, and brace your core.

EXECUTION

Initiate the movement by driving your butt backward. Allow your gaze to follow the path of your upper body as you hip hinge downward. Continue downward until the weights are just past your knees and you feel a gentle stretch in your hamstrings. Hold for a moment, then reverse the motion by driving your hips forward. Contract your glutes and hamstrings at the top of the movement, taking care not to overextend your low back by leaning backward.

CUES

Brace your core, bend your knees slightly, and push your butt back.

COMMON MISTAKES

- Overextending your neck during the eccentric phase by gazing straight ahead instead of letting your gaze follow the path of movement.
- Using the low back muscles to drive the movement instead of the glutes and hamstrings.
- Letting the low back round at the bottom and hyperextend at the top (instead of staying neutral).

VARIATIONS

- **Single Leg Dumbbell RDL:** The single leg variation involves lifting one leg off the ground and extending it behind you. This variation requires much lighter weights and is primarily a balance exercise.
- **Isometric RDL:** The Isometric RDL involves holding the bottom position of the RDL for several seconds before completing the repetition. This variation brings awareness into your body mechanics at the end range of motion.

SUBSTITUTES

- **Band Good Morning:** The Band Good Morning is a convenient at-home or travel option because it requires only the use of a single heavy loop band. To set this variation up, step onto one side of a heavy loop band with both feet. Then, grasp each side of the band outside your foot, choosing a spot on the band that provides significant tension as you stand up. Then, perform the exercise as described above. *TIP: If you want to add even more glute activation to this move, try wrapping a hip band around your legs just above the knees.*

Single Leg Dumbbell RDL

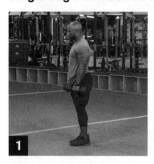
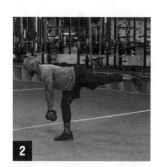

Single Leg Dumbbell RDL (Body Weight)

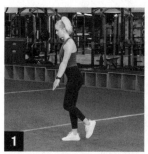
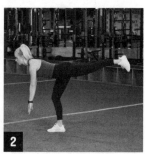

Band Good Morning

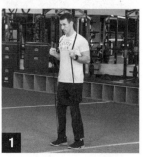
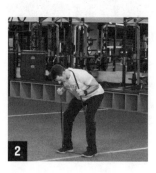

LOWER BODY PULL

Swiss Ball Leg Curl

More than any other exercise, you only get out what you put in with the Swiss Ball Leg Curl. That's because you can easily get lazy with form and cheat, and because the amount of force your hamstrings exert is up to you. The harder you press your legs into the Swiss ball, the more you will feel it. I have been doing this exercise for years, and to this day I can still create an intense burn with several concentrated repetitions. The Swiss Ball Leg Curl is my favorite knee-dominant hamstring exercise because force production is maximized at the end range of motion, where people are often weak and tight. Resistance band leg curls and machine leg curls tend to favor maximum force in the contracted position. The key to this exercise is contracting hard at the end range of motion. When executed properly, you will build hamstring power, eccentric control, and functional mobility.

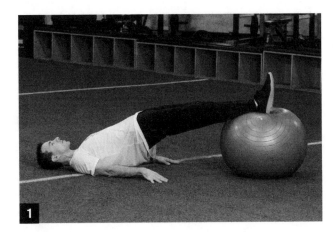

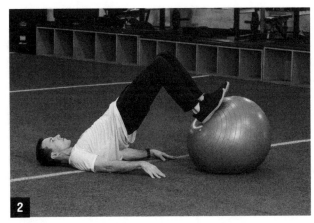

SETUP

Lie on your back with your feet elevated onto a Swiss ball. Place your hands on the ground to stabilize your body. Roll the ball directly under your calves with straight legs to set up the exercise. Though it will be tempting to flex your neck upward and watch what is going on, do your best to keep the back of your head down against the floor.

EXECUTION

Contract your glutes and extend your hips upward. Then, contract your hamstrings hard into the Swiss ball (before anything else moves). Maintaining the hamstring contraction, bring the ball closer to your body until your knees are bent to 90 degrees and the ball is under the soles of your feet. At this point, your hips will be elevated further off the ground. In this knees-bent position, check to make sure your hips are not sagging. Then slowly straighten your knees, never losing the hamstring contraction. Continue until your legs are fully straightened.

CUES

Hips high, active hamstrings, contract hard at the end range.

COMMON MISTAKES

- Failing to accurately set up the placement of your legs on the ball to begin the exercise.
- Stopping the range of motion before your knees are fully extended.
- Losing hamstring tension during the movement.
- Letting the hips sag downward in the knees-extended position.

Continued on next page

VARIATIONS

- **Single Leg Swiss Ball Curl:** For this variation, only one leg is placed on the Swiss ball while the other is planted on the ground for balance. While this version is easier to balance, it allows you to put more hamstring force into the ball. Which you'll feel.

- **Single Leg Slide Disc Curl** (not pictured): If you don't have access to a large Swiss ball (or you lack the required balance to perform it currently), you can perform a single leg curl variation with a slide disc. A paper plate works well, too. To perform this variation, plant one foot firmly on the ground with the heel of the other leg on the slide disc. Raise your hips as you would in the normal variation, then contract the hamstrings as you slide the disc through 90 degrees of knee flexion and extension.

Single-Leg Swiss Ball Curl

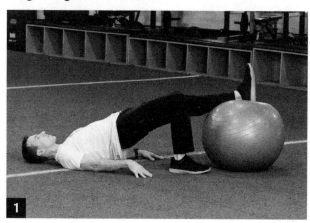

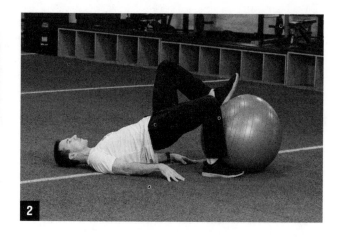

LOWER BODY PULL

Barbell Hip Thrust

The Barbell Hip Thrust will fire up your glutes unlike any other exercise. As glute training expert Bret Conteras points out, it's the lower body equivalent of a bench press—utilizing gravity and enabling three points of supportive contact for stable, compound movement. But it's not just for powerlifters and bikini competitors. If you have struggled with low back pain when performing deadlifts or other hip hinges in the past, the Barbell Hip Thrust is a solid substitute. It also works well as a muscle activator before doing hip hinge exercises to reduce low back strain. The only problem is how difficult it is to get into position. If you are lucky enough to belong to a gym with a specialized hip thruster bench, then take advantage and use that machine. If not, it's still worth the few minutes required to set this movement up with a normal weight bench. Even if you do not use the barbell variation mentioned below, you can still build muscle and endurance using only your body weight, resistance bands, and dumbbells. Start with your body weight and work up through the variations as your strength and endurance increases.

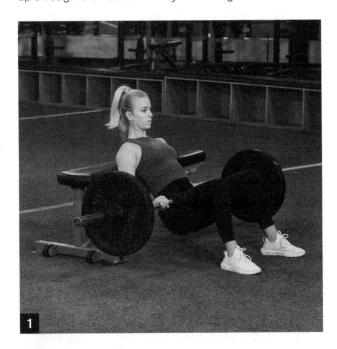

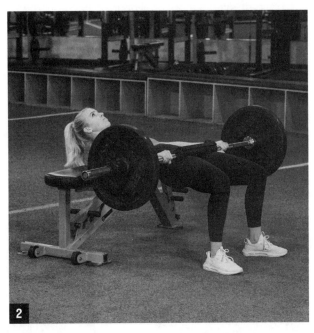

SETUP

Unlike a glute bridge, the hip thrust begins from a position of hip flexion. You can achieve this by lying perpendicular across a flat bench, with your upper back in contact with the bench. Bend your knees to 90 degrees and place your feet firmly on the ground.

EXECUTION

Push your heels into the ground and thrust your hips upward until they are in line with your knees. Forcefully contract your glutes at the top of the motion before slowly lowering your hips back down. Execution is relatively simple. The real challenge is getting into this position with a barbell or dumbbell (see variations below).

CUES

Tuck your chin and push through your heels. Squeeze your glutes at the top.

COMMON MISTAKES

- Overextending your hips at the top of the motion, stressing your low back.
- Failing to align your knees directly over your heels.
- Failing to contract your glutes at the top of the hip extension.

Continued on next page

VARIATIONS

- **Body-Weight Hip Thrust:** Start with body weight only and progress through each subsequent variation below as your strength increases.
- **Hip Band Hip Thrust:** Perform the hip thrust with a hip band looped around your legs just above your knees.
- **Dumbbell Hip Thrust:** Place a dumbbell sideways just below your waistline. Hold it in place with your hands as you perform the hip thrust.
- **Single Leg Hip Thrust (Body Weight):** Raise one leg a few inches off the ground, increasing the mechanical load on the exercising leg. This adds a balance element as well.
- **Barbell Glute Bridge:** After mastering the dumbbell hip thrust, switch to a glute bridge on flat ground. Perform this variation with a barbell anchored just below your waistline. Use both hands to keep the bar firmly in place throughout the movement. For heavy weights, use a pad or cushioned mat between the weight and your upper legs. See "Roll Up Setup" below on how to get the barbell into position.

- **Barbell Hip Thrust—Roll Up Setup:** To get the barbell in the starting position for a Barbell Hip Thrust, sit down in front of a flat bench with legs straight. Then, roll a loaded barbell over your legs, positioning it just below your hip bones. Grab the bar with both hands and thrust upward to anchor your back against the bench. You may have to shimmy around a bit to get the bar balanced and your back positioned. Because it's such a pain to get into, I recommend starting with light weight, slow tempos, and high-repetition sets.

Body-Weight Hip Thrust

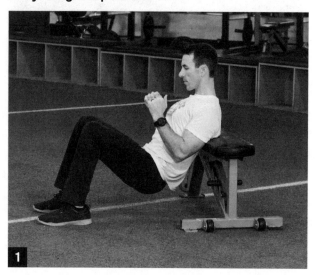
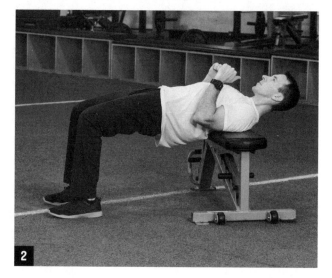

Hip Band Hip Thrust

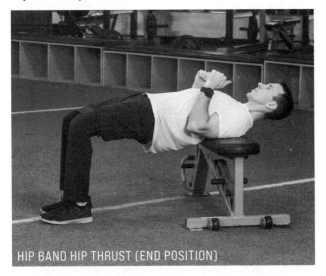

HIP BAND HIP THRUST (END POSITION)

Dumbbell Hip Thrust

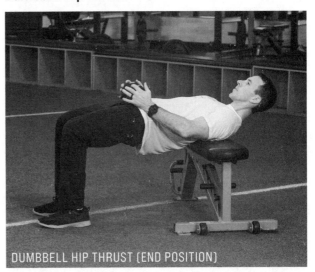

DUMBBELL HIP THRUST (END POSITION)

Single Leg Hip Thrust (Body Weight)

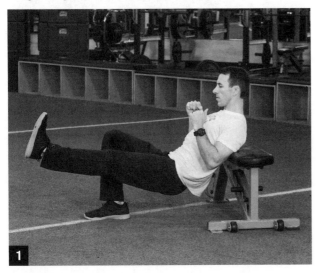

1

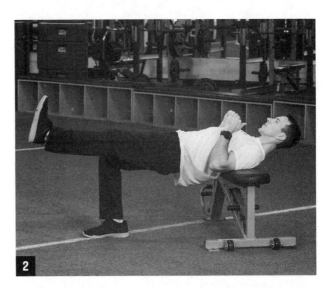

2

Barbell Glute Bridge

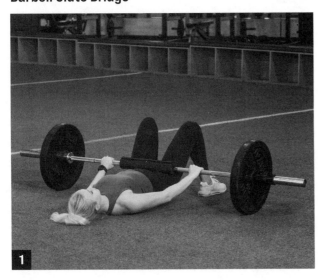

1

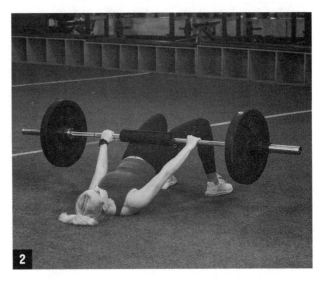

2

LOWER BODY ACCESSORY
Ankle Glides

Just as forearm tendon glides improve tendon and nerve flow through the principle of irradiation, so do ankle tendon glides for the lower leg. This exercise is deceiving because you might not feel anything during the first few reps. But after a few repetitions, if you are flexing and extending through your ankles' full range of motion, you will feel a neural stretch throughout your lower leg compartment. You will also feel fatigue in the often-neglected muscles on the front of your lower leg (e.g. tibilais anterior) that counteract the forces of the large calf muscles. This exercise provides a safe, active stretch for the calves, develops strength in the supportive muscles of the ankle, and gives a nice neural massage to your lower legs, working out kinks and knots in the tight fascia sheaths surrounding your calves. This is one exercise where I find it especially helpful to foam roll prior to loosen up muscle knots and tight fascia.

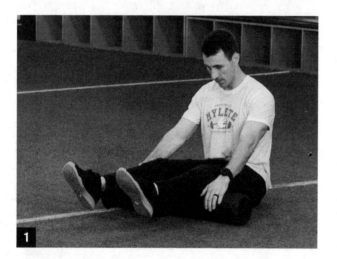
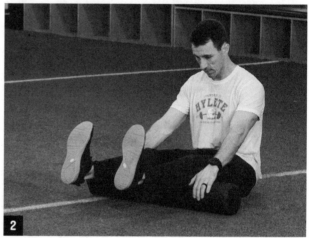

SETUP

From a seated position, place a foam roller perpendicular to your legs, anchored just below your knee pit where the gastrocnemius inserts into the knee joint. There's usually a tender spot here at the top of your calf muscles. Straighten your legs and lean forward until you can grasp the foam roller in both hands. Push down with your legs on the foam roller and simultaneously pull back gently with your arms, creating shear force that pulls against your calf and surrounding connective tissue. You may feel a tug or kink in the top of your calves from this pressure (indicating tight fascia points).

EXECUTION

Lean forward and slowly point your toes and flex your calf muscles, as if you are performing a calf raise. Hold the contraction for a moment, then reverse the motion and pull your toes toward your head, stretching your calves and contracting the muscles on the front of your shins forcefully. You should feel tension from your toes to your hips. That completes one repetition.

CUES

Point, flex.

COMMON MISTAKES

- Not fully extending and flexing the ankles (lazy repetitions).
- Failing to set up the foam roll anchor in the right position (just below your knee pits).

VARIATIONS

If you do not have access to a foam roller, you can perform this exercise from a seated position on the floor with a block or pillow placed under your knee pits to elevate your feet. This allows you to extend and flex your ankles without hitting the ground.

LOWER BODY ACCESSORY

Standing Straight Leg Calf Raise

Even if you have no desire to train your calf muscles, the ankle joint needs your attention. Weak ankles destabilize every joint that sits on top of them. In addition, training your calves and Achilles tendon to contract at maximum forces with sustained contractions can help prevent the dreaded Achilles tendinopathy—one of the most common and difficult to resolve connective tissue injuries.

Even with all the fancy calf training equipment available, I've found that body weight and a sturdy wall are still the best therapeutic tools for your lower legs. Instead of thinking of calf raises as muscle-building exercises, think of them as a way to build lower leg endurance, resilience, and athleticism. For those of you who loathe calf training, hopefully this helps.

Focus on expanding your range of motion (by actively stretching in the bottom position) and maximizing motor unit recruitment (by holding an intense isometric contraction at the top of the motion).

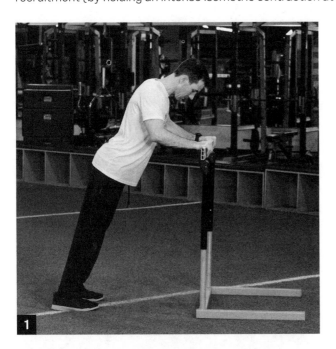

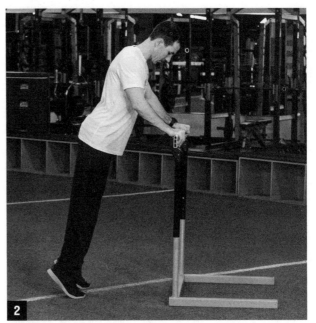

SETUP (FOR THE STANDING STRAIGHT LEG VARIATION)

Place your hands against a sturdy wall. Walk your feet backward, knees extended, until you feel a stretch in your calf muscles. Position your hips, knees, and ankles in a straight line. This is your starting position.

EXECUTION

Raise up on your toes, contracting your calf muscles forcefully at the top. Hold for a moment before slowly lowering back down. Try to incrementally expand your range of motion at the bottom of the movement with each repetition. To add resistance, push harder against the wall with your hands.

CUES

Contract hard at the top, expand at the bottom.

COMMON MISTAKES

- Not forcefully contracting your calf muscles at the top of the range of motion.
- Failing to set up the starting position in a way that actively stretches your calves during the movement.
- Using a fast-paced tempo that does not allow you to feel the exercise working.

Continued on next page

VARIATIONS

- **Standing Bent Leg Calf Raise:** This variation is performed in the same manner but with knees slightly bent. Whereas the straight leg variation targets the large gastrocnemius muscle, bent leg variations develop the underlying soleus—an important muscle for posture.

- **Standing Single Leg Calf Raise:** By raising one leg off the ground, you double the mechanical load of each repetition. If two-legged calf raises feel too easy, do this variation. Complete all repetitions on one leg before switching to the opposite.

- **Calf Raise from Block:** You can intensify body-weight calf raises by performing them with your exercising leg elevated on a block. This allows you to drop your heel below parallel, making the exercise more difficult and expanding your functional range of motion.

Standing Bent Leg Calf Raise

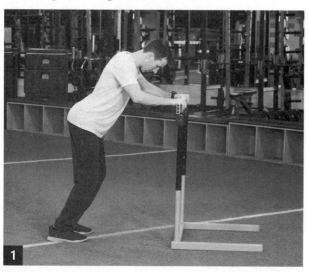
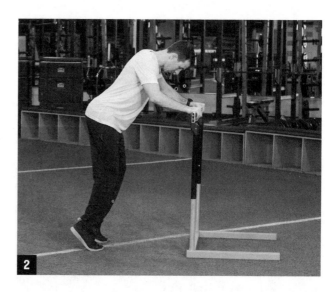

Standing Single Leg Calf Raise

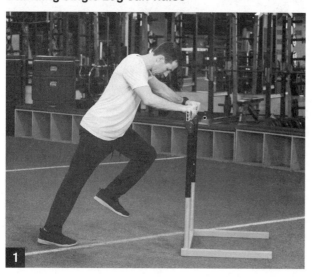
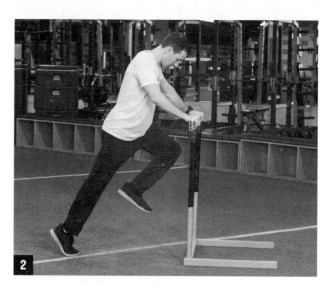

Calf Raise from Block (Straight Leg)

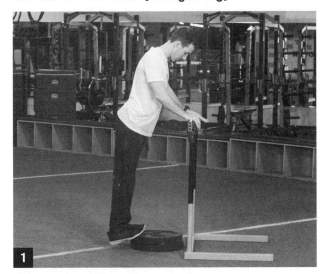

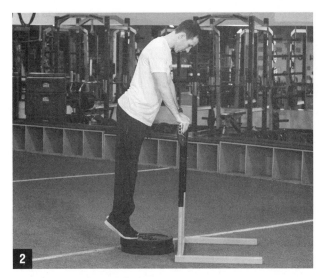

Calf Raise from Block (Single Leg, Bent Knee)

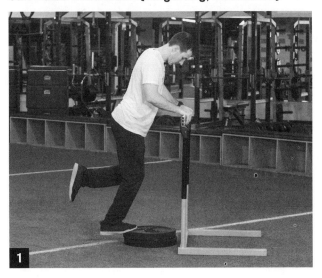

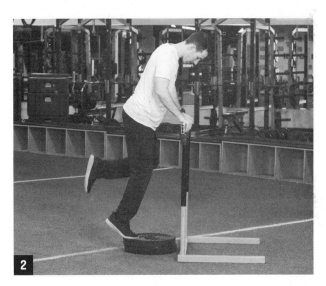

The BFB Training Program

Training is designed to improve athletes, not break them down.
— Peter Reaburn and David Jenkins, in *Training for Speed and Endurance*

Here's my challenge to the main groups that make up this book's readership:

- **Masters athlete**: A "masters athlete" is typically defined as 35 years or older, because that's when cardiovascular issues become a greater cause of morbidity. Depressing as this definition is, being a master doesn't have to slow you down. Whether you're in your 30s, 40s, 50s, 60s or beyond—this program will show you that an experienced body can make dramatic improvements in strength, muscle, joint function, and overall fitness.

- **Novice**: If you're a novice or new to intense training, challenge yourself to build skill around the movements in this program. Don't worry about how much weight you are lifting—focus solely on mastering the movements. You'll be blown away by what your body can do in just a few short weeks.

- **Recreational fitness enthusiast**: If you exercise primarily to look good and feel good, you may not value the functional side of fitness as much as an athlete would. Even so, this program will give you a rock-solid platform for building more muscle, increasing strength, losing body fat, and increasing your overall health and well-being.

- **Seasoned weightlifter**: If you are a weightlifter with constant joint and muscle pain, follow this program for at least eight weeks (two 4-week mesocycles). It will be a crucial stepping-stone to beating your weightlifting PRs without damaging your body.

- **Endurance athlete**: If you are an endurance athlete or use a cross-training approach to fitness, forgo or cut back on your normal endurance training for eight weeks while you follow this program. Afterward, you'll be more resilient as you take on long runs, swims, and bike rides.

- **Skill athlete**: Use this as your primary conditioning program for eight weeks as you continue skill work training. You'll be amazed how fast these exercises translate to better performance in your sport.

Enough preamble. Let's do this. This chapter lays out the exact warm-up and exercise routines for three different training programs: beginner, intermediate, and advanced. Here's an overview of how each training session is structured. The exact daily training templates you'll follow are listed in table form in the appendix of this book.

Workout Structure

- Dynamic Warm-up & Mobility Training (10–15 minutes)
- Resistance Training (30–45 minutes)
- Active Isolated Stretching (AIS) (2–3 minutes)

Beginner Program: Two Days per Week

The beginner program is designed for

- Complete beginners without any resistance training experience.
- Novices who have *not* been lifting weights consistently for at least six months.
- More experienced trainees who have taken a break from weightlifting or otherwise are not accustomed to lifting weights at least three days per week.
- Athletes, recreational fitness enthusiasts, or other activity-based hobbyists who want to build muscle and connective tissue health with minimal time commitment.

Although the beginner program is designed to ramp you up to three days of training per week (and eventually four days per week), you could follow this schedule indefinitely. The set and repetition schemes are designed to build tissue load tolerance and resilience, focusing on slow, controlled movements and perfect execution of the exercise. For masters athletes and seniors who want to maintain muscle mass and connective tissue with the absolute minimum effective dose of exercise, this program fits the bill. Studies show novice trainees who work out two times per week can achieve 80% of the strength gains of those who train three days per week.[283]

Example training schedule

- Day 1 (Monday): **Resistance training—full body**
- Day 2 (Tuesday): Active recovery*
- Day 3 (Wednesday): Active recovery*

- Day 4 (Thursday): Active recovery*
- Day 5 (Friday): **Resistance training—full body**
- Day 6 (Saturday): Active recovery*
- Day 7 (Sunday): Rest day (You don't have to lie around all day, but avoid high-intensity exercise that stresses your CNS or joints.)

Includes varied movement, low-intensity exercise, manual therapy, mobility training, recreational sports, and active hobbies.

Program Notes

- While the intermediate and advanced programs more aggressively address common muscle imbalances, the beginner program is primarily designed to establish healthy motor patterns, build connective tissue load tolerance, and establish a baseline level of muscle conditioning.
- Intensity must be high on each set performed to get results when training only two days per week. You need to push yourself to the brink of technical failure on each set, where you can only perform one more repetition without sacrificing form. For safety reasons, some exercises allow you to push intensity to near failure while you must be more cautious with others. For example, you don't want to reach muscular failure when performing squats because you'll fall down with a weight slamming on top of you.

Criteria for Progressing to Intermediate Program

- Completion of at least one beginner program four-week mesocycle without injury, increases in joint pain, or debilitating soreness from training two days per week. Beginners typically should complete at least two cycles (eight weeks total) of the beginner program before moving to the intermediate program.
- A desire to build significant muscle mass, strength, or functional movement capabilities.
- Ability to commit to three hours of training per week (one hour on three nonconsecutive days).

Intermediate Program: Three Days per Week

The intermediate program is designed for

- Experienced lifters who are not able to commit to four-day training weeks or who have not been training at least three days per week consistently for at least six months.

- Athletes or recreational fitness enthusiasts who train with other modalities a few days per week.

- Novices who have just completed the beginner program (two days per week) successfully without experiencing injuries, increases in joint pain, extreme fatigue, or debilitating soreness from training two days per week.

- Advanced trainees may also want to cycle back and forth between the intermediate program and advanced program.

Although it's designed to help you ramp up to four training days per week, many people thrive with three-day training weeks. It lowers the time commitment and gives you more total rest days, which often translates to greater increases in strength. Depending on your age, goals, and injury history you may find that the three-day training week allows you to perform your best while still feeling great outside the gym.

Example training schedule

- Day 1 (Monday): **Resistance training—lower body**
- Day 2 (Tuesday): Active recovery*
- Day 3 (Wednesday): **Resistance training—upper body**
- Day 4 (Thursday): Active recovery*
- Day 5 (Friday): **Resistance training—full body**
- Day 6 (Saturday): Active recovery*
- Day 7 (Sunday): Rest day (You don't have to lie around all day, but avoid high-intensity exercise that stresses your CNS or joints.)

Includes varied movement, low-intensity exercise, manual therapy, mobility training, recreational sports, and active hobbies.

Criteria for Progressing to Advanced Program

- Baseline level of comfort with the exercises and repetition schemes (you feel relatively comfortable performing the movements listed in the intermediate program).

- Completion of at least one four-week cycle of the intermediate program without injury, increases in joint pain, extreme fatigue, or debilitating soreness from training three days per week. Novices who advanced through the beginner program should also complete at least two cycles of the intermediate program before starting the advanced program.

- A desire to build significant muscle mass, strength, and functional movement capabilities.

- Ability to commit to four hours of training per week (one-hour sessions four days per week).

Advanced Program

The advanced program is designed for

- Experienced lifters who have been training at least three days per week consistently for at least six months.

- Trainees who have just completed the intermediate program successfully without experiencing injuries, increases in joint pain, extreme fatigue, or debilitating soreness from training three days per week.

Example training schedule

Although you can schedule your training days and off days to fit your schedule each week, I recommend the following schedule:

- Day 1 (Monday): **Resistance training—upper body**
- Day 2 (Tuesday): **Resistance training—lower body**
- Day 3 (Wednesday): Active recovery*
- Day 4 (Thursday): **Resistance training—upper body**
- Day 5 (Friday): **Resistance training—lower body**
- Day 6 (Saturday): Active recovery*
- Day 7 (Sunday): Rest day (You don't have to lie around all day, but avoid high-intensity exercise that stresses your CNS or joints.

Includes varied movement, low-intensity exercise, manual therapy, mobility training, recreational sports, and active hobbies.

This setup allows for two or three days of connective tissue healing between joint-specific training days and full muscle recovery between sessions, and it still provides enough frequency to realize significant strength gains. Although you can make progress by training on two or three days per week, studies show a four-day training schedule results in more muscle growth and reduced body fat levels.[284]

For those of you who are novices or are not accustomed to training several days per week, this program will be intense. You'll find the movements challenging (especially as you learn new exercises), the workouts will test your endurance, and you'll experience some muscle soreness. For athletes and experienced lifters, this might be less overall volume than you are used to during the first few training sessions. That's OK. Remember that the goal of training isn't to destroy your body but to build it up. The success of your workout should be judged based on how well you improve from one training session to the next.

Three Days per Week

If you're ready for the advanced program but are only able to train three days per week, you can cycle through the workouts as follows:

- Week 1: Workouts ABC (e.g. Monday, Wednesday, Friday)
- Week 2: Workouts DAB
- Week 3: Workouts CDA
- Week 4: Workouts BCD

Refer to the workout routines section in the appendix to view workouts A, B, C, and D.

On this schedule, you would cycle through each workout a total of three times every four weeks. At the end of four weeks, you can move on to the next mesocycle (skipping the lighter endurance week). Because total work volume is relatively low at three sessions per week, your body likely won't need a deload week. The other option is to finish all the prescribed workouts, extending each mesocycle timeframe from four weeks to about five and a half weeks. Although you will see faster progress with a four-day training week, the advanced program can be successfully implemented on this schedule. You will just have to adjust your own calendar and timelines since each phase will take longer. Again, if possible, shoot for four sessions per week. You'll be glad you did.

Program Notes

- Each training week consists of four sessions: two upper body days and two lower body days.

- If you complete the advanced program four-week mesocycle more than once, switch up the exercises while following the same template for movement category selection.

- If you find yourself overthinking the repetition speeds, take a step back and look at the intention of the exercise. Is it slow and controlled all the way through? Slow only on the eccentric phase with a faster concentric phase? Or is it a faster, more natural tempo with one-second rep speeds to build strength? If you understand the intention of the exercise, you'll be able to successfully complete the set even if the rep speeds aren't perfect. Remember that these metrics serve as guidelines only. Perfection is not required.

Workout Routines

- Beginner Program: 2 Days per Week, page 293
- Intermediate Program: 3 Days per Week, page 295
- Advanced Program: 4 Days per Week, page 298

What's Next?

After you complete the advanced program, you have a few options:

1. **Do it again.** Repeat the 4-week training block at least once (for a total of eight weeks). There's nothing wrong with repeating it continually. It's designed for that very purpose. You'll find that with each subsequent cycle, your movement skill has improved and you're able to safely increase the load—which means a greater metabolic response, increased strength, and better results. During each subsequent cycle, you can also play with exercise alternatives, further challenging your body by adding new and different movement challenges.

2. **Repeat and modify.** Another option is to repeat the program with some modifications to suit your needs. You can keep the idea of goal-specific, themed weeks, but change up other factors like exercise selection, training frequency, or set/rep/rest schemes.

3. **Cycle up and down the other training programs.** Depending on your goals, you may want to alternate between the two-, three-, and four-day training plans.

4. **Move on to another program or type of training.** The goal of this book isn't to chain you to one type of training (and thinking). It's to show you the principles that allow you to customize a program for yourself when injuries, pain, limitations, and other individual factors change the dynamic. My ultimate hope is for you to eventually follow a more intuitive fitness program without all the micromanagement, using your knowledge of corrective exercise programming to adapt as necessary.

Building Your Workout—Customizable Training Templates

You can build your own custom program around the Built from Broken principles. When assembling your periodized training schedule, prioritize these principles:

1. **Vary your training intensity and repetition schemes from week to week.** This is proven to produce better results than simple linear progression. Example repetition scheme for four-week mesocycle:
   - **Week 1:** Connective tissue remodeling: 2× 7 reps, 5151 tempo
   - **Week 2:** Hypertrophy with heavy slow resistance training (HSR): 3× 8–12 reps, 3131 tempo
   - **Week 3:** Strength training: 3× 5–7 reps, 3111 tempo
   - **Week 4:** Neuromuscular endurance training: 3× 15 reps, 1010 tempo
   - Repeat

2. **Incorporate all the major training approaches that address muscle strength, size, endurance, and connective tissue health.** This includes

   - Heavy resistance that you can only complete 5–7 times before technical failure

   - Hypertrophy-focused training in the 8–12 repetition range

   - Slow, eccentric-biased movement and HSR with rep speeds of 3–5 seconds

   - Muscular endurance training with 15–20 repetitions per set

   - Power and agility training with a focus on low-repetition sets of explosive movements with longer rest periods

   NOTE: Don't try to train all these styles at once.

3. **Deload.** Every four to eight weeks, strategically reduce the overall load (especially if you have been training with heavy weights).

4. **Prioritize corrective exercise.** Don't fall into the trap of thinking you don't need corrective exercise because you no longer have pain. And don't use corrective exercise only when you're hurt. Make it a priority. The most common weak points that require some extra attention include the shoulder rotator cuff, upper back, entire posterior chain (hamstrings, glutes, low back), and wrist extensors and wrist supinators (rotating your hand to pinky side). Commonly tight muscles that create imbalances include the hamstrings, hip flexors, thoracic spine, anterior shoulder complex, lats, and wrist flexors.

5. **Use a dynamic warm-up before each workout.** Spend at least five minutes working on dynamic stretches that target your full body, with special attention to joint systems you'll be working that day.

6. **Incorporate nontraditional exercises that challenge core stability, balance, coordination, and endurance.** Train like an athlete. Be wary of machines and isolation movements. Make the bulk of your training compound movements with free weight resistance or those that use your own body weight as resistance.

Workout Routine

- Beginner Program: 2 Days per Week (Build Your Own), page 302
- Intermediate Program: 3 Days per Week (Build Your Own), page 304
- Advanced Program: 4 Days per Week (Build Your Own), page 307

At-Home and Travel Training

At-Home Training Plan—Minimalist Equipment

For the at-home training plan below, you will need the following equipment:

- Exercise band set
- Hip band
- 1 light kettlebell
- 1 heavy kettlebell
- Set (2) of light dumbbells
- Foam roller or Swiss ball
- Box, chair, or stool
- Stopwatch

At-Home Exercise Routine, page 311

Travel Training Plan

When traveling or otherwise stuck without exercise equipment, you can still get a solid training session in if you have the following:

- Exercise band set
- Hip band
- Box, chair, or stool
- Stopwatch

Travel Exercise Routine, page 315

SETTING UP THE DOMINOS

Success is sequential, not simultaneous.

—Gary Keller, founder of Keller Williams and author of *The One Thing*

Success is sequential, not simultaneous. Nowhere is this truer than in fitness. When you see someone who has achieved the peak of their physical potential, it's easy to assume they won the genetic lottery or somehow developed all the tools necessary to self-actualize in one shining moment. But for most, even for athletes at the peak of the bell curve in terms of physical gifts, success was built slowly and sequentially.

Before Adam Archuleta was a first-round pick in the 2001 NFL Draft who went on to play seven seasons in the National Football League, he was a skinny high schooler who couldn't get the attention of any college recruiters.

If you've ever seen Archuleta, or watched him play, that's hard to imagine. At 26 years old, he was bench pressing 531 pounds, squatting over 630 pounds, leaping 39 inches off the floor, and running the 40-yard dash in 4.37 seconds with a neck wider than the crown of his head. But he wasn't born that way. And it didn't happen all at once.

While still in high school, Archuleta developed a six-year plan to reach the NFL under the tutelage of a local trainer. The first step focused solely on building strength in his hamstrings—the most important muscle for speed and lower body power. Then, he worked on building mass so he could compete with the big boys. Finally, he switched gears to developing maximum power using plyometrics and painful electrical stimulation sessions. When he was drafted into the NFL, Archuleta was called the new "prototype" of the NFL physique.[285] People assumed he was a genetic phenom, but the truth is he built his body up using a long-term, disciplined, sequential training plan.

Before Arnold Schwarzenegger was the Terminator, he was Mr. Universe. Before moving to the U.S., he was an ambitious young Austrian with the dream of dominating the bodybuilding world, becoming a famous actor, and eventually going into politics. Arnold knew before any of that could happen, he needed to develop a base of strength to build his body (and career) on top of. So before becoming a bodybuilder, he spent years competing as a powerlifter. This early base of strength allowed him to build the Herculean physique we all have burned into our minds, which earned him a ticket to America where he became Mr. Universe, which he parlayed into one of the most successful acting careers of all time, businesses opportunities, and eventually the seat as governor of California.

When you dig into the lives of people who have achieved massive success, you see the same sequential process. Especially in fitness. Maybe you don't have aspirations of being an NFL defensive back or the Terminator, but the model of long-term, sequential, step-by-step focus still applies. In Gary Keller's best-selling book *The One Thing*, he calls this the domino effect.[286] Not only can dominos be arranged in a sequence to topple each other over in mass quantities, "a single domino is capable of bringing down another domino that is actually 50 percent larger.… Getting extraordinary results is all about creating a domino effect in your life," says Keller.

The implications of domino physics are powerful. The trick is to start with the end in mind, work your way backward to the *first* domino, then whack away at it until it falls. This makes it easier to knock over the next domino, and the next, and so on. This concept works in the field of goal achievement with mathematical predictability. But most people don't have the vision necessary to see the dominos, nor the discipline to stay focused on the first domino. Instead, they skip to the 10th domino without adequately mastering the fundamentals. This is usually driven by ego or impatience.

To rebuild your body from the ground up, you have to start at the ground. While it may seem painstaking to use lighter weights and go back to mastering basic movement patterns like the row and lunge, you'll quickly see that this creates an opportunity for exponential progress. Building core stability, mobility, and connective tissue resilience will translate to more strength, a better body, and pain-free movement faster than you might think. It just takes a little vision, and enough discipline to do the first thing first. Then the next thing, then the next. Do this long enough to see your first substantial leap in progress, and you'll be hooked.

Built from Broken Dominoes

1. Take the road less traveled by.

Two roads diverged in a wood, and I—
I took the one less traveled by,
And that has made all the difference.

— "The Road Not Taken," by Robert Frost

Just for a moment, scrap all the weightlifting dogma, single-minded ideologies, and groupthink that you've been exposed to on your fitness journey. While you're at it, chuck your ego out the window and think about what you are really trying to accomplish long-term. Develop a clear picture of what kind of body you want to inhabit a year from now, 5 years from now, 10, 20…. Got it?

Now, think about your friends, acquaintances at the gym, and even elite fitness professionals of a certain age. Are they pain-free? Or have they damaged the vehicle that is their body beyond repair? The sad truth is that most people don't make much progress on their quest to attain peak fitness levels. If they're lucky, they will plateau and maintain a stable level of strength and function (for a while, at least). But often, people start going downhill once they hit middle age. First slowly, then quickly when a precipitating event such as an injury knocks them backward. This can be avoided, but it requires the uncomfortable acceptance that you have glaring weaknesses. Possibly the biggest mistake you can make is to avoid weaknesses instead of addressing them. Develop a mindset around the idea that a chain is only as strong as its weakest link, and apply it accordingly when you exercise.

If you don't believe that the well-worn path of heavy lifting, boring cardio workouts, bloated egos, painful joints, and declining mobility is the best path to travel on, then take the road less traveled by. It'll make all the difference.

2. Weave habits into your daily routine that support optimal posture, mobility, and varied movement.

Here are three of the most important habits to implement for a pain-free, mobile lifestyle:

- **Work on your posture:** This means constantly striving to stay aware and improve the way you sit, stand, and move. Awareness is key. If you can get to the point that you recognize when you're slumped over, fixing it becomes that much easier.

- **Move in the morning:** Build a habit of moving first thing in the morning. It doesn't have to be a formal exercise routine—just something that brings movement into your body and greases your joints. A short walk, a stretching routine, a bike ride, or a quick circuit of lightweight resistance movements. (Refer to the Morning Mobility Routine listed in the appendix.)

- **Commit to the walking habit:** Carve out 10–20 minutes every day for walking. Make it interesting so you'll be more likely to prioritize it. Listen to your favorite music, an audiobook, or find a spot in nature you enjoy being in.

3. Establish your fitness priorities.

Though you don't always act like it, being healthy (specifically, NOT in a state of disease) is always your number one priority. Without a minimum of overall health, nothing else really matters. For those of you who have suffered a life-changing injury, you know how quickly such an event can bring your real priorities into focus. You can quickly go from worrying about your body fat levels to just wanting the ability to walk again. There's a certain level of overall health and functional movement capability that is so fundamental to life that everything else is secondary. This includes being able to move freely through your day without pain, being able to walk moderate distances, and having the ability to bend and lift small objects.

4. Lay out a periodized exercise program.

This is where you turn pro. It takes surprisingly little time and attention to set up a periodized training plan. It's something you can do quarterly or less often. The real challenge is simply remembering to do it and preventing yourself from drifting through the weeks and months without checking in. Instead of relying on your memory, leverage the power of systems. I've found two simple tactics that virtually guarantee the successful implementation of a periodized plan.

First, set a reminder. It doesn't matter if you use a calendar, app, or journal. Just set a reminder somewhere you won't miss it. Assuming you've established at least an eight-week plan after reading this book, set yourself a reminder for exactly eight weeks from now. When the date arrives, review your progress and spend some time planning out what you want to accomplish for the next eight weeks, or whatever long-term time range works for you.

Second, track your workouts. You can write down every set and rep if you want, or just simply create a journal of when you have exercised with a few highlights. All of the dramatic weight-loss-transformation clients I've coached in the last several years (i.e. 80+ pounds weight loss) were dedicated to tracking their nutrition and fitness activity. While many of them only micromanaged nutrition in the beginning, all of them kept a detailed exercise log.

Third, be adaptable. Don't force-feed your body exercises it isn't ready for or needs a break from. As you familiarize yourself with new exercises and understand their purpose, you'll be able to discern when it makes sense to skip a movement or find an alternative.

5. Resolve painful joints.

Stop the bleeding before going any further. You now know that working through joint pain means that you are actively fraying connective tissue fibers and damaging nerves. It's not OK to work through joint pain. Toughing it out is dumb. Plain and simple. So before worrying about your beach body or how you will deadlift 600 pounds, work on establishing a baseline of pain-free movement capability.

6. Prioritize muscle imbalance correction.

Virtually everyone you meet at the gym is building a house of cards. Impressive lifts and piles of muscle built on top of imbalances is the rule, not the exception. And it's a recipe for imminent disaster. Unless you address muscle imbalances first, any fitness improvements you make will be short-term only.

7. Improve motor control in the basic human movements.

You should be able to push, pull, squat, lunge, hinge, rotate, and carry objects under load without pain or injury. If you can't do all of these movements, you're at risk of developing debilitating pain. I've seen powerlifters who can't balance on one leg. Lifters who can bench press 300+ pounds but can't touch their toes. Long-distance runners who are not able to perform a simple weighted row without their shoulders dumping forward. Some specialty athletes know about these glaring weaknesses and they don't care because it doesn't seem to affect their performance.

What these athletes don't realize is that all these categories are interrelated. Lunging requires hip stability, which transfers over to more power in bilateral movements like the squat. The ability to stabilize your core in various positions translates to more power-generating capabilities. Upper back strength is not only important for rowing and pressing but also for maintaining optimal running posture. These seven movements make up the complete human movement experience. So it makes sense to be proficient at all of them.

8. Build a scaffolding of strong, resilient connective tissue.

Joint health isn't something that comes naturally then declines gradually over time. You can influence it just like you can influence muscle strength and endurance. Traditional muscle building plans and steady-state aerobic exercise like running and biking are not sufficient. Make eccentric-biased strength training, HSR, endurance exercise, and even power and agility training part of your routine. Value your collagen health as much as you value muscle health. Not only will your body work better, you will be more resilient to injury and your body will age better.

9. Establish a baseline of full body mobility.

The science of stretching, as it turns out, is quite a stretch. To say the least, static stretching underperforms in clinical studies. But that doesn't mean mobility isn't important. It just means that you need to change the way you think about it. Prioritize dynamic stretching and full body movements that challenge and expand your pain-free ranges of motion. This should be planned, tracked, and reviewed as diligently as weight training or sport-specific exercise. You don't have to become a yogi or master the split. You just need enough mobility to keep your body in alignment at rest and while exercising.

10. Build foundational (and functional) strength.

Functional strength doesn't mean you can lift a kettlebell over your head with eyes closed while standing on a BOSU ball. It means strength that directly translates to real life. You may not have the sport-specific needs of an athlete, but you should still train like one. You never know when your body will be called into action. It could be something dramatic like lifting a dresser off your neighbor's dog, or as simple as twisting to catch a vase before it topples and shatters on the floor. More commonly, your body will have to protect itself against accidents and falls that lead to injury. Fitness becomes a lot more fun once you start seeing your body this way. When you look for the carryover of exercise into real life, it's not hard to find. This reinforces the *why* of fitness. Even if all you care about is looking good naked, challenging your body with functional movements is the best way to protect your ability to continue exercising without injuries and setbacks that put you on the sidelines.

The Final Domino

I keep a running list of commonalities among the weight loss transformation clients I've worked with over the years. I've always been fascinated by what it takes to make that kind of shift. Losing even 10 to 15 pounds is a victory for someone who is overweight and wants to change that. But losing 70 or 80 pounds is absolutely life altering. When I get the opportunity to speak with someone who has achieved that kind of transformation, I always ask: "How has this changed your life?" The answers would knock you out of your chair. One particularly memorable client came to us after her doctor recommended a double knee replacement. She suffered from bilateral knee arthritis and could barely get around. She was more than 100 pounds overweight, and had been for most of her adult life.

To say this client was motivated to lose weight is an understatement. (Which, by the way, is another commonality among all dramatic transformation clients I've interviewed. In every case, a precipitating event like an injury or poor health report jolted them into action.) Fast-forward a year later, and this client had dropped over 80 pounds. And kept it off.

What I found most memorable about her was how much a student of fitness and nutrition she became during her weight loss journey, and how relaxed and intuitive she was about managing her health several months later when we caught up. In the beginning, she journaled every meal, tracked every workout, experimented with new healthy recipes and read newsletters to stay informed on the latest in exercise science. As time went on, she moved to a less restrictive way of eating and moving. She used her historical records as templates, sure, but there was also an element of intuition in maintaining her results.

In almost all cases of major body transformations, there is a transition where the client moves from micromanagement to macromanagement. They use their knowledge and experience almost like a background operating system to maintain their results. Since tracking every calorie and counting every second of every repetition tempo isn't sustainable, I believe this process is fundamental to achieving remarkable results that stick.

Numbers to Leave Numbers

The chess prodigy and martial artist Josh Waitzkin describes this process in his book *The Art of Learning*. He refers to it as "numbers to leave numbers," where technical information is integrated into what feels like natural intelligence. Waitzkin uses the example of a novice chess player's first lesson. Initially, the player will count the values of each chess piece in their heads or on their fingers before making their move. "In time, they will stop counting," Waitzkin explains. "The pieces will achieve a more flowing and integrated value system…. What was once seen mathematically is now felt intuitively."[287]

I believe that internalizing the principles in this book and mastering the movements recommended will provide results not only over the few weeks you follow the program but for a lifetime. This is why reading books is more effective for learning than reading short articles. The case studies, lessons, and multiple angles of explanation in a well-written book allow for a thorough understanding of the topic. Short, pithy blog articles may give you the same advice, but the impact isn't the same. It's why professional athletes break down movements of their sport into the most basic components, mastering them one at a time. If at any point during this book you have asked yourself why such a granular level of detail is described, it's because I believe a deep understanding of the component parts is necessary to see the whole picture. This deep understanding is also needed to graduate to a more intuitive, sustainable way of moving through life.

You've made it through a lot of dense reading material. So you've earned the right to take a break from journal articles and metastudies. Avoid the trap of information overload, where you are frozen in place by the infinite variety of opinions on the best ways to improve fitness. For the next four to eight weeks, focus on applying the principles on these pages. There is much more to fitness and longevity than can be captured in one book. But for right now, focus on action. Jump in with both feet and start rebuilding.

Conclusion

Thank you for taking the time to read *Built from Broken*. This book has been a passion project spanning the last several years. I hope my enthusiasm and curiosity for the subject comes through in this text. And I hope you have gained insight that will help you prevent injuries, build stronger joints, and use your body to its full potential for years to come.

If you enjoyed this book, I would love to hear from you. Feel free to share your questions or notes about your progress by emailing **help@saltwrap.com**. You can also help support the book by leaving an honest review on Amazon .com or anywhere *Built from Broken* is sold.

About SaltWrap: I founded SaltWrap to serve as an online resource for managing injuries, healing with natural ingredients, and improving fitness longevity. To learn more about therapeutic sports nutrition, visit our blog at **saltwrap.com/blog**. To view our selection of natural, therapeutic sports nutrition supplements which I personally formulated, visit our store at **shop.saltwrap.com.**

Appendix: Workout Routines

BEGINNER PROGRAM: 2 Days per Week

DAY 1: Workout A — Full Body

Dynamic Warm-up Exercise	Repetitions
a Supine Drawing In	10 contractions
b Cat-Cow	20
c World's Greatest Stretch	10 rotations (each side)
d Thoracic Extension on Foam Roller	15
e Swimmer's Stretch	15
f Glute Bridge with Hip Band	20 repetitions + 10-second hold (top of last rep)
g Band High Pull Apart with External Rotation	25

Exercise	Week 1 Connective Tissue Remodeling	Week 2 Hypertrophy	Week 3 Strength	Week 4 Endurance Plus Energy Loading
Rest between sets (seconds)	60	90	120	30–60
1 Dual Dumbbell Row, Bent Over 45 Degrees	2 × 7, 5151	3 × 8–12, 3131	3 × 5–7, 3111	3 × 15, 1010
2 Incline Dumbbell Fly Press	2 × 7, 5151	3 × 8–12, 3311	3 × 5–7, 3311	3 × 15, 1010
3 Bulgarian Split Squat	2 × 7, 5151	3 × 8–12, 3131	3 × 5–7, 3111	3 × 15, 1010
4 Dumbbell Romanian Deadlift (RDL) with Hip Band	2 × 7, 5151	3 × 8–12, 3131	3 × 5–7, 3111	3 × 15, 1010
5 Cossack Squat (each side)	2 × 7, 5151	3 × 8–12, 3131	3 × 5–7, 3111	3 × 15, 1010

Active Isolated Stretching (AIS)

Cossack Squat: 2 sets of 10 repetitions, each side (2-second hold in stretched position)

DAYS 2–3: Rest/Active Recovery

Continued on next page

BEGINNER PROGRAM: 2 Days per Week *(continued)*

DAY 4: Workout B—Full Body

Dynamic Warm-up Exercise	Repetitions
a World's Greatest Stretch	10 rotations (each side)
b Hinge to Squat	15
c Glute Bridge (with Isometric Groin Squeeze)	20 repetitions + 10-second hold (top of last rep)
d Ankle Glides	20
e Band Facepull	25
f Swimmer's Stretch	15
g Forearm Tendon Glides	20

	Week 1	Week 2	Week 3	Week 4
	Connective Tissue Remodeling	Hypertrophy	Strength	Endurance Plus Energy Loading
Exercise				
Rest between sets (seconds)	60	90	120	30–60
1 Box Stepdown	3 × 10, 3131	3 × 15, 3131	3 × 10, 3111	3 × 15, 1010
2 Dumbbell Goblet Squat	2 × 7, 5151	3 × 8–12, 3111	3 × 5–7, 3111	3 × 15, 1010
3 Seated Cable High Facepull	2 × 7, 5151	3 × 8–12, 3131	3 × 5–7, 3111	3 × 15, 1010
4 Bottoms-Up Kettlebell Press	2 × 7, 5151	3 × 8–12, 3131	3 × 5–7, 3111	3 × 15, 1010
5 Single Arm Dumbbell Row, Strict Variation (Knee on Bench)	2 × 7, 5151	3 × 8–12, 3131	3 × 5–7, 3111	3 × 15, 1010

Active Isolated Stretching (AIS)

Anchored Lat Stretch: 2 sets of 10 repetitions (2-second hold in stretched position)

DAY 5–7: Rest/Active Recovery

INTERMEDIATE PROGRAM: 3 Days per Week

DAY 1: Workout A—Lower Body (Low Back/Posterior Chain Focus)

Dynamic Warm-up Exercise

		Repetitions
a	Supine Drawing In	10 contractions
b	Cat-Cow	20
c	World's Greatest Stretch	10 rotations (each side)
d	Bird Dog	20 (each side)
e	Fire Hydrant	25 (each side)
f	Glute Bridge with Hip Band	20 repetitions + 10-second hold (top of last rep)
g	Single Leg Romanian Deadlift—Body Weight	10 (each side)

		Week 1	Week 2	Week 3	Week 4
		Connective Tissue Remodeling	Hypertrophy	Strength	Endurance Plus Energy Loading
Exercise					
Rest between sets (seconds)		60	90	120	30-60
1	Cable Pull Through	2x7, 5151	3 x 8-12, 3131	3 x 5-7, 3111	3 x 15, 1010
2	Bulgarian Split Squat	2x7, 5151	3 x 8-12, 3131	3 x 5-7, 3111	3 x 15, 1010
3	Dumbbell Romanian Deadlift (RDL)	2x7, 5151	3 x 8-12, 3311	3 x 5-7, 3311	3 x 15, 1010
4	Cossack Squat (each side)	2x7, 5151	3 x 8-12, 3131	3 x 5-7, 3111	3 x 15, 1010
5	Single Leg Calf Raise from Block, Straight Knee	2x7, 5151	3 x 8-12, 3131	3 x 15, 3111	3 x 15, 1010

Active Isolated Stretching (AIS)

Cossack Squat: 2 sets of 10 repetitions, each side (2-second hold in stretched position)

DAY 2: Rest/Active Recovery

Continued on next page

INTERMEDIATE PROGRAM: 3 Days per Week *[continued]*

DAY 3: Workout B—Upper Body [Horizontal Focus]

Dynamic Warm-up Exercise	Repetitions
a Cat-Cow	20
b Band Pass Through	15
c Thoracic Extension on Foam Roller	15
d Anchored Lat Stretch	10-10-10*
e Swimmer's Stretch	15
f Pronation/Supination, Bent Elbow Variation	20 [each way]
g Band High Pull Apart with External Rotation	25

Exercise	Week 1 Connective Tissue Remodeling	Week 2 Hypertrophy	Week 3 Strength	Week 4 Endurance Plus Energy Loading
Rest between sets [seconds]	60	90	120	30-60
1 Suspension Trainer High Row with Straight Arm Eccentric**	2 x 7, 5151	3 x 8-12, 3131	3 x 5-7, 3111	3 x 15, 1010
2 Push-up Plus with Band	2 x 5-7, 5555	3 x 8-12, 1515	2 x 5-7, 5555	3 x 15, 1010
3 Incline Dumbbell Row	2 x 7, 5151	3 x 8-12, 3131	3 x 5-7, 3111	3 x 15, 1010
4 Incline Dumbbell Fly Press	2 x 7, 5551	3 x 8-12, 3311	3 x 5-7, 3311	3 x 15, 1010
5 Alternating Dumbbell Curl with Supination	2 x 7, 5151	3 x 8-12, 3131	3 x 5-7, 3111	3 x 15, 1010

Active Isolated Stretching [AIS]

Anchored Lat Stretch: 2 sets of 10 repetitions [2-second hold in stretched position]

DAY 4: Rest/Active Recovery

*10-second gentle stretch, 10 stretch pulses, 10-second stretch hold

**Perform a high row, then straighten your arms and slowly lower back to the starting position.

INTERMEDIATE PROGRAM: 3 Days per Week *(continued)*

DAY 5: Workout C—Full Body (Lower Anterior Chain + Shoulder Stability)

Dynamic Warm-up Exercise	Repetitions
a World's Greatest Stretch	10 rotations (each side)
b Hinge to Squat	15
c Glute Bridge (with Isometric Groin Squeeze)	20 repetitions + 10-second hold (top of last rep)
d Ankle Glides	20
e Band High Pull Apart with External Rotation	25
f Swimmer's Stretch	15
g Forearm Tendon Glides	20

Exercise	Week 1 Connective Tissue Remodeling	Week 2 Hypertrophy	Week 3 Strength	Week 4 Endurance Plus Energy Loading
Rest between sets (seconds)	60	90	120	30–60
1 Box Stepdown	3 x 10, 3131	3 x 15, 3131	3 x 10, 3111	3 x 15, 1010
2 Dumbbell Goblet Squat	2 x 7, 5151	3 x 8–12, 3131	3 x 5–7, 3111	3 x 15, 1010
3 Seated Cable High Facepull	2 x 7, 5151	3 x 8–12, 3131	3 x 5–7, 3111	3 x 15, 1010
4 Bottoms-Up Kettlebell Press	2 x 7, 5151	3 x 8–12, 3131	3 x 5–7, 3111	3 x 15, 1010
5 Single Arm Dumbbell Row, Strict Variation (Staggered Stance)	2 x 7, 5151	3 x 8–12, 3131	3 x 5–7, 3111	3 x 15, 1010

Active Isolated Stretching (AIS)

Pigeon Stretch: 2 sets of 10 repetitions, each side (2 second hold in stretched position)

DAYS 6–7: Rest/Active Recovery

ADVANCED PROGRAM: 4 Days per Week

DAY 1: Workout A — Lower Body (Low Back/Posterior Chain Focus)

Dynamic Warm-up Exercise	Repetitions
a Supine Drawing In	**10 contractions**
b Cat-Cow	**20**
c World's Greatest Stretch	**10 rotations (each side)**
d Bird Dog	**20 (each side)**
e Fire Hydrant	**25 (each side)**
f Glute Bridge with Hip Band	**20 repetitions + 10-second hold (top of last rep)**
g Single Leg Romanian Deadlift—Body Weight	**10 (each side)**

	Week 1	Week 2	Week 3	Week 4
	Connective Tissue Remodeling	Hypertrophy	Strength	Endurance Plus Energy Loading
Exercise				
Rest between sets (seconds)	60	90	120	30–60
1 Cable Pull Through	2 x 7, 5151	3 x 8–12, 3131	3 x 5–7, 3111	3 x 15, 1010
2 Bulgarian Split Squat	2 x 7, 5151	3 x 8–12, 3131	3 x 5–7, 3111	3 x 15, 1010
3 Dumbbell Romanian Deadlift (RDL)*	2 x 7, 5151	3 x 8–12, 3311	3 x 5–7, 3311	3 x 15, 1010
4 Cossack Squat (each side)	2 x 7, 5151	3 x 8–12, 3131	3 x 5–7, 3111	3 x 15, 1010
5 Single Leg Calf Raise from Block, Straight Knee	2 x 7, 5151	3 x 8–12, 3131	3 x 15, 3111	3 x 15, 1010

Active Isolated Stretching (AIS)

Cossack Squat: 2 sets of 10 repetitions, each side (2-second hold in stretched position)

Weeks 1–2: use hip band variation (band anchored above knees).

ADVANCED PROGRAM: 4 Days per Week *(continued)*

DAY 2: Workout B—Upper Body (Horizontal Focus)

Dynamic Warm-up Exercise	Repetitions
a World's Greatest Stretch	10 rotations (each side)
b Band Pass Through	15
c Thoracic Extension on Foam Roller	15
d Anchored Lat Stretch	10-10-10*
e Swimmer's Stretch	15
f Pronation/Supination, Bent Elbow Variation	20 (each way)
g Band High Facepull	25

	Week 1	Week 2	Week 3	Week 4
	Connective Tissue Remodeling	Hypertrophy	Strength	Endurance Plus Energy Loading
Exercise				
Rest between sets (seconds)	60	90	120	30-60
1 Suspension Trainer High Row with Straight Arm Eccentric**	2 x 7, 5151	3 x 8-12, 3131	3 x 5-7, 3111	3 x 15, 1010
2 Push-up Plus with Band	2 x 5-7, 5555	3 x 8-12, 1515	2 x 5-7, 5555	3 x 15, 1010
3 Incline Dumbbell High Row	2 x 7, 5151	3 x 8-12, 3131	3 x 5-7, 3111	3 x 15, 1010
4 Incline Dumbbell Fly Press	2 x 7, 5551	3 x 8-12, 3311	3 x 5-7, 3311	3 x 15, 1010
5 Alternating Dumbbell Curl with Supination	2 x 7, 5151	3 x 8-12, 3131	3 x 5-7, 3111	3 x 15, 1010

Active Isolated Stretching (AIS)

Anchored Lat Stretch: 2 sets of 10 repetitions (2-second hold in stretched position)

DAY 3: Rest/Active Recovery

*10-second gentle stretch, 10 stretch pulses, 10-second stretch hold
** Perform a high row, then straighten your arms and slowly lower back to the starting position.

Continued on next page

ADVANCED PROGRAM: 4 Days per Week *(continued)*

DAY 4: Workout C—Lower Body [Knee/Anterior Chain Focus]

Dynamic Warm-up Exercise	Repetitions
a Supine Drawing In	10 contractions
b Cat-Cow	20
c World's Greatest Stretch	10 rotations (each side)
d Bird Dog	20 (each side)
e Hinge to Squat	15
f Glute Bridge (with Isometric Groin Squeeze)	20 repetitions + 10-second hold (top of last rep)
g Ankle Glides	20

Exercise	Week 1 Connective Tissue Remodeling	Week 2 Hypertrophy	Week 3 Strength	Week 4 Endurance Plus Energy Loading
Rest between sets (seconds)	60	90	120	30–60
1 Box Stepdown	3 x 10, 3131	3 x 15, 3131	3 x 10, 3111	3 x 15, 1010
2 Spanish Squat	2 x 10, 5555	3 x 8–12, 3333	3 x 15, 1115	3 x 20, 1010
3 Swiss Ball Leg Curl	2 x 5–7, 5555	3 x 8–12, 3311	3 x 10, 3111	3 x 20, 1010
4 Dumbbell Goblet Squat	2 x 7, 5151	3 x 8–12, 3111	3 x 5–7, 3111	3 x 15, 1010
5 Single Leg Calf Raise from Block, Bent Knee	2 x 7, 5151	3 x 8–12, 3131	3 x 15, 3111	3 x 15, 1010

Active Isolated Stretching (AIS)

Pigeon Stretch: 2 sets of 10 repetitions, each side (2-second hold in stretched position)

ADVANCED PROGRAM: 4 Days per Week [continued]

DAY 5: Workout D – Upper Body [Shoulder Stability Focus]

Dynamic Warm-up Exercise	Repetitions
a Band Pass Through	15
b Thoracic Extension on Foam Roller	15
c Anchored Lat Stretch	10-10-10
d Swimmer's Stretch	15
e Forearm Tendon Glides	25
f Band High Pull Apart with External Rotation	25
g Scapular Pull-up	15

	Week 1	Week 2	Week 3	Week 4
	Connective Tissue Remodeling	Hypertrophy	Strength	Endurance Plus Energy Loading
Exercise				
Rest between sets [seconds]	60	90	120	30-60
1 Seated Cable High Facepull	2 x 7, 5151	3 x 8-12, 3131	3 x 5-7, 3111	3 x 15, 1010
2 Scapula Plane Dumbbell Raise	2 x 7, 5151	3 x 8-12, 3131	3 x 5-7, 3111	3 x 15, 1010
3 Single Arm Dumbbell Row, Strict Variation [Split Stance]	2 x 7, 5151	3 x 8-12, 3131	3 x 5-7, 3111	3 x 15, 1010
4 Bottoms-Up Kettlebell Press	2 x 7, 5151	3 x 8-12, 3131	3 x 5-7, 3111	3 x 15, 1010
5 Reverse Grip Cable Pulldown	2 x 7, 5151	3 x 8-12, 3131	3 x 5-7, 3111	3 x 15, 1010

Active Isolated Stretching [AIS]

Scapular Pull-up: 2 sets of 10 repetitions [2-second hold in stretched position]

DAYS 6–7: Rest/Active Recovery

BEGINNER PROGRAM: 2 Days per Week [Build Your Own]

DAY 1: Workout A—Full Body

Dynamic Warm-up Exercise	Repetitions
a	Supine Drawing In	**10 contractions**
b	Cat-Cow	**20**
c	World's Greatest Stretch	**10 rotations [each side]**
d	Thoracic Extension on Foam Roller	**15**
e	Swimmer's Stretch	**15**
f	Glute Bridge with Hip Band	**20 repetitions + 10-second hold [top of last rep]**
g	Band High Pull Apart with External Rotation	**25**

Exercise	Week 1 Connective Tissue Remodeling	Week 2 Hypertrophy	Week 3 Strength	Week 4 Endurance Plus Energy Loading
Rest between sets [seconds]	60	90	120	30–60
1 Upper Body Pull, Posterior Shoulder Focus	2 x 7, 5151	3 x 8–12, 3131	3 x 5–7, 3111	3 x 15, 1010
2 Upper Body Push	2 x 7, 5551	3 x 8–12, 3311	3 x 5–7, 3311	3 x 15, 1010
3 Lower Body Push, Single Leg	2 x 7, 5151	3 x 8–12, 3131	3 x 5–7, 3111	3 x 15, 1010
4 Lower Body Pull	2 x 7, 5151	3 x 8–12, 3131	3 x 5–7, 3111	3 x 15, 1010
5 Lower Body Push	2 x 7, 5151	3 x 8–12, 3131	3 x 5–7, 3111	3 x 15, 1010

Active Isolated Stretching [AIS]

Cossack Squat: 2 sets of 10 repetitions, each side [2-second hold in stretched position]

DAYS 2–3: Rest/Active Recovery

BEGINNER PROGRAM: 2 Days per Week [Build Your Own] *(continued)*

DAY 4: Workout B—Full Body

Dynamic Warm-up Exercise	Repetitions
a World's Greatest Stretch	10 rotations (each side)
b Hinge to Squat	15
c Glute Bridge (with Isometric Groin Squeeze)	20 repetitions + 10-second hold (top of last rep)
d Ankle Glides	20
e Band Facepull	25
f Swimmer's Stretch	15
g Forearm Tendon Glides	20

Exercise	Week 1 Connective Tissue Remodeling	Week 2 Hypertrophy	Week 3 Strength	Week 4 Endurance Plus Energy Loading
Rest between sets (seconds)	60	90	120	30–60
1 Lower Body Push, Single Leg	2 x 7, 5151	3 x 8–12, 3111	3 x 5–7, 3111	3 x 15, 1010
2 Lower Body Push	2 x 7, 5151	3 x 8–12, 3111	3 x 5–7, 3111	3 x 15, 1010
3 Upper Body Pull, Posterior Shoulder Focus	2 x 7, 5151	3 x 8–12, 3131	3 x 5–7, 3111	3 x 15, 1010
4 Shoulder Stability	2 x 7, 5151	3 x 8–12, 3131	3 x 5–7, 3111	3 x 15, 1010
5 Upper Body Pull, Single Arm	2 x 7, 5151	3 x 8–12, 3131	3 x 5–7, 3111	3 x 15, 1010

Active Isolated Stretching [AIS]

Anchored Lat Stretch: 2 sets of 10 repetitions (2-second hold in stretched position)

DAYS 5–7: Rest/Active Recovery

INTERMEDIATE PROGRAM: 3 Days per Week [Build Your Own]

DAY 1: Workout A — Lower Body [Low Back/Posterior Chain Focus]

Dynamic Warm-up Exercise

		Repetitions
a	Supine Drawing In	10 contractions
b	Cat-Cow	20
c	World's Greatest Stretch	10 rotations (each side)
d	Bird Dog	20 (each side)
e	Fire Hydrant	25 (each side)
f	Glute Bridge with Hip Band	20 repetitions + 10-second hold [top of last rep]
g	Single Leg Romanian Deadlift—Body Weight	10 (each side)

	Week 1	Week 2	Week 3	Week 4
	Connective Tissue Remodeling	Hypertrophy	Strength	Endurance Plus Energy Loading
Exercise				
Rest between sets (seconds)	60	90	120	30–60
1 Lower Body Pull	2 x 7, 5151	3 x 8–12, 3131	3 x 5–7, 3111	3 x 15, 1010
2 Lower Body Push, Single Leg	2 x 7, 5151	3 x 8–12, 3131	3 x 5–7, 3111	3 x 15, 1010
3 Lower Body Pull	2 x 7, 5151	3 x 8–12, 3131	3 x 5–7, 3111	3 x 15, 1010
4 Lower Body Push, Single Leg	2 x 7, 5151	3 x 8–12, 3131	3 x 5–7, 3111	3 x 15, 1010
5 Lower Body Accessory	2 x 7, 5151	3 x 8–12, 3131	3 x 5–7, 3111	3 x 15, 1010

Active Isolated Stretching [AIS]

Cossack Squat: 2 sets of 10 repetitions, each side (2-second hold in stretched position)

DAY 2: Rest/Active Recovery

INTERMEDIATE PROGRAM: 3 Days per Week [Build Your Own] [continued]

DAY 3: Workout B — Upper Body [Horizontal Focus]

Dynamic Warm-up Exercise	Repetitions
a	Cat-Cow	20
b	Band Pass Through	15
c	Thoracic Extension on Foam Roller	15
d	Anchored Lat Stretch	10-10-10*
e	Swimmer's Stretch	15
f	Pronation/Supination, Bent Elbow Variation	20 (each way)
g	Band High Pull Apart with External Rotation	25

	Week 1	Week 2	Week 3	Week 4
	Connective Tissue Remodeling	Hypertrophy	Strength	Endurance Plus Energy Loading
Exercise				
Rest between sets (seconds)	60	90	120	30-60
1 Upper Body Pull, Posterior Shoulder Focus	2 x 7, 5151	3 x 8-12, 3131	3 x 5-7, 3111	3 x 15, 1010
2 Upper Body Push	2 x 7, 5151	3 x 8-12, 3131	3 x 5-7, 3111	3 x 15, 1010
3 Upper Body Pull	2 x 7, 5151	3 x 8-12, 3131	3 x 5-7, 3111	3 x 15, 1010
4 Upper Body Push	2 x 7, 5151	3 x 8-12, 3131	3 x 5-7, 3111	3 x 15, 1010
5 Upper Body Accessory	2 x 7, 5151	3 x 8-12, 3131	3 x 5-7, 3111	3 x 15, 1010

Active Isolated Stretching (AIS)

Anchored Lat Stretch: 2 sets of 10 repetitions (2-second hold in stretched position)

DAY 4: Rest/Active Recovery

*10-second gentle stretch, 10 stretch pulses, 10-second stretch hold

Continued on next page

INTERMEDIATE PROGRAM: 3 Days per Week [Build Your Own] *(continued)*

DAY 5: Workout C—Fully Body [Lower Anterior Chain + Shoulder Stability]

Dynamic Warm-up Exercise	Repetitions
a World's Greatest Stretch	10 rotations (each side)
b Hinge to Squat	15
c Glute Bridge (with Isometric Groin Squeeze)	20 repetitions + 10-second hold (top of last rep)
d Ankle Glides	20
e Band High Pull Apart with External Rotation	25
f Swimmer's Stretch	15
g Forearm Tendon Glides	20

	Week 1	Week 2	Week 3	Week 4
	Connective Tissue Remodeling	Hypertrophy	Strength	Endurance Plus Energy Loading
Exercise				
Rest between sets (seconds)	60	90	120	30–60
1 Lower Body Push, Single Leg	2 x 7, 5151	3 x 8–12, 3111	3 x 5–7, 3111	3 x 15, 1010
2 Lower Body Push	2 x 7, 5151	3 x 8–12, 3111	3 x 5–7, 3111	3 x 15, 1010
3 Upper Body Pull, Posterior Shoulder Focus	2 x 7, 5151	3 x 8–12, 3131	3 x 5–7, 3111	3 x 15, 1010
4 Shoulder Stability	2 x 7, 5151	3 x 8–12, 3131	3 x 5–7, 3111	3 x 15, 1010
5 Upper Body Pull, Single Arm	2 x 7, 5151	3 x 8–12, 3131	3 x 5–7, 3111	3 x 15, 1010

Active Isolated Stretching [AIS]

Pigeon Stretch: 2 sets of 10 repetitions, each side (2-second hold in stretched position)

DAYS 6–7: Rest/Active Recovery

ADVANCED PROGRAM: 4 Days per Week (Build Your Own)

DAY 1: Workout A—Lower Body (Low Back/Posterior Chain Focus)

Dynamic Warm-up Exercise	Repetitions
a Supine Drawing In	10 contractions
b Cat-Cow	20
c World's Greatest Stretch	10 rotations (each side)
d Bird Dog	20 (each side)
e Fire Hydrant	25 (each side)
f Glute Bridge with Hip Band	20 repetitions + 10-second hold (top of last rep)
g Single Leg Romanian Deadlift—Body Weight	10 (each side)

Exercise	Week 1 Connective Tissue Remodeling	Week 2 Hypertrophy	Week 3 Strength	Week 4 Endurance Plus Energy Loading
Rest between sets (seconds)	60	90	120	30–60
1 Lower Body Pull	2 x 7, 5151	3 x 8-12, 3131	3 x 5-7, 3111	3 x 15, 1010
2 Lower Body Push, Single Leg	2 x 7, 5151	3 x 8-12, 3131	3 x 5-7, 3111	3 x 15, 1010
3 Lower Body Pull	2 x 7, 5151	3 x 8-12, 3311	3 x 5-7, 3311	3 x 15, 1010
4 Lower Body Push, Single Leg	2 x 7, 5151	3 x 8-12, 3131	3 x 5-7, 3111	3 x 15, 1010
5 Lower Body Accessory	2 x 7, 5151	3 x 8-12, 3131	3 x 5-7, 3111	3 x 15, 1010

Active Isolated Stretching (AIS)

Cossack Squat: 2 sets of 10 repetitions, each side (2-second hold in stretched position)

Continued on next page

ADVANCED PROGRAM: 4 Days per Week [Build Your Own] *[continued]*

DAY 2: Workout B—Upper Body [Horizontal Focus]

Dynamic Warm-up Exercise	Repetitions
a World's Greatest Stretch	10 rotations [each side]
b Band Pass Through	15
c Thoracic Extension on Foam Roller	15
d Anchored Lat Stretch	10-10-10*
e Swimmer's Stretch	15
f Pronation/Supination, Bent Elbow Variation	20 [each way]
g Band High Facepull	25

Exercise	Week 1 Connective Tissue Remodeling	Week 2 Hypertrophy	Week 3 Strength	Week 4 Endurance Plus Energy Loading
Rest between sets (seconds)	60	90	120	30-60
1 Upper Body Pull, Posterior Shoulder Focus	2 x 7, 5151	3 x 8-12, 3131	3 x 5-7, 3111	3 x 15, 1010
2 Upper Body Push	2 x 7, 5151	3 x 8-12, 3131	3 x 5-7, 3111	3 x 15, 1010
3 Upper Body Pull	2 x 7, 5151	3 x 8-12, 3131	3 x 5-7, 3111	3 x 15, 1010
4 Upper Body Push	2 x 7, 5151	3 x 8-12, 3131	3 x 5-7, 3111	3 x 15, 1010
5 Upper Body Accessory	2 x 7, 5151	3 x 8-12, 3131	3 x 5-7, 3111	3 x 15, 1010

Active Isolated Stretching [AIS]

Anchored Lat Stretch: 2 sets of 10 repetitions [2-second hold in stretched position]

DAY 3: Rest/Active Recovery

*10-second gentle stretch, 10 stretch pulses, 10-second stretch hold

ADVANCED PROGRAM: 4 Days per Week (Build Your Own) *(continued)*

DAY 4: Workout C—Lower Body (Knee/Anterior Chain Focus) *(continued)*

Dynamic Warm-up Exercise	Repetitions
a Supine Drawing In	10 contractions
b Cat-Cow	20
c World's Greatest Stretch	10 rotations (each side)
d Bird Dog	20 (each side)
e Hinge to Squat	15
f Glute Bridge (with Isometric Groin Squeeze)	20 repetitions + 10-second hold (top of last rep)
g Ankle Glides	20

Exercise		Week 1 Connective Tissue Remodeling	Week 2 Hypertrophy	Week 3 Strength	Week 4 Endurance Plus Energy Loading
Rest between sets (seconds)		60	90	120	30–60
1	Lower Body Push, Single Leg	2 x 7, 5151	3 x 8–12, 3111	3 x 5–7, 3111	3 x 15, 1010
2	Lower Body Push	2 x 7, 5151	3 x 8–12, 3111	3 x 5–7, 3111	3 x 15, 1010
3	Lower Body Pull	2 x 7, 5151	3 x 8–12, 3111	3 x 5–7, 3111	3 x 15, 1010
4	Lower Body Push	2 x 7, 5151	3 x 8–12, 3111	3 x 5–7, 3111	3 x 15, 1010
5	Lower Body Accessory	2 x 7, 5151	3 x 8–12, 3111	3 x 5–7, 3111	3 x 15, 1010

Active Isolated Stretching (AIS)

Pigeon Stretch: 2 sets of 10 repetitions, each side (2-second hold in stretched position)

Continued on next page

ADVANCED PROGRAM: 4 Days per Week [Build Your Own] *[continued]*

DAY 5: Workout D — Upper Body [Shoulder Stability Focus]

Dynamic Warm-up Exercise	Repetitions
a Band Pass Through	15
b Thoracic Extension on Foam Roller	15
c Anchored Lat Stretch	10-10-10*
d Swimmer's Stretch	15
e Forearm Tendon Glides	25
f Band High Pull Apart with External Rotation	25
g Scapular Pull-up	15

	Week 1	Week 2	Week 3	Week 4
Exercise	**Connective Tissue Remodeling**	**Hypertrophy**	**Strength**	**Endurance Plus Energy Loading**
Rest between sets (seconds)	60	90	120	30–60
1 Upper Body Pull, Posterior Shoulder Focus	2 x 7, 5151	3 x 8-12, 3131	3 x 5-7, 3111	3 x 15, 1010
2 Shoulder Stability	2 x 7, 5151	3 x 8-12, 3131	3 x 5-7, 3111	3 x 15, 1010
3 Upper Body Pull, Single Arm	2 x 7, 5151	3 x 8-12, 3131	3 x 5-7, 3111	3 x 15, 1010
4 Shoulder Stability	2 x 7, 5151	3 x 8-12, 3131	3 x 5-7, 3111	3 x 15, 1010
5 Upper Body Pull, Vertical Focus**	2 x 7, 5151	3 x 8-12, 3131	3 x 5-7, 3111	3 x 15, 1010

Active Isolated Stretching (AIS)

Scapular Pull-up: 2 sets of 10 repetitions (2-second hold in stretched position)

DAY 6–7: Rest/Active Recovery

*10-second gentle stretch, 10 stretch pulses, 10-second stretch hold

**Choose a top-down vertical pull exercise, such as a pull-up or cable machine lat pulldown.

AT-HOME TRAINING PLAN — Minimalist Equipment (4 Days per Week)

DAY 1: Workout A — Lower Body (Low Back/Posterior Chain Focus)

Dynamic Warm-up Exercise

	Exercise	Repetitions
a	Supine Drawing In	10 contractions
b	Cat-Cow	20
c	World's Greatest Stretch	10 rotations (each side)
d	Bird Dog	20 (each side)
e	Fire Hydrant	25 (each side)
f	Glute Bridge with Hip Band	20 repetitions + 10-second hold (top of last rep)
g	Single Leg Romanian Deadlift — Body Weight	10 (each side)

		Week 1	Week 2	Week 3	Week 4
		Connective Tissue Remodeling	Hypertrophy	Strength	Endurance Plus Energy Loading
	Exercise				
	Rest between sets (seconds)	60	90	120	30–60
1	Band Pull Through	2 x 7, 5151	3 x 8–12, 3131	3 x 5–7, 3111	3 x 15, 1010
2	Bulgarian Split Squat with Heavy Kettlebell (Contralateral)*	2 x 7, 5151	3 x 8–12, 3131	3 x 5–7, 3111	3 x 15, 1010
3	Kettlebell Romanian Deadlift with Hip Band**	2 x 7, 5151	3 x 8–12, 3131	3 x 5–7, 3111	3 x 15, 1010
4	Kettlebell Cossack Squat (each side)	2 x 7, 5151	3 x 8–12, 3131	3 x 5–7, 3111	3 x 15, 1010
5	Single Leg Calf Raise from Block, Straight Knee	2 x 7, 5151	3 x 8–12, 3131	3 x 5–7, 3111	3 x 15, 1010

Active Isolated Stretching (AIS)

Cossack Squat: 2 sets of 10 repetitions, each side (2-second hold in stretched position)

* Hold weight in opposite hand of exercising leg.
** Place hip band just above knees. Hold a heavy kettlebell with both hands.

Continued on next page

AT-HOME TRAINING PLAN — Minimalist Equipment [4 Days per Week] *[continued]*

DAY 2: Workout B — Upper Body [Horizontal Focus]

Dynamic Warm-up Exercise	Repetitions
a	World's Greatest Stretch	10 rotations [each side]
b	Band Pass Through	15
c	Thoracic Extension on Foam Roller	15
d	Anchored Lat Stretch	10-10-10*
e	Swimmer's Stretch	15
f	Pronation/Supination, Bent Elbow Variation	20 [each way]
g	Band High Facepull	25

		Week 1	Week 2	Week 3	Week 4
		Connective Tissue Remodeling	Hypertrophy	Strength	Endurance Plus Energy Loading
Exercise					
Rest between sets (seconds)		60	90	120	30-60
1	Band Facepull	2 x 7, 5151	3 x 8-12, 3131	3 x 5-7, 3111	3 x 15, 1010
2	Push-up Plus with Band	2 x 5-7, 5555	3 x 8-12, 1515	2 x 5-7, 5555	3 x 15, 1010
3	Single Arm Kettlebell Row, Split Stance Variation	2 x 7, 5151	3 x 8-12, 3131	3 x 5-7, 3111	3 x 15, 1010
4	Standing Kettlebell Pullover [Light Kettlebell]	2 x 7, 5551	3 x 8-12, 3311	3 x 5-7, 3311	3 x 15, 1010
5	Dumbbell Zottman Curl	2 x 7, 5151	3 x 8-12, 3131	3 x 5-7, 3111	3 x 15, 1010

Active Isolated Stretching [AIS]

Anchored Lat Stretch: 2 sets of 10 repetitions [2-second hold in stretched position]

DAY 3: Rest/Active Recovery

*10-second gentle stretch, 10 stretch pulses, 10-second stretch hold

AT-HOME TRAINING PLAN — Minimalist Equipment (4 Days per Week) *(continued)*

DAY 4: Workout C — Lower Body (Knee/Anterior Chain Focus)

Dynamic Warm-up Exercise	Repetitions
a Supine Drawing In	10 contractions
b Cat-Cow	20
c World's Greatest Stretch	10 rotations (each side)
d Bird Dog	20 (each side)
e Hinge to Squat	15
f Glute Bridge (with Isometric Groin Squeeze)	20 repetitions + 10-second hold (top of last rep)
g Ankle Glides	20

Exercise	Week 1 Connective Tissue Remodeling	Week 2 Hypertrophy	Week 3 Strength	Week 4 Endurance Plus Energy Loading
Rest between sets (seconds)	60	90	120	30-60
1 Box Stepdown	3 x 10, 3131	3 x 15, 3131	3 x 10, 3111	3 x 15, 1010
2 Spanish Squat	2 x 10, 5555	3 x 8-12, 3333	3 x 15, 1115	3 x 20, 1010
3 Single Leg Romanian Deadlift, Light Dumbbells	2 x 5-7, 5555	3 x 8-12, 2311	3 x 10, 3111	3 x 20, 1010
4 Kettlebell Goblet Squat	2 x 7, 5151	3 x 8-12, 3111	3 x 5-7, 3111	3 x 15, 1010
5 Single Leg Calf Raise from Block, Bent Knee	2 x 7, 5151	3 x 8-12, 3131	3 x 15, 3111	3 x 15, 1010

Active Isolated Stretching (AIS)

Pigeon Stretch: 2 sets of 10 repetitions, each side (2-second hold in stretched position)

Continued on next page

AT-HOME TRAINING PLAN — Minimalist Equipment (4 Days per Week) *(continued)*

DAY 5: Workout D — Upper Body (Shoulder Stability Focus)

Dynamic Warm-up Exercise	Repetitions
a Band Pass Through	15
b Thoracic Extension on Foam Roller	15
c Anchored Lat Stretch	10-10-10*
d Swimmer's Stretch	15
e Forearm Tendon Glides	25
f Banded W	25
g Scapular Pull-up	15

	Week 1	Week 2	Week 3	Week 4
Exercise	Connective Tissue Remodeling	Hypertrophy	Strength	Endurance Plus Energy Loading
Rest between sets (seconds)	60	90	120	30-60
1 Anchored Band Pull Apart	2 x 7, 5151	3 x 8-12, 3131	3 x 5-7, 3111	3 x 15, 1010
2 Scapular Plane Dumbbell Raises	2 x 7, 5151	3 x 8-12, 3131	3 x 5-7, 3111	3 x 15, 1010
3 Single Arm Kettlebell Row, Strict Variation	2 x 7, 5151	3 x 8-12, 3131	3 x 5-7, 3111	3 x 15, 1010
4 Bottoms-Up Kettlebell Press	2 x 7, 5151	3 x 8-12, 3131	3 x 5-7, 3111	3 x 15, 1010
5 Dumbbell Pronation/Supination, Straight Arm Variation	2 x 7, 5151	3 x 8-12, 3131	3 x 5-7, 3111	3 x 15, 1010

Active Isolated Stretching (AIS)

Scapular Pull-up: 2 sets of 10 repetitions (2-second hold in stretched position)

DAY 6-7: Rest/Active Recovery

* 10-second gentle stretch, 10 stretch pulses, 10-second stretch hold

TRAVEL TRAINING PLAN: 4 Days per Week

DAY 1: Workout A — Lower Body [Low Back/Posterior Chain Focus]

Dynamic Warm-up Exercise	Repetitions
a Supine Drawing In	10 contractions
b Cat-Cow	20
c World's Greatest Stretch	10 rotations [each side]
d Bird Dog	20 [each side]
e Fire Hydrant	25 [each side]
f Glute Bridge with Hip Band	20 repetitions + 10-second hold [top of last rep]
g Single Leg Romanian Deadlift—Body Weight	10 [each side]

	Week 1	Week 2	Week 3	Week 4
Exercise	Connective Tissue Remodeling	Hypertrophy	Strength	Endurance Plus Energy Loading
Rest between sets [seconds]	60	90	120	30–60
1 Band Pull Through	2 x 7, 5151	3 x 8–12, 3131	3 x 5–7, 3111	3 x 15, 1010
2 Bulgarian Split Squat—Body Weight	2 x 7, 5151	3 x 8–12, 3131	3 x 5–7, 3111	3 x 15, 1010
3 Romanian Deadlift with Hip Band*	2 x 7, 5151	3 x 8–12, 3131	3 x 5–7, 3111	3 x 15, 1010
4 Cossack Squat [each side]	2 x 7, 5151	3 x 8–12, 3131	3 x 5–7, 3111	3 x 15, 1010
5 Single Leg Calf Raise from Block, Straight Knee	2 x 7, 5151	3 x 8–12, 3131	3 x 5–7, 3111	3 x 15, 1010

Active Isolated Stretching [AIS]

Cossack Squat: 2 sets of 10 repetitions, each side [2-second hold in stretched position]

Place hip band just above knees.

Continued on next page

TRAVEL TRAINING PLAN: 4 Days per Week *(continued)*

DAY 2: Workout B — Upper Body [Horizontal Focus]

Dynamic Warm-up Exercise	Repetitions
a	World's Greatest Stretch	10 rotations (each side)
b	Band Pass Through	15
c	Thoracic Extension on Foam Roller*	15
d	Anchored Lat Stretch	10-10-10**
e	Swimmer's Stretch	15
f	Pronation/Supination, Bent Elbow Variation	20 (each way)
g	Band High Facepull	25

	Week 1	Week 2	Week 3	Week 4
	Connective Tissue Remodeling	Hypertrophy	Strength	Endurance Plus Energy Loading
Exercise				
Rest between sets (seconds)	60	90	120	30-60
1 Band Facepull	2 x 7, 5151	3 x 8-12, 3131	3 x 5-7, 3111	3 x 15, 1010
2 Push-up Plus with Band	2 x 5-7, 5555	3 x 8-12, 1515	2 x 5-7, 5555	3 x 15, 1010
3 Anchored Band Pull Apart	2 x 7, 5151	3 x 8-12, 3131	3 x 5-7, 3111	3 x 15, 1010
4 Scapula Plane Band Raise	2 x 7, 5551	3 x 8-12, 3311	3 x 5-7, 3311	3 x 15, 1010
5 Band Zottman Curl	2 x 7, 5151	3 x 8-12, 3131	3 x 5-7, 3111	3 x 15, 1010

Active Isolated Stretching [AIS]

Anchored Lat Stretch: 2 sets of 10 repetitions (2-second hold in stretched position)

DAY 3: Rest/Active Recovery

Substitute any ball or object you can slide across the floor (e.g. pillow) while extending your arms outward.

**10-second gentle stretch, 10 stretch pulses, 10-second stretch hold*

TRAVEL TRAINING PLAN: 4 Days per Week *(continued)*

DAY 4: Workout C—Lower Body [Knee/Anterior Chain Focus]

Dynamic Warm-up Exercise	Repetitions
a Supine Drawing In	10 contractions
b Cat-Cow	20
c World's Greatest Stretch	10 rotations (each side)
d Bird Dog	20 (each side)
e Hinge to Squat	15
f Glute Bridge (with Isometric Groin Squeeze)	20 repetitions + 10-second hold (top of last rep)
g Ankle Glides	20

Exercise	Week 1 Connective Tissue Remodeling	Week 2 Hypertrophy	Week 3 Strength	Week 4 Endurance Plus Energy Loading
Rest between sets (seconds)	60	90	120	30-60
1 Box Stepdown	3 x 10, 3131	3 x 15, 3131	3 x 10, 3111	3 x 15, 1010
2 Spanish Squat	2 x 10, 5555	3 x 8-12, 3333	3 x 15, 1115	3 x 20, 1010
3 Single Leg Romanian Deadlift, body weight	2 x 5-7, 5555	3 x 8-12, 3311	3 x 10, 3111	3 x 20, 1010
4 Split Squat, body weight	2 x 7, 5151	3 x 8-12, 3111	3 x 5-7, 3111	3 x 15, 1010
5 Single Leg Calf Raise from Block, bent knee	2 x 7, 5151	3 x 8-12, 3131	3 x 15, 3111	3 x 15, 1010

Active Isolated Stretching [AIS]

Pigeon Stretch: 2 sets of 10 repetitions, each side (2-second hold in stretched position)

Continued on next page

TRAVEL TRAINING PLAN: 4 Days per Week *[continued]*

DAY 5: Workout D—Upper Body [Shoulder Stability Focus]

Dynamic Warm-up Exercise	Repetitions
a	Band Pass Through	15
b	Thoracic Extension on Foam Roller	15
c	Anchored Lat Stretch	10-10-10*
d	Swimmer's Stretch	15
e	Forearm Forearm Tendon Glides	25
f	Banded W	25
g	Scapular Pull-up	15

Exercise	Week 1 Connective Tissue Remodeling	Week 2 Hypertrophy	Week 3 Strength	Week 4 Endurance Plus Energy Loading
Rest between sets (seconds)	60	90	120	30-60
1 Anchored Band Pull Apart	2 x 7, 5151	3 x 8-12, 3131	3 x 5-7, 3111	3 x 15, 1010
2 Scapula Plane Band Raise	2 x 7, 5151	3 x 8-12, 3131	3 x 5-7, 3111	3 x 15, 1010
3 Band High Row	2 x 7, 5151	3 x 8-12, 3131	3 x 5-7, 3111	3 x 15, 1010
4 Band Zottman Curl	2 x 7, 5151	3 x 8-12, 3131	3 x 5-7, 3111	3 x 15, 1010
5 Push-up Plus with Band	2 x 7, 5151	3 x 8-12, 3131	3 x 5-7, 3111	3 x 15, 1010

Active Isolated Stretching [AIS]

Scapular Pull-up: 2 sets of 10 repetitions [2-second hold in stretched position]

DAY 6-7: Rest/Active Recovery

*10-second gentle stretch, 10 stretch pulses, 10-second stretch hold

MORNING MOBILITY ROUTINE
Perform one set of each exercise listed below every morning.

Body Weight Mobility Sequence

Perform five slow and controlled repetitions of each dynamic stretch. Then, hold the stretched (end) position of each movement for five seconds.

Exercise

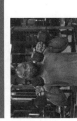 **1.** Cat-Cow

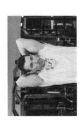 **2.** World's Greatest Stretch

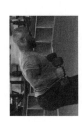 **3.** Glute Bridge

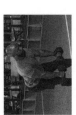 **4.** Hinge to Squat

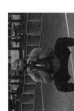 **5.** Cossack Squat

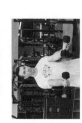 **6.** Band Pass Through

Weighted Mobility Sequence

Perform ten repetitions of each exercise. Allow 1–2 seconds to lift the weight and 1–2 seconds to lower the weight.

Exercise

 1. Dumbbell Zottman Curl

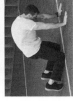 **2.** Standing Dumbbell Pullover

 3. Bent Over Dumbbell Row

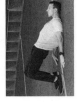 **4.** Dumbbell Romanian Deadlift

 5. Dumbbell Goblet Squat

  6. Dumbbell Pronation/Supination

References

1. Torgovnik May, K. (2012). *7 powerful stories of recovery after injury*. TEDBlog. https://blog.ted.com/7-powerful-stories-of-recovery-after-injury/

2. "Mechanotransduction." Nature.com. https://www.nature.com/subjects/mechanotransduction

3. Artero, E. G., D. C. Lee, C. J. Lavie, España-Romero, V., Sui, X., Church, T. S., & Blair, S. N. (2012). Effects of muscular strength on cardiovascular risk factors and prognosis. *Journal of cardiopulmonary rehabilitation and prevention*, *32*(6), 351–358. https://doi.org/10.1097/HCR.0b013e3182642688

4. Schoenfeld, B. J., Contreras, B., Vigotsky, A. D., & Peterson, M. (2016). Differential effects of heavy versus moderate loads on measures of strength and hypertrophy in resistance-trained men. *Journal of Sports Science & Medicine*, *15*(4), 715–722.

5. Levangie, P. K., & Norkin, C. C. (2011). *Joint Structure and Function: A Comprehensive Analysis*, 5th ed. Philadelphia: F. A. Davis.

6. Hong, A. R., & Kim, S. W. (2018). Effects of resistance exercise on bone health. *Endocrinology and Metabolism (Seoul, Korea)*, *33*(4), 435–444. https://doi.org/10.3803/EnM.2018.33.4.435

7. Li, R., Xia, J., Zhang, X. I., Gathirua-Mwangi, W. G., Guo, J., Li, Y., et al. (2018). Associations of muscle mass and strength with all-cause mortality among US older adults. *Medicine and Science in Sports and Exercise*, *50*(3), 458–467. https://doi.org/10.1249/MSS.0000000000001448

8. Wang, H., Hai, S., Liu, Y., Liu, Y, & Dong, B. (2019). Skeletal muscle mass as a mortality predictor among nonagenarians and centenarians: A prospective cohort study. *Scientific Reports*, *9*, 2420. https://doi.org/10.1038/s41598-019-38893-0

9. Abbasi, J. (2016, April 20). Strength training helps older adults live longer. *Penn State News*. https://news.psu.edu

10. Broadhouse, K. M., Singh, M. F., Suo, C., Gates, N., Wen, W., Brodaty, H., et al. (2020). Hippocampal plasticity underpins long-term cognitive gains from resistance exercise in MCI. *NeuroImage. Clinical*, *25*, 102182. https://doi.org/10.1016/j.nicl.2020.102182

11. McKendry, J., Shad, B. J., Smeuninx, B., Oikawa, S. Y., Wallis, G., Greig, C., et al. (2019). Comparable rates of integrated myofibrillar protein synthesis between endurance-trained master athletes and untrained older individuals. *Frontiers in Physiology*, *10*, 1084. https://doi.org/10.3389/fphys.2019.01084

12. MacDougall, J. D., Gibala, M. J., Tarnopolsky, M. A., MacDonald, J. R., Interisano, S. A., & Yarasheski, K. E. (1995). The time course for elevated muscle protein synthesis following heavy resistance exercise. *Canadian Journal of Applied Physiology*, *20*(4), 480–486. https://doi.org/10.1139/h95-038

13. Peterson, M. D., & Gordon, P. M. (2011). Resistance exercise for the aging adult: Clinical implications and prescription guidelines. *The American Journal of Medicine*, *124*, 194–198. https://doi.org/10.1016/j.amjmed.2010.08.020

14. Mazzone, M. F., & McCue, T. (2002). Common conditions of the Achilles tendon. *American Family Physician*, *65*(9), 1805–1810.

15. Zhou, B., Zhou, Y., & Tang, K. (2014). An overview of structure, mechanical properties, and treatment for age-related tendinopathy. *The Journal of Nutrition, Health & Aging*, *18*(4), 441–448. https://doi.org/10.1007/s12603-014-0026-2

16. Centers for Disease Control and Prevention. (2008). QuickStats: Percentage of adults reporting joint pain or stiffness, National Health Interview Survey, United States, 2006. *Morbidity and Mortality Weekly Report*, *57*(17), 467. https://www.cdc.gov/mmwr/preview/mmwrhtml/mm5717a9.htm

17. Nguyen, U. S., Zhang, Y., Zhu, Y., Niu, J., Zhang, B., & Felson, D. T. (2011). Increasing prevalence of knee pain and symptomatic knee osteoarthritis: Survey and cohort data. *Annals of Internal Medicine*, *155*(11), 725–732. https://doi.org/10.7326/0003-4819-155-11-201112060-00004

18. Mundell, E. J. (2016, October 6). *Number of Americans with severe joint pain rising*. WebMD News from HealthDay. https://www.webmd.com/arthritis/news/20161006/number-of-americans-with-severe-joint-pain-keeps-rising

19. Kwon, Y., Kim, J. W., Heo, J. H., Jeon, H. M., Choi, E. B., & Eom, G. M. (2018). The effect of sitting posture on the loads at cervico-thoracic and lumbosacral joints. *Technology and Health Care: Official Journal of the European Society for Engineering and Medicine*, *26*(S1), 409–418. https://doi.org/10.3233/THC-174717

20. Singla, D., & Veqar, Z. (2017). Association between forward head, rounded shoulders, and increased thoracic kyphosis: A review of the literature. *Journal of Chiropractic Medicine*, *16*(3), 220–229. https://doi.org/10.1016/j.jcm.2017.03.004

21. Zemková E. (2016). Instability resistance training for health and performance. *Journal of Traditional and Complementary Medicine, 7*(2), 245–250. https://doi.org/10.1016/j.jtcme.2016.05.007

22. McGill S. (2015). *Back mechanic: The secrets to a healthy spine your doctor isn't telling you.* Stuart McGill.

23. Smith, C. (2018, April 27). *Study: 29 of 32 NFL first round picks were multisport high school athletes.* USA Today High School Sports. https://usatodayhss.com/2018/study-29-of-32-nfl-first-round-picks-were-multisport-high-school-athletes

24. Gardner, B., & Jones, T. (2018, May). *Report: Multisport athletes injured less often.* Spokane Spokesman Review. Accessed on AthleticBusiness.com, https://www.athleticbusiness.com/athlete-safety/report-multisport-athletes-injured-less-often.html

25. Kay, A. D., & Blazevich, A. J. (2012). Effect of acute static stretch on maximal muscle performance: A systematic review. *Medicine and Science in Sports and Exercise, 44*(1), 154–164. https://doi.org/10.1249/MSS.0b013e318225cb27

26. Young, W. B. (2007). The use of static stretching in warm-up for training and competition. *International Journal of Sports Physiology and Performance, 2*(2), 212–216. https://doi.org/10.1123/ijspp.2.2.212

27. Witvrouw, E., Mahieu, N., Danneels, L., & McNair, P. (2004). Stretching and injury prevention: An obscure relationship. *Sports Medicine, 34*(7), 443–449. https://doi.org/10.2165/00007256-200434070-00003

28. Koh, T. J., & DiPietro, L. A. (2011). Inflammation and wound healing: The role of the macrophage. *Expert Reviews in Molecular Medicine, 13*, e23. https://doi.org/10.1017/S1462399411001943

29. Centers for Disease Control and Prevention. (2020). *How CDC improves quality of life for people with arthritis.* https://www.cdc.gov/chronicdisease/resources/publications/factsheets/arthritis.htm

30. King, L. K., March, L., & Anandacoomarasamy, A. (2013). Obesity & osteoarthritis. *The Indian Journal of Medical Research, 138*(2), 185–193. https://www.ncbi.nlm.nih.gov/pmc/articles/PMC3788203/

31. Watson, S. (2012). *Staying active with osteoarthritis.* WebMD. https://www.webmd.com/osteoarthritis/features/staying-active-with-oa#1

32. Cleveland Clinic. (2019). *Connective tissue diseases.* https://my.clevelandclinic.org/health/diseases/14803-connective-tissue-diseases

33. Johns Hopkins Arthritis Center. (n.d.). *Role of body weight in osteoarthritis.* https://www.hopkinsarthritis.org/patient-corner/disease-management/role-of-body-weight-in-osteoarthritis/

34. Shahidi, B., & Maluf, K. S. (2017). Adaptations in evoked pain sensitivity and conditioned pain modulation after development of chronic neck pain. *BioMed Research International, 2017*, 8985398. https://doi.org/10.1155/2017/8985398

35. Benzon, H., Raja, S. N., Fishman, S., Liu, S., Cohen, S. P. (2017). *Essentials of pain medicine,* 4th ed. Elsevier.

36. Government of Western Australia, Department of Health (n.d.). Pain types. painHEALTH. https://painhealth.csse.uwa.edu.au/pain-module/pain-types/

37. Warren, S. (2019). *The pain relief secret: How to retrain your nervous system, heal your body, and overcome chronic pain.* TCK Publishing.

38. Zhaoyang, R., Martire, L. M., & Darnall, B. D. (2020). Daily pain catastrophizing predicts less physical activity and more sedentary behavior in older adults with osteoarthritis. *Pain, 161*, 2603–2610. doi: 10.1097/j.pain.0000000000001959

39. Lautenbacher, S., Kunz, M., Strate, P., Nielsen, J., & Arendt-Nielsen, L. (2005). Age effects on pain thresholds, temporal summation and spatial summation of heat and pressure pain. *Pain, 115*(3), 410–418. https://doi.org/10.1016/j.pain.2005.03.025

40. Seidman, A. J., Limaiem, F. (2020). *Synovial fluid analysis.* StatPearls. https://www.ncbi.nlm.nih.gov/books/NBK537114/

41. Kisiel, J. (2018). *Winning the injury game: How to stop chronic pain and achieve peak performance.* Moab, UT: The Pain Free Athlete.

42. Askenase, M. H., & Sansing, L. H. (2016). Stages of the inflammatory response in pathology and tissue repair after intracerebral hemorrhage. *Seminars in Neurology, 36*(3), 288–297. https://doi.org/10.1055/s-0036-1582132

43. Hunter, P. (2012). The inflammation theory of disease: The growing realization that chronic inflammation is crucial in many diseases opens new avenues for treatment. *EMBO Reports, 13*(11), 968–970. https://doi.org/10.1038/embor.2012.142

44. Pahwa, R., Goyal, A., Bansal, P., & Jialal, I. (2020). *Chronic inflammation.* StatPearls. https://www.ncbi.nlm.nih.gov/books/NBK493173/

45. Rees, J. D., Stride, M., & Scott, A. (2014). Tendons: Time to revisit inflammation. *British Journal of Sports Medicine, 48*(21), 1553–1557. https://doi.org/10.1136/bjsports-2012-091957

46. Franceschi, C., & Campisi, J. (2014). Chronic inflammation (inflammaging) and its potential contribution to age-associated diseases. *The Journals of Gerontology: Series A, 69*, S4–S9. https://doi.org/10.1093/gerona/glu057

47. Ellulu, M. S., Patimah, I., Khaza'ai, H., Rahmat, A., & Abed, Y. (2017). Obesity and inflammation: The linking mechanism and the complications. *Archives of Medical Science, 13*(4), 851–863. https://doi.org/10.5114/aoms.2016.58928

48. Liu, Y. Z., Wang, Y. X., & Jiang, C. L. (2017). Inflammation: The common pathway of stress-related diseases. *Frontiers in Human Neuroscience, 11,* 316. https://doi.org/10.3389/fnhum.2017.00316

49. Elsevier. (2008, September 4). Loss of sleep, even for a single night, increases inflammation in the body. *ScienceDaily.* www.sciencedaily.com/releases/2008/09/080902075211.htm

50. Lee, J., Taneja, V., & Vassallo, R. (2012). Cigarette smoking and inflammation: Cellular and molecular mechanisms. *Journal of Dental Research, 91*(2), 142–149. https://doi.org/10.1177/0022034511421200

51. Doux, J. D., Bazar, K. A., Lee, P. Y., & Yun, A. J. (2005). Can chronic use of anti-inflammatory agents paradoxically promote chronic inflammation through compensatory host response? *Medical Hypotheses, 65*(2), 389–391. https://doi.org/10.1016/j.mehy.2004.12.021

52. Minihane, A. M., Vinoy, S., Russell, W. R., Baka, A., Roche, H. M., Tuohy, K. M., et al. (2015). Low-grade inflammation, diet composition and health: Current research evidence and its translation. *The British Journal of Nutrition, 114*(7), 999–1012. https://doi.org/10.1017/S0007114515002093

53. Bianchi, V. E. (2018). Weight loss is a critical factor to reduce inflammation. *Clinical Nutrition ESPEN, 28,* 21–35. https://doi.org/10.1016/j.clnesp.2018.08.007

54. Messier, S. P., Gutekunst, D. J., Davis, C., & DeVita, P. (2005). Weight loss reduces knee-joint loads in overweight and obese older adults with knee osteoarthritis. *Arthritis & Rheumatism, 52,* 2026-2032. https://doi.org/10.1002/art.21139

55. Ziltener, J. L., Leal, S., & Fournier, P. E. (2010). Non-steroidal anti-inflammatory drugs for athletes: An update. *Annals of Physical and Rehabilitation Medicine, 53*(4), 278–288. https://doi.org/10.1016/j.rehab.2010.03.001

56. Carroll C. C. (2016). Analgesic drugs alter connective tissue remodeling and mechanical properties. *Exercise and Sport Sciences Reviews, 44*(1), 29–36. https://doi.org/10.1249/JES.0000000000000067

57. Greer, T. (2019, March 22). *Study: Low-carb diet provides relief from knee osteoarthritis.* UAB News. https://www.uab.edu/news/health/item/10316-study-low-carb-diet-provides-relief-from-knee-osteoarthritis

58. Sun, Q., Li, J., & Gao, F. (2014). New insights into insulin: The anti-inflammatory effect and its clinical relevance. *World Journal of Diabetes, 5*(2), 89–96. https://doi.org/10.4239/wjd.v5.i2.89

59. Calder P. C. (2010). Omega-3 fatty acids and inflammatory processes. *Nutrients, 2*(3), 355–374. https://doi.org/10.3390/nu2030355

60. Dimitrov, S., Hulteng, E., & Hong, S. (2017). Inflammation and exercise: Inhibition of monocytic intracellular TNF production by acute exercise via β_2-adrenergic activation. *Brain, Behavior, and Immunity, 61,* 60–68. https://doi.org/10.1016/j.bbi.2016.12.017

61. Mullington, J. M., Simpson, N. S., Meier-Ewert, H. K., & Haack, M. (2010). Sleep loss and inflammation. *Best Practice & Research. Clinical Endocrinology & Metabolism, 24*(5), 775–784. https://doi.org/10.1016/j.beem.2010.08.014

62. Walker, M. (2018). *Why we sleep: Unlocking the power of sleep and dreams.* New York: Scribner.

63. Tolahunase, M., Sagar, R., & Dada, R. (2017). Impact of yoga and meditation on cellular aging in apparently healthy individuals: A prospective, open-label single-arm exploratory study. *Oxidative Medicine and Cellular Longevity, 2017,* 7928981. https://doi.org/10.1155/2017/7928981

64. Laukkanen, J., & Laukkanen, T. (2017). Sauna bathing and systemic inflammation. *European Journal of Epidemiology, 33.* 10.1007/s10654-017-0335-y

65. Ciubotaru, I., Lee, Y. S., & Wander, R. C. (2003). Dietary fish oil decreases C-reactive protein, interleukin-6, and triacylglycerol to HDL-cholesterol ratio in postmenopausal women on HRT. *The Journal of Nutritional Biochemistry, 14*(9), 513–521. https://doi.org/10.1016/s0955-2863(03)00101-3

66. Filaire, E., Massart, A., Portier, H., Rouveix, M., Rosado, F., Bage, A. S., et al. (2010). Effect of 6 Weeks of n-3 fatty-acid supplementation on oxidative stress in Judo athletes. *International Journal of Sport Nutrition and Exercise Metabolism, 20*(6), 496–506. https://doi.org/10.1123/ijsnem.20.6.496

67. Kelley, D. S., Taylor, P. C., Nelson, G. J., Schmidt, P. C., Ferretti, A., Erickson, K. L., et al. (1999). Docosahexaenoic acid ingestion inhibits natural killer cell activity and production of inflammatory mediators in young healthy men. *Lipids, 34*(4), 317–324. https://doi.org/10.1007/s11745-999-0369-5

68. Kuptniratsaikul, V., Dajpratham, P., Taechaarpornkul, W., Buntragulpoontawee, M., Lukkanapichonchut, P., Chootip, C., et al. (2014). Efficacy and safety of Curcuma domestica extracts compared with ibuprofen in patients with knee osteoarthritis: a multicenter study. *Clinical Interventions in Aging, 9,* 451–458. https://doi.org/10.2147/CIA.S58535

69. Sahebkar, A., Serban, M.-C., Ursoniu, S., & Banach, M. (2015). Effect of curcuminoids on oxidative stress: A systematic review and meta-analysis of randomized controlled trials. *Atherosclerosis, 241,* e189–e190. doi: 10.1016/j.atherosclerosis.2015.04.931.

70. Rahimnia, A. R., Panahi, Y., Alishiri, G., Sharafi, M., & Sahebkar, A. (2015). Impact of supplementation with curcuminoids on systemic inflammation in patients with knee osteoarthritis: Findings from a randomized double-blind placebo-controlled trial. *Drug Research, 65*(10), 521–525. https://doi.org/10.1055/s-0034-1384536

71. Daily, J. W., Yang, M., & Park, S. (2016). Efficacy of turmeric extracts and curcumin for alleviating the symptoms of joint arthritis: A systematic review and meta-analysis of randomized clinical trials. *Journal of Medicinal Food, 19*(8), 717–729. https://doi.org/10.1089/jmf.2016.3705

72. Shoba, G., Joy, D., Joseph, T., Majeed, M., Rajendran, R., & Srinivas, P. S. (1998). Influence of piperine on the pharmacokinetics of curcumin in animals and human volunteers. *Planta Medica, 64*(4), 353–356. https://doi.org/10.1055/s-2006-957450

73. Siddiqui M. Z. (2011). Boswellia serrata, a potential antiinflammatory agent: An overview. *Indian Journal of Pharmaceutical Sciences, 73*(3), 255–261. https://doi.org/10.4103/0250-474X.93507

74. Sengupta, K., Krishnaraju, A. V., Vishal, A. A., Mishra, A., Trimurtulu, G., Sarma, K. V., et al. (2010). Comparative efficacy and tolerability of 5-Loxin and Aflapin against osteoarthritis of the knee: A double blind, randomized, placebo controlled clinical study. *International Journal of Medical Sciences, 7*(6), 366–377. https://doi.org/10.7150/ijms.7.366

75. Gerbeth, K., Hüsch, J., Fricker, G., Werz, O., Schubert-Zsilavecz, M., & Abdel-Tawab, M. (2013). In vitro metabolism, permeation, and brain availability of six major boswellic acids from Boswellia serrata gum resins. *Fitoterapia, 84,* 99–106.

76. Lugo, J. P., Saiyed, Z. M., Lau, F. C., Molina, J. P., Pakdaman, M. N., Shamie, A. N., & Udani, J. K. (2013). Undenatured type II collagen (UC-II®) for joint support: A randomized, double-blind, placebo-controlled study in healthy volunteers. *Journal of the International Society of Sports Nutrition, 10*(1), 48. https://doi.org/10.1186/1550-2783-10-48

77. Maggio, M., De Vita, F., Lauretani, F., Buttò, V., Bondi, G., Cattabiani, C., et al. (2013). IGF-1, the cross road of the nutritional, inflammatory and hormonal pathways to frailty. *Nutrients, 5*(10), 4184–4205. https://doi.org/10.3390/nu5104184

78. Sokolove, J., & Lepus, C. M. (2013). Role of inflammation in the pathogenesis of osteoarthritis: Latest findings and interpretations. *Therapeutic Advances in Musculoskeletal Disease, 5*(2), 77–94. https://doi.org/10.1177/1759720X12467868

79. Bass E. (2012). Tendinopathy: Why the difference between tendinitis and tendinosis matters. *International Journal of Therapeutic Massage & Bodywork, 5*(1), 14–17. https://doi.org/10.3822/ijtmb.v5i1.153

80. Khan, K. M., Cook, J. L., Kannus, P., Maffulli, N., & Bonar, S. F. (2002). Time to abandon the "tendinitis" myth. *BMJ (Clinical Research Ed.), 324*(7338), 626–627. https://doi.org/10.1136/bmj.324.7338.626

81. Cook, J. L., & Purdam, C. R. (2009). Is tendon pathology a continuum? A pathology model to explain the clinical presentation of load-induced tendinopathy. *British Journal of Sports Medicine, 43*(6), 409–416. https://doi.org/10.1136/bjsm.2008.051193

82. Khan, K. M., & Maffulli, N. (1998). Tendinopathy: An Achilles' heel for athletes and clinicians. *Clinical Journal of Sport Medicine: Official Journal of the Canadian Academy of Sport Medicine, 8*(3), 151–154.

83. Stahl, S., & Kaufman, T. (1997). The efficacy of an injection of steroids for medial epicondylitis. A prospective study of sixty elbows. *The Journal of Bone and Joint Surgery. American Volume, 79*(11), 1648–1652. https://doi.org/10.2106/00004623-199711000-00006

84. Cook, J. L., Rio, E., Purdam, C. R., et al. (2016). Revisiting the continuum model of tendon pathology: What is its merit in clinical practice and research? *British Journal of Sports Medicine, 50,* 1187–1191.

85. Docking, S. I., & Cook, J. (2019). How do tendons adapt? Going beyond tissue responses to understand positive adaptation and pathology development: A narrative review. *Journal of Musculoskeletal & Neuronal Interactions, 19*(3), 300–310.

86. Wertz, J., Galli, M., & Borchers, J. R. (2013). Achilles tendon rupture: Risk assessment for aerial and ground athletes. *Sports Health, 5*(5), 407–409. https://doi.org/10.1177/1941738112472165

87. Hefti, F., & Stoll, T. M. (1995). Heilung von Ligamenten und Sehnen [Healing of ligaments and tendons]. *Der Orthopade, 24*(3), 237–245.

88. Killian, M. L., Cavinatto, L., Galatz, L. M., & Thomopoulos, S. (2012). The role of mechanobiology in tendon healing. *Journal of Shoulder and Elbow Surgery, 21*(2), 228–237. https://doi.org/10.1016/j.jse.2011.11.002

89. Mersmann, F., Bohm, S., & Arampatzis, A. (2017). Imbalances in the development of muscle and tendon as risk factor for tendinopathies in youth athletes: A review of current evidence and concepts of prevention. *Frontiers in Physiology, 8,* 987. https://doi.org/10.3389/fphys.2017.00987

90. Davenport, T. E., Kulig, K., Matharu, Y., & Blanco, C. E. (2005). The EdUReP model for nonsurgical management of tendinopathy. *Physical Therapy, 85,* 1093–1103. https://doi.org/10.1093/ptj/85.10.1093

91. Mascaró, A., Cos, M. Á., Morral, A., Roig, A., Purdam, C., & Cook, J. (2018). Load management in tendinopathy: Clinical progression for Achilles and patellar tendinopathy. *Apunts Sports Medicine, 53,* 19–27. doi: 10.1016/j.apunts.2017.11.005

92. Witvrouw, E., Mahieu, N., Roosen, P., & McNair, P. (2007). The role of stretching in tendon injuries. *British Journal of Sports Medicine, 41*(4), 224–226. https://doi.org/10.1136/bjsm.2006.034165

93. Activity could help keep knees lubricated. (2015, October 21). *ScienceDaily.* www.sciencedaily.com/releases/2015/10/151021104419.htm

94. Healio. (2005, June 8). Decreased synovial fluid lubrication linked with cartilage damage. www.healio.com

95. Punzi, L., Galozzi, P., Luisetto, R., Favero, M., Ramonda, R., Oliviero, F., & Scanu, A. (2016). Post-traumatic arthritis: Overview on pathogenic mechanisms and role of inflammation. *RMD Open, 2*(2), e000279. https://doi.org/10.1136/rmdopen-2016-000279

96. Pitsillides, A. A., Skerry, T. M., & Edwards, J.C.W. (1999). Joint immobilization reduces synovial fluid hyaluronan concentration and is accompanied by changes in the synovial intimal cell populations. *Rheumatology, 38*(11) 1108–1112. https://doi.org/10.1093/rheumatology/38.11.1108

97. Millar, P. J., McGowan, C. L., Cornelissen, V. A., Araujo, C. G., & Swaine, I. L. (2014). Evidence for the role of isometric exercise training in reducing blood pressure: Potential mechanisms and future directions. *Sports Medicine, 44*(3), 345–356. https://doi.org/10.1007/s40279-013-0118-x

98. Anwer, S., & Alghadir, A. (2014). Effect of isometric quadriceps exercise on muscle strength, pain, and function in patients with knee osteoarthritis: A randomized controlled study. *Journal of Physical Therapy Science, 26*(5), 745–748. https://doi.org/10.1589/jpts.26.745

99. Zhang, S. L., Liu, H. Q., Xu, X. Z., Zhi, J., Geng, J. J., & Chen, J. (2013). Effects of exercise therapy on knee joint function and synovial fluid cytokine levels in patients with knee osteoarthritis. *Molecular Medicine Reports, 7*(1), 183–186. https://doi.org/10.3892/mmr.2012.1168

100. Bear, T., Philipp, M., Hill, S. & Mündel, T. (2016). A preliminary study on how hypohydration affects pain perception. *Psychophysiology, 53,* 605–610. https://doi.org/10.1111/psyp.12610

101. International Cartilage Regeneration & Joint Preservation Society. (n.d.). What is cartilage? https://cartilage.org/patient/about-cartilage/what-is-cartilage/

102. Zhu, X., Sang, L., Wu, D., Rong, J., & Jiang, L. (2018). Effectiveness and safety of glucosamine and chondroitin for the treatment of osteoarthritis: A meta-analysis of randomized controlled trials. *Journal of Orthopaedic Surgery and Research, 13*(1), 170. https://doi.org/10.1186/s13018-018-0871-5

103. Poole, A. R., Kobayashi, M., Yasuda, T., et al. (2002). Type II collagen degradation and its regulation in articular cartilage in osteoarthritis. *Annals of the Rheumatic Diseases, 61,* ii78–ii81.

104. Baar, K. (2015, April). Training and nutrition to prevent soft tissue injuries and accelerate return to play. Sports Science Exchange #142, Gatorade Sports Science Institute. https://www.gssiweb.org

105. Feeley, B. T., Kennelly, S., Barnes, R. P., Muller, M. S., Kelly, B. T., Rodeo, S. A., & Warren, R. F. (2008). Epidemiology of National Football League training camp injuries from 1998 to 2007. *The American Journal of Sports Medicine, 36*(8), 1597–1603. https://doi.org/10.1177/0363546508316021

106. Paterno, M. V., Taylor-Haas, J. A., Myer, G. D., & Hewett, T. E. (2013). Prevention of overuse sports injuries in the young athlete. *The Orthopedic Clinics of North America, 44*(4), 553–564. https://doi.org/10.1016/j.ocl.2013.06.009

107. Sheu, Y., Chen, L.-H., & Hedegaard, H. (2016). Sports-and recreation-related injury episodes in the United States, 2011–2014. *National Health Statistics Reports, 99.* https://www.cdc.gov/nchs/data/nhsr/nhsr099.pdf

108. Lodish, H., Berk, A., Zipursky, S. L., Matsudaira, P., Baltimore, & D., Darnell, J. (2000). Collagen: The fibrous proteins of the matrix. In *Molecular cell biology* (4th ed., sec. 22.3). New York: W. H. Freeman. https://www.ncbi.nlm.nih.gov/books/NBK21582/

109. Varani, J., Dame, M. K., Rittie, L., Fligiel, S. E., Kang, S., Fisher, G. J., & Voorhees, J. J. (2006). Decreased collagen production in chronologically aged skin: Roles of age-dependent alteration in fibroblast function and defective mechanical stimulation. *The American Journal of Pathology, 168*(6), 1861–1868. https://doi.org/10.2353/ajpath.2006.051302

110. Babraj, J. A., Cuthbertson, D.J.R., Smith, K., Langberg, H., Miller, B., Krogsgaard, M. R., et al. (2005). Collagen synthesis in human musculoskeletal tissues and skin. *American Journal of Physiology—Endocrinology and Metabolism, 289*, E864–869. https://doi.org/10.1152/ajpendo.00243.2005

111. Dressler, P., Gehring, D., Zdzieblik, D., Oesser, S., Gollhofer, A., & König, D. (2018). Improvement of functional ankle properties following supplementation with specific collagen peptides in athletes with chronic ankle instability. *Journal of Sports Science & Medicine, 17*(2), 298–304.

112. Deyl, Z., Macek, K., Horáková, M., & Adam, M. (1981). The effect of food restriction and low protein diet upon collagen type I and III ratio in rat skin. *Physiologia Bohemoslov, 30*(3), 243–250.

113. Kothapalli, C. R., & Ramamurthi, A. (2009). Lysyl oxidase enhances elastin synthesis and matrix formation by vascular smooth muscle cells. *J Tissue Eng Regen Med., 3*(8), 655–661. doi: 10.1002/term.214. PMID: 19813219; PMCID: PMC2828049.

114. Xue, M., & Jackson, C. J. (2015). Extracellular matrix reorganization during wound healing and its impact on abnormal scarring. *Advances in Wound Care, 4*(3), 119–136. https://doi.org/10.1089/wound.2013.0485

115. McAnulty, R. J., & Laurent, G. J. (1987). Collagen synthesis and degradation in vivo. Evidence for rapid rates of collagen turnover with extensive degradation of newly synthesized collagen in tissues of the adult rat. *Collagen and Related Research, 7*(2), 93–104. https://doi.org/10.1016/s0174-173x(87)80001-8

116. Ramaswamy, K. S., Palmer, M. L., van der Meulen, J. H., Renoux, A., Kostrominova, T. Y., Michele, D. E., & Faulkner, J. A. (2011). Lateral transmission of force is impaired in skeletal muscles of dystrophic mice and very old rats. *The Journal of Physiology, 589*(Pt 5), 1195–1208. https://doi.org/10.1113/jphysiol.2010.201921

117. Kongsgaard, M., Kovanen, V., Aagaard, P., Doessing, S., Hansen, P., Laursen, A. H., et al. (2009). Corticosteroid injections, eccentric decline squat training and heavy slow resistance training in patellar tendinopathy. *Scandinavian Journal of Medicine & Science in Sports, 19*(6), 790–802. https://doi.org/10.1111/j.1600-0838.2009.00949.x

118. Langberg, H., Ellingsgaard, H., Madsen, T., Jansson, J., Magnusson, S. P., Aagaard, P., & Kjaer, M. (2007). Eccentric rehabilitation exercise increases peritendinous type I collagen synthesis in humans with Achilles tendinosis. *Scandinavian Journal of Medicine & Science in Sports, 17*(1), 61–66.

119. Rio, E., Kidgell, D., Purdam, C., Gaida, J., Moseley, G. L., Pearce, A. J., & Cook, J. (2015). Isometric exercise induces analgesia and reduces inhibition in patellar tendinopathy. *British Journal of Sports Medicine, 49*(19), 1277–1283. https://doi.org/10.1136/bjsports-2014-094386

120. Ward, T. (n.d.). Tendinopathy: New thinking on an old problem. *Sports Injury Bulletin.* https://www.sportsinjurybulletin.com/tendinopathy-new-thinking-on-an-old-problem/

121. Yousefi, M. R., Ahmad, N., Abbaszadeh, M. R., & Rokhsati, S. (2012). The effect of isometric training on prevention of bone density reduction in injured limbs during an immobilization period. *Research in Medicine, 35* (4), 195–199. http://pejouhesh.sbmu.ac.ir/article-1-971-en.html

122. Gerber, J. P., Marcus, R. L., Leland, E. D., & Lastayo, P. C. (2009). The use of eccentrically biased resistance exercise to mitigate muscle impairments following anterior cruciate ligament reconstruction: A short review. *Sports Health, 1*(1), 31–38. https://doi.org/10.1177/1941738108327531

123. Lorenz, D., & Reiman, M. (2011). The role and implementation of eccentric training in athletic rehabilitation: Tendinopathy, hamstring strains, and ACL reconstruction. *International Journal of Sports Physical Therapy, 6*(1), 27–44.

124. Arampatzis, A., Karamanidis, K., & Albracht, K. (2007). Adaptational responses of the human Achilles tendon by modulation of the applied cyclic strain magnitude. *The Journal of Experimental Biology, 210*(Pt 15), 2743–2753. https://doi.org/10.1242/jeb.003814

125. Reichel, T., Mitnacht, M., Fenwick, A., Meffert, R., Hoos, O., & Fehske, K. (2019). Incidence and characteristics of acute and overuse injuries in elite powerlifters. *Cogent Medicine, 6*(1), doi: 10.1080/2331205X.2019.1588192

126. Sophia Fox, A. J., Bedi, A., & Rodeo, S. A. (2009). The basic science of articular cartilage: Structure, composition, and function. *Sports Health, 1*(6), 461–468. https://doi.org/10.1177/1941738109350438

127. Docking, S. I., Girdwood, M. A., Cook, J., Fortington, L. V., & Rio, E. (2020). Reduced levels of aligned fibrillar structure are not associated with Achilles and patellar tendon symptoms. *Clinical Journal of Sport Medicine: Official Journal of the Canadian Academy of Sport Medicine, 30*(6), 550–555. https://doi.org/10.1097/JSM.0000000000000644

128. Magnusson, S. P., Langberg, H., & Kjaer, M. (2010). The pathogenesis of tendinopathy: Balancing the response to loading. *Nature Reviews. Rheumatology, 6*(5), 262–268. https://doi.org/10.1038/nrrheum.2010.43

129. Kim, E., Dear, A., Ferguson, S. L., Seo, D., & Bemben, M. G. (2011). Effects of 4 weeks of traditional resistance training vs. superslow strength training on early phase adaptations in strength, flexibility, and aerobic capacity in college-aged women. *Journal of Strength and Conditioning Research, 25*(11), 3006–3013. https://doi.org/10.1519/JSC.0b013e318212e3a2

130. Wikipedia contributors. (2019). *Super slow.* https://en.wikipedia.org/wiki/Super_Slow

131. Macaluso, F., Isaacs, A. W., & Myburgh, K. H. (2012). Preferential type II muscle fiber damage from plyometric exercise. *Journal of Athletic Training, 47*(4), 414–420. https://doi.org/10.4085/1062-6050-47.4.13

132. Wilson, G. J., Wood, G. A., & Elliott, B. C. (1991). Optimal stiffness of series elastic component in a stretch-shorten cycle activity. *Journal of Applied Physiology, 70*(2), 825–833. https://doi.org/10.1152/jappl.1991.70.2.825

133. Kubo, K., Ishigaki, T., & Ikebukuro, T. (2017). Effects of plyometric and isometric training on muscle and tendon stiffness in vivo. *Physiological Reports, 5*(15), e13374. https://doi.org/10.14814/phy2.13374

134. Turner, A. N., & Jeffreys, I. (2010). The stretch-shortening cycle: Proposed mechanisms and methods for enhancement. *Strength and Conditioning Journal, 32*, 87–99. doi: 10.1519/SSC.0b013e3181e928f9

135. Timmins, R. G., Opar, D. A., Williams, M. D., Schache, A. G., Dear, N. M., & Shield, A. J. (2014). Reduced biceps femoris myoelectrical activity influences eccentric knee flexor weakness after repeat sprint running. *Scandinavian Journal of Medicine & Science in Sports, 24*(4), e299–e305. https://doi.org/10.1111/sms.12171

136. Smeets, J.S.J., Horstman, A.M.H., Vles, G. F., Emans, P. J., Goessens, J.P.B., Gijsen, A. P., et al. (2019). Protein synthesis rates of muscle, tendon, ligament, cartilage, and bone tissue *in vivo* in humans. *PLoS ONE, 14*(11), e0224745. https://doi.org/10.1371/journal.pone.0224745

137. Leitman, D. C., Benson, S. C., & Johnson, L. K. (1984). Glucocorticoids stimulate collagen and noncollagen protein synthesis in cultured vascular smooth muscle cells. *Journal of Cell Biology, 98*, 541–549. https://rupress.org/jcb/article-pdf/98/2/541/1390360/541.pdf

138. Baar, K. (2017). Minimizing injury and maximizing return to play: Lessons from engineered ligaments. *Sports Medicine, 47*(Suppl 1), 5–11. https://doi.org/10.1007/s40279-017-0719-x

139. Nutt, J. J. (2009). *Diseases and deformities of the foot.* BiblioLife.

140. Murakami, H., Shimbo, K., Inoue, Y., Takino, Y., & Kobayashi, H. (2012). Importance of amino acid composition to improve skin collagen protein synthesis rates in UV-irradiated mice. *Amino Acids 42*, 2481–2489. https://doi.org/10.1007/s00726-011-1059-z

141. Ganceviciene, R., Liakou, A. I., Theodoridis, A., Makrantonaki, E., & Zouboulis, C. C. (2012). Skin anti-aging strategies. *Dermato-endocrinology, 4*(3), 308–319. https://doi.org/10.4161/derm.22804

142. Leblanc, D. R., Schneider, M., Angele, P., Vollmer, G., & Docheva, D. (2017). The effect of estrogen on tendon and ligament metabolism and function. *Journal of Steroid Biochemistry and Molecular Biology, 172*, 106–116. https://doi.org/10.1016/j.jsbmb.2017.06.008

143. Hunt, T. K., Knighton, D. R., Thakral, K. K., Goodson, W. H., 3rd, & Andrews, W. S. (1984). Studies on inflammation and wound healing: Angiogenesis and collagen synthesis stimulated in vivo by resident and activated wound macrophages. *Surgery, 96*(1), 48–54.

144. Goldring, M. B., & Otero, M. (2011). Inflammation in osteoarthritis. *Current Opinion in Rheumatology, 23*(5), 471–478. https://doi.org/10.1097/BOR.0b013e328349c2b1

145. Certain lifestyle habits can contribute to collagen loss and premature aging. (2016, April 29). Technology.org. https://www.technology.org/2016/04/29/certain-lifestyle-habits-can-contribute-collagen-loss-premature-aging/

146. National Sleep Foundation. (n.d.) *How sleep improves your skin.* https://www.sleep.org/articles/how-sleep-improves-your-skin/

147. Chojkier, M., Spanheimer, R., & Peterkofsky, B. (1983). Specifically decreased collagen biosynthesis in scurvy dissociated from an effect on proline hydroxylation and correlated with body weight loss. In vitro studies in guinea pig calvarial bones. *The Journal of Clinical Investigation, 72*(3), 826–835. https://doi.org/10.1172/JCI111053

148. Spanheimer, R. G., & Peterkofsky, B. (1984). A specific decrease in collagen synthesis in acutely fasted, vitamin C–supplemented, guinea pigs. *Journal of Biological Chemistry, 260*, 3855–3962.

149. Briese, V., & Hopp, H. (1989). Somatomedine--Insulinähnliche Wachstumsfaktoren [Somatomedins--insulin-like growth factors]. *Zentralblatt fur Gynakologie, 111*(15), 1017–1024. https://pubmed.ncbi.nlm.nih.gov/2554621/

150. Goldstein, R. H., Poliks, C. F., Pilch, P. F., Smith, B. D., & Fine, A. (1989). Stimulation of collagen formation by insulin and insulin-like growth factor I in cultures of human lung fibroblasts. *Endocrinology, 124*(2), 964–970. https://doi.org/10.1210/endo-124-2-964

151. Woods, J. (2015, May). *What does estrogen have to do with belly fat?* Obstetrics & Gynecology: Menopause [Blog]. https://www.rochester.edu

152. Ronon, C. (2001). The use of massage to influence collagen synthesis in the hand: A physiological justification. *The British Journal of Hand Therapy, 6*(3), 95–99. https://doi.org/10.1177/175899830100600305

153. Lee, K. O., Kim, S. N., & Kim, Y. C. (2014). Anti-wrinkle effects of water extracts of teas in hairless mouse. *Toxicological Research, 30*(4), 283–289. https://doi.org/10.5487/TR.2014.30.4.283

154. Farup, J., Rahbek, S. K., Vendelbo, M. H., Matzon, A., Hindhede, J., Bejder, et al. (2014). Whey protein hydrolysate augments tendon and muscle hypertrophy independent of resistance exercise contraction mode. *Scandinavian Journal of Medicine & Science in Sports, 24*(5), 788–798. https://doi.org/10.1111/sms.12083

155. Banaszek, A., Townsend, J. R., Bender, D., Vantrease, W. C., Marshall, A. C., & Johnson, K. D. (2019). The effects of whey vs. pea protein on physical adaptations following 8-weeks of high-intensity functional training (HIFT): A pilot study. *Sports, 7*(1), 12. https://doi.org/10.3390/sports7010012

156. Bukhari, S. S., Phillips, B. E., Wilkinson, D. J., Limb, M. C., Rankin, D., Mitchell, W. K., et al. (2015). Intake of low-dose leucine-rich essential amino acids stimulates muscle anabolism equivalently to bolus whey protein in older women at rest and after exercise. *American Journal of Physiology: Endocrinology and Metabolism, 308*(12), E1056–E1065. https://doi.org/10.1152/ajpendo.00481.2014

157. Park, S., Church, D. D., Azhar, G. et al. (2020). Anabolic response to essential amino acid plus whey protein composition is greater than whey protein alone in young healthy adults. *J Int Soc Sports Nutr, 17*, 9 (2020). https://doi.org/10.1186/s12970-020-0340-5

158. Shaw, G., Lee-Barthel, A., Ross, M. L., Wang, B., & Baar, K. (2017). Vitamin C-enriched gelatin supplementation before intermittent activity augments collagen synthesis. *The American Journal of Clinical Nutrition, 105*(1), 136–143. https://doi.org/10.3945/ajcn.116.138594

159. Figueres Juher, T., & Basés Pérez, E. (2015). Revisión de los efectos beneficiosos de la ingesta de colágeno hidrolizado sobre la salud osteoarticular y el envejecimiento dérmico [An overview of the beneficial effects of hydrolysed collagen intake on joint and bone health and on skin ageing]. *Nutricion Hospitalaria, 32 Suppl 1*, 62–66. https://doi.org/10.3305/nh.2015.32.sup1.9482

160. DePhillipo, N. N., Aman, Z. S., Kennedy, M. I., Begley, J. P., Moatshe, G., & LaPrade, R. F. (2018). Efficacy of vitamin c supplementation on collagen synthesis and oxidative stress after musculoskeletal injuries: A systematic review. *Orthopaedic Journal of Sports Medicine, 6*(10), 2325967118804544. https://doi.org/10.1177/2325967118804544

161. Bakilan, F., Armagan, O., Ozgen, M., Tascioglu, F., Bolluk, O., & Alatas, O. (2016). Effects of native type II collagen treatment on knee osteoarthritis: A randomized controlled trial. *The Eurasian Journal of Medicine, 48*(2), 95–101. https://doi.org/10.5152/eurasianjmed.2015.15030

162. Barnett, M. L., Kremer, J. M., St Clair, E. W., Clegg, D. O., Furst, D., Weisman, M., et al. (1998). Treatment of rheumatoid arthritis with oral type II collagen: Results of a multicenter, double-blind, placebo-controlled trial. *Arthritis and Rheumatism, 41*(2), 290–297. https://doi.org/10.1002/1529-0131(199802)41:2<290::AID-ART13>3.0.CO;2-R

163. Paul, C., Leser, S., & Oesser, S. (2019). Significant amounts of functional collagen peptides can be incorporated in the diet while maintaining indispensable amino acid balance. *Nutrients, 11*(5), 1079. https://doi.org/10.3390/nu11051079

164. Paxton, J. Z., Hagerty, P., Andrick, J. J., & Baar, K. (2012). Optimizing an intermittent stretch paradigm using ERK1/2 phosphorylation results in increased collagen synthesis in engineered ligaments. *Tissue Engineering. Part A, 18*(3-4), 277–284. https://doi.org/10.1089/ten.TEA.2011.0336

165. Marlowe, F.W. (2010). *The Hadza: Hunter-gatherers of Tanzania.* University of California Press.

166. Raichlen, D. A., Wood, B. M., Gordon, A. D., Mabulla, A. Z., Marlowe, F. W., & Pontzer, H. (2014). Evidence of Lévy walk foraging patterns in human hunter-gatherers. *Proceedings of the National Academy of Sciences of the United States of America, 111*

167. Bowman, K. (2017). *Move your DNA: Restore your health through natural movement.* Propriometrics Press.

168. Luttrell, M. (2013). *Lone survivor: The eyewitness account of Operation Redwing and the lost heroes of SEAL Team 10.* Little, Brown and Company.

169. Gabbett, T. (2016). The training-injury prevention paradox: Should athletes be training smarter and harder? *British Journal of Sports Medicine, 50.* doi:10.1136/bjsports-2015-095788

170. Bowen, L., Gross, A. S., Gimpel M., Bruce-Low, S., & Li, F.-X. (2020). Spikes in acute:chronic workload ratio (ACWR) associated with a 5–7 times greater injury rate in English Premier League football players: A comprehensive 3-year study. *British Journal of Sports Medicine, 54,* 731–738. http://dx.doi.org/10.1136/bjsports-2018-099422

171. Gabbett, T. J. (2020). Debunking the myths about training load, injury and performance: Empirical evidence, hot topics and recommendations for practitioners. *British Journal of Sports Medicine, 54*(1), 58–66. https://doi.org/10.1136/bjsports-2018-099784

172. Gabbett, T. J., Kennelly, S., Sheehan, J., Hawkins, R., Milsom, J., King, E., et al. (2016). If overuse injury is a 'training load error', should undertraining be viewed the same way? *British Journal of Sports Medicine, 50*(17), 1017–1018. https://doi.org/10.1136/bjsports-2016-096308

173. Ferrell, B. A., Josephson, K. R., Pollan, A. M., Loy, S., & Ferrell, B. R. (1997). A randomized trial of walking versus physical methods for chronic pain management. *Aging (Milan, Italy), 9*(1-2), 99–105. https://doi.org/10.1007/BF03340134

174. Kovar, P. A., Allegrante, J. P., MacKenzie, C. R., Peterson, M. G., Gutin, B., & Charlson, M. E. (1992). Supervised fitness walking in patients with osteoarthritis of the knee. A randomized, controlled trial. *Annals of Internal Medicine, 116*(7), 529–534. https://doi.org/10.7326/0003-4819-116-7-529

175. Vanti, C., Andreatta, S., Borghi, S., Guccione, A. A., Pillastrini, P., & Bertozzi, L. (2019). The effectiveness of walking versus exercise on pain and function in chronic low back pain: A systematic review and meta-analysis of randomized trials. *Disability and Rehabilitation, 41*(6), 622–632. https://doi.org/10.1080/09638288.2017.1410730

176. Polaski, A. M., Phelps, A. L., Szucs, K. A., Ramsey, A. M., Kostek, M. C., & Kolber, B. J. (2019). The dosing of aerobic exercise therapy on experimentally-induced pain in healthy female participants. *Scientific Reports, 9*(1), 14842. doi:10.1038/s41598-019-51247-0

177. Hlaváček, M. (1999). Lubrication of the human ankle joint in walking with the synovial fluid filtrated by the cartilage with the surface zone worn out: Steady pure sliding motion. *Journal of Biomechanics, 32*(10), 1059–1069. https://doi.org/10.1016/s0021-9290(99)00095-0

178. Lee, J. S., & Kang, S. J. (2016). The effects of strength exercise and walking on lumbar function, pain level, and body composition in chronic back pain patients. *Journal of Exercise Rehabilitation, 12*(5), 463–470. https://doi.org/10.12965/jer.1632650.325

179. Ridge, S. T., Olsen, M. T., Bruening, D. A., Jurgensmeier, K., Griffin, D., Davis, I. S., & Johnson, A. W. (2019). Walking in minimalist shoes is effective for strengthening foot muscles. *Medicine and Science in Sports and Exercise, 51*(1), 104–113. https://doi.org/10.1249/MSS.0000000000001751

180. Hackford, J., Mackey, A., & Broadbent, E. (2019). The effects of walking posture on affective and physiological states during stress. *Journal of Behavior Therapy and Experimental Psychiatry, 62,* 80–87. https://doi.org/10.1016/j.jbtep.2018.09.004.

181. Krall, E. A., & Dawson-Hughes, B. (1994). Walking is related to bone density and rates of bone loss. *The American Journal of Medicine, 96*(1), 20–26. https://doi.org/10.1016/0002-9343(94)90111-2

182. Bond Brill, J., Perry, A. C., Parker, L., Robinson, A., & Burnett, K. (2002). Dose-response effect of walking exercise on weight loss. How much is enough? *International Journal of Obesity and Related Metabolic Disorders, 26*(11), 1484–1493. https://doi.org/10.1038/sj.ijo.0802133

183. Gordon, R., & Bloxham, S. (2016). A systematic review of the effects of exercise and physical activity on non-specific chronic low back pain. *Healthcare (Basel, Switzerland), 4*(2), 22. https://doi.org/10.3390/healthcare4020022

184. Ahmad, A. H., & Zakaria, R. (2015). Pain in times of stress. *The Malaysian Journal of Medical Sciences, 22*(Spec. Issue), 52–61.

185. Oschman, J. L., Chevalier, G., & Brown, R. (2015). The effects of grounding (earthing) on inflammation, the immune response, wound healing, and prevention and treatment of chronic inflammatory and autoimmune diseases. *Journal of Inflammation Research*, 8, 83–96. https://doi.org/10.2147/JIR.S69656

186. Alghadir, A. H., Anwer, S., Sarkar, B., Paul, A. K., & Anwar, D. (2019). Effect of 6-week retro or forward walking program on pain, functional disability, quadriceps muscle strength, and performance in individuals with knee osteoarthritis: A randomized controlled trial (retro-walking trial). *BMC Musculoskeletal Disorders*, 20(1), 159. https://doi.org/10.1186/s12891-019-2537-9

187. Olugbade, T., Bianchi-Berthouze, N., Williams, A. (2019). The relationship between guarding, pain, and emotion. *PAIN Reports*, 4, e770. doi: 10.1097/PR9.0000000000000770

188. Levine, J. A. (2002). Non-exercise activity thermogenesis (NEAT). *Best Practice & Research. Clinical Endocrinology & Metabolism*, 16(4), 679–702. https://doi.org/10.1053/beem.2002.0227

189. Krivickas, L. S., & Feinberg, J. H. (1996). Lower extremity injuries in college athletes: Relation between ligamentous laxity and lower extremity muscle tightness. *Archives of Physical Medicine and Rehabilitation*, 77(11), 1139–1143. https://doi.org/10.1016/s0003-9993(96)90137-9

190. Yeung, J., Cleves, A., Griffiths, H., & Nokes, L. (2016). Mobility, proprioception, strength and FMS as predictors of injury in professional footballers. *BMJ Open Sport & Exercise Medicine*, 2(1), e000134. https://doi.org/10.1136/bmjsem-2016-000134

191. Knobloch, K., Martin-Schmitt, S., Gösling, T., Jagodzinski, M., Zeichen, J., & Krettek, C. (2005). Prospektives Propriozeptions- und Koordinationstraining zur Verletzungsreduktion im professionellen Frauenfussballsport [Prospective proprioceptive and coordinative training for injury reduction in elite female soccer]. *Sportverletzung Sportschaden : Organ der Gesellschaft fur Orthopadisch-Traumatologische Sportmedizin*, 19(3), 123–129. https://doi.org/10.1055/s-2005-858345

192. Lauersen, J. B., Bertelsen, D. M., Andersen, L. B. (2014). The effectiveness of exercise interventions to prevent sports injuries: A systematic review and meta-analysis of randomised controlled trials. *British Journal of Sports Medicine*, 48, 871–877.

193. Sadigursky, D., Braid, J. A., De Lira, D., Machado, B., Carneiro, R., & Colavolpe, P. O. (2017). The FIFA 11+ injury prevention program for soccer players: A systematic review. *BMC Sports Science, Medicine & Rehabilitation*, 9, 18. https://doi.org/10.1186/s13102-017-0083-z

194. Blazevich, A. J., Cannavan, D., Waugh, C. M., Miller, S. C., Thorlund, J. B., Aagaard, P., & Kay, A. D. (2014). Range of motion, neuromechanical, and architectural adaptations to plantar flexor stretch training in humans. *Journal of Applied Physiology*, 117(5), 452–462. https://doi.org/10.1152/japplphysiol.00204.2014

195. Aquino, C. F., Fonseca, S. T., Gonçalves, G. G., Silva, P. L., Ocarino, J. M., & Mancini, M. C. (2010). Stretching versus strength training in lengthened position in subjects with tight hamstring muscles: A randomized controlled trial. *Manual Therapy*, 15(1), 26–31. https://doi.org/10.1016/j.math.2009.05.006

196. Page, P., Frank, C., & Lardner, R. (2010). *Assessment and treatment of muscle imbalance: The Janda approach*. Human Kinetics

197. Winters, T. M., Takahashi, M., Lieber, R. L., & Ward, S. R. (2011). Whole muscle length-tension relationships are accurately modeled as scaled sarcomeres in rabbit hindlimb muscles. *Journal of Biomechanics*, 44(1), 109–115. https://doi.org/10.1016/j.jbiomech.2010.08.033

198. Zöllner, A. M., Abilez, O. J., Böl, M., & Kuhl, E. (2012). Stretching skeletal muscle: chronic muscle lengthening through sarcomerogenesis. *PloS One*, 7(10), e45661. https://doi.org/10.1371/journal.pone.0045661

199. Page, P. (2011). Shoulder muscle imbalance and subacromial impingement syndrome in overhead athletes. *International Journal of Sports Physical Therapy*, 6(1), 51–58.

200. Betts, J. G., Young, K. A., Wise, J. A., Johnson, E., Poe, B., Kruse, D. H., et al. (2013). *Anatomy and physiology*. OpenStax.

201. Tsepis, E., Vagenas, G., Giakas, G., & Georgoulis, A. (2004). Hamstring weakness as an indicator of poor knee function in ACL-deficient patients. *Knee Surgery, Sports Traumatology, Arthroscopy*, 12(1), 22–29. https://doi.org/10.1007/s00167-003-0377-4

202. Physopedia contributors. (2020, December 8). *Cardinal planes and axes of movement*. Physopedia. https://www.physio-pedia.com/Cardinal_Planes_and_Axes_of_Movement

203. McGill, S. (2007). *Low back disorders: Evidence-based prevention and rehabilitation*, 2nd ed. Human Kinetics.

204. Weppler, C. H., & Magnusson, S. P. (2010). Increasing muscle extensibility: A matter of increasing length or modifying sensation? *Physical Therapy, 90*, 438–449. https://doi.org/10.2522/ptj.20090012

205. Miller, K. C., & Burne, J. A. (2014). Golgi tendon organ reflex inhibition following manually applied acute static stretching. *Journal of Sports Sciences, 32*(15), 1491–1497. https://doi.org/10.1080/02640414.2014.899708

206. Park, H. K., Jung, M. K., Park, E., Lee, C. Y., Jee, Y. S., Eun, D., et al. (2018). The effect of warm-ups with stretching on the isokinetic moments of collegiate men. *Journal of Exercise Rehabilitation, 14*(1), 78–82. https://doi.org/10.12965/jer.1835210.605

207. Hindle, K. B., Whitcomb, T. J., Briggs, W. O., & Hong, J. (2012). Proprioceptive neuromuscular facilitation (PNF): Its mechanisms and effects on range of motion and muscular function. *Journal of Human Kinetics, 31*, 105–113. https://doi.org/10.2478/v10078-012-0011-y

208. Kukkonen, P. T. (2019). Scientific basis of active isolated stretching: A review. *Journal of Exercise Physiology Online, 22*, 58–70. https://www.asep.org/asep/asep/JEPonlineAPRIL2019_Kukkonen.pdf

209. Franklin, N. C., Ali, M. M., Robinson, A. T., Norkeviciute, E., & Phillips, S. A. (2014). Massage therapy restores peripheral vascular function after exertion. *Archives of Physical Medicine and Rehabilitation, 95*, 1127–1134. https://doi.org/10.1016/j.apmr.2014.02.007

210. Wiewelhove, T., Döweling, A., Schneider, C., Hottenrott, L., Meyer, T., Kellmann, M., et al. (2019). A meta-analysis of the effects of foam rolling on performance and recovery. *Frontiers in Physiology, 10*, 376. https://doi.org/10.3389/fphys.2019.00376

211. Penney, S. (2013, August 21). Foam rolling: Applying the technique of self-myofascial release [Blog]. https://nasm.org

212. Beardsley, C., & Škarabot, J. (2015). Effects of self-myofascial release: A systematic review. *Journal of Bodywork & Movement Therapies, 19*, 747–758. http://dx.doi.org/10.1016/j.jbmt.2015.08.007

213. Wheeler, M. J., Green, D. J., Ellis, K. A., et al. (2020). Distinct effects of acute exercise and breaks in sitting on working memory and executive function in older adults: A three-arm, randomised cross-over trial to evaluate the effects of exercise with and without breaks in sitting on cognition. *British Journal of Sports Medicine, 54*, 776–781. https://bjsm.bmj.com/content/early/2019/04/24/bjsports-2018-100168

214. Crone C. (1993). Reciprocal inhibition in man. *Danish Medical Bulletin, 40*(5), 571–581. https://www.ncbi.nlm.nih.gov/pubmed/8299401

215. Wright, P., Drysdale, I. (2008). A comparison of post-isometric relaxation (PIR) and reciprocal inhibition (RI) muscle energy techniques applied to piriformis. *International Journal of Osteopathic Medicine, 11*, 158–159. https://doi.org/10.1016/j.ijosm.2008.08.015

216. Boyle, M. (n.d.). *Advances in functional training* excerpt. On Target Publications. https://www.otpbooks.com

217. Contreras, B., & Cordoza, G. (2019). *Glute lab: The art and science of strength and physique training.* Victory Belt Publishing.

218. Kim, K. H., Cho, S. H., Goo, B. O., & Baek, I. H. (2013). Differences in transversus abdominis muscle function between chronic low back pain patients and healthy subjects at maximum expiration: Measurement with real-time ultrasonography. *Journal of Physical Therapy Science, 25*(7), 861–863. https://doi.org/10.1589/jpts.25.861

219. Lynders, C. (2019). The critical role of development of the transversus abdominis in the prevention and treatment of low back pain. *HSS Jrnl, 15*, 214–220. https://doi.org/10.1007/s11420-019-09717-8

220. Tajiri, K., Huo, M., & Maruyama, H. (2014). Effects of co-contraction of both transverse abdominal muscle and pelvic floor muscle exercises for stress urinary incontinence: A randomized controlled trial. *Journal of Physical Therapy Science, 26*(8), 1161–1163. https://doi.org/10.1589/jpts.26.1161

221. Takimoto, R., Kimura, M., Yokoba, M., Ichikawa, T., & Matsunaga A. (2016). Relationship between abdominal pressure and diaphragmatic movement in abdominal breathing. *European Respiratory Journal, 48*, PA1372. doi: 10.1183/13993003.congress-2016.PA1372

222. Abdelraouf, O. R., & Abdel-Aziem, A. A. (2016). The relationship between core endurance and back dysfunction in collegiate male athletes with and without nonspecific low back pain. *International Journal of Sports Physical Therapy, 11*(3), 337–

223. O'Sullivan, P. B., Mitchell, T., Bulich, P., Waller, R., & Holte, J. (2006). The relationship between posture and back muscle endurance in industrial workers with flexion-related low back pain. *Manual Therapy, 11*(4), 264–271. https://doi.org/10.1016/j.math.2005.04.004

224. Smith, A. J., O'Sullivan, P. B., Campbell, A. C., & Straker, L. M. (2010). The relationship between back muscle endurance and physical, lifestyle, and psychological factors in adolescents. *Journal of Orthopedic & Sports Physical Therapy, 40*(8), 517–523.

225. McGill, S. (n.d.). *Designing back exercise: From rehabilitation to enhancing performance.* https://www.backfitpro.com/documents/RehabtoEnhancing.pdf

226. Physiopedia contributors. (2020). *Lumbar multifidus.* https://www.physio-pedia.com

227. Kolber M. J., & Beekhuizen, K. (2007). Lumbar stabilization: An evidence-based approach for the athlete with low back pain. *Strength and Conditioning Journal, 29,* 26–37

228. Chang, L. R., Anand, P., Varacallo, M. (2020). *Anatomy, shoulder and upper limb, glenohumeral joint.* StatPearls. https://www.ncbi.nlm.nih.gov/books/NBK537018/

229. Paine, R., & Voight, M. L. (2013). The role of the scapula. *International Journal of Sports Physical Therapy, 8*(5), 617–629.

230. van der Windt, D. A., Koes, B. W., de Jong, B. A., & Bouter, L. M. (1995). Shoulder disorders in general practice: Incidence, patient characteristics, and management. *Annals of the Rheumatic Diseases, 54*(12), 959–964. https://doi.org/10.1136/ard.54.12.959

231. Kromer, T. O., Tautenhahn, U. G., de Bie, R. A., Staal, J. B., & Bastiaenen, C.H.G. (2009). Effects of physiotherapy in patients with shoulder impingement syndrome: A systematic review of the literature. *Journal of Rehabilitation Medicine, 41,* 870–880. doi: 10.2340/16501977-0453

232. Mihata, T., Gates, J., McGarry, M. H., Lee, J., Kinoshita, M., & Lee, T. Q. (2009). Effect of rotator cuff muscle imbalance on forceful internal impingement and peel-back of the superior labrum: A cadaveric study. *The American Journal of Sports Medicine, 37*(11), 2222–2227. https://doi.org/10.1177/0363546509337450

233. Sadeghifar, A., Ilka, S., Dashtbani, H., & Sahebozamani, M. (2014). A comparison of glenohumeral internal and external range of motion and rotation strength in healthy and individuals with recurrent anterior instability. *The Archives of Bone and Joint Surgery, 2*(3), 215–219.

234. Malliou, P. C., Giannakopoulos, K., Beneka, A. G., et al. (2004). Effective ways of restoring muscular imbalances of the rotator cuff muscle group: A comparative study of various training methods. *British Journal of Sports Medicine, 38,* 766–772.

235. Physiopedia contributors. (2021). *Scapulohumeral rhythm.* https://www.physio-pedia.com/Scapulohumeral_Rhythm

236. Ludewig, P. M., & Cook, T. M. (2000). Alterations in shoulder kinematics and associated muscle activity in people with symptoms of shoulder impingement. *Physical Therapy, 80*(3), 276–291.

237. Samuels, V. (2018). *Foundations in kinesiology and biomechanics.* F. A. Davis.

238. Nicolini, A. P., de Carvalho, R. T., Matsuda, M. M., Sayum, J. F., & Cohen, M. (2014). Common injuries in athletes' knee: Experience of a specialized center. *Acta Ortopedica Brasileira, 22*(3), 127–131. https://doi.org/10.1590/1413-78522014220300475

239. Mullaney, M. J., & Fukunaga, T. (2016). Current concepts and treatment of patellofemoral compressive issues. *International Journal of Sports Physical Therapy, 11*(6), 891–902.

240. Halabchi, F., Abolhasani, M., Mirshahi, M., & Alizadeh, Z. (2017). Patellofemoral pain in athletes: Clinical perspectives. *Open Access Journal of Sports Medicine, 8,* 189–203. https://doi.org/10.2147/OAJSM.S127359

241. Sharma, L. (2007). The role of varus and valgus alignment in knee osteoarthritis. [Editorial]. *Arthritis & Rheumatism, 56,* 1044–1047. doi 10.1002/art.22514

242. Ferber, R., D. Kendall, K. D., Farr, L. (2011). Changes in knee biomechanics after a hip-abductor strengthening protocol for runners with patellofemoral pain syndrome. *J Athl Train, 46*(2), 142–149. doi: https://doi.org/10.4085/1062-6050-46.2.142

243. Hibbert, O., Cheong, K., Grant, A., Beers, A., & Moizumi, T. (2008). A systematic review of the effectiveness of eccentric strength training in the prevention of hamstring muscle strains in otherwise healthy individuals. *North American Journal of Sports Physical Therapy, 3*(2), 67–81.

244. Proske, U., Morgan, D. L., Brockett, C. L., & Percival, P. (2004). Identifying athletes at risk of hamstring strains and how to protect them. *Clinical and Experimental Pharmacology & Physiology, 31*(8), 546–550. https://doi.org/10.1111/j.1440-1681.2004.04028.x

245. Ferber, R., Bolgla, L., Earl-Boehm, J. E., Emery, C., & Hamstra-Wright, K. (2015). Strengthening of the hip and core versus knee muscles for the treatment of patellofemoral pain: A multicenter randomized controlled trial. *Journal of Athletic Training, 50*(4), 366–377. https://doi.org/10.4085/1062-6050-49.3.70

246. Kim, S. H., Kwon, O. Y., Park, K. N., Jeon, I. C., & Weon, J. H. (2015). Lower extremity strength and the range of motion in relation to squat depth. *Journal of Human Kinetics, 45,* 59–69. https://doi.org/10.1515/hukin-2015-0007

247. Landrum, E. L., Kelln, C. B., Parente, W. R., Ingersoll, C. D., & Hertel, J. (2008). Immediate effects of anterior-to-posterior talocrural joint mobilization after prolonged ankle immobilization: A preliminary study. *Journal of Manual & Manipulative Therapy, 16*(2), 100–105. https://doi.org/10.1179/106698108790818413

248. Gross, K. D., Felson, D. T., Niu, J., Hunter, D. J., Guermazi, A., Roemer, F. W., et al. (2011). Association of flat feet with knee pain and cartilage damage in older adults. *Arthritis Care & Research, 63*(7), 937–944. https://doi.org/10.1002/acr.20431

249. Goo, Y. M., Kim, T. H., & Lim, J. Y. (2016). The effects of gluteus maximus and abductor hallucis strengthening exercises for four weeks on navicular drop and lower extremity muscle activity during gait with flatfoot. *Journal of Physical Therapy Science, 28*(3), 911–915. https://doi.org/10.1589/jpts.28.911

250. Dupuy, O., Douzi, W., Theurot, D., Bosquet, L., & Dugué, B. (2018). An evidence-based approach for choosing post-exercise recovery techniques to reduce markers of muscle damage, soreness, fatigue, and inflammation: A systematic review with meta-analysis. *Frontiers in Physiology, 9*, 403. https://doi.org/10.3389/fphys.2018.00403

251. Mirkin, G. (2015, September 16). *Why ice delays recovery*. https://www.drmirkin.com/fitness/why-ice-delays-recovery.html

252. Khan, K. M., Scott, A. (2009). Mechanotherapy: How physical therapists' prescription of exercise promotes tissue repair. *British Journal of Sports Medicine, 43*, 247–252.

253. van den Bekerom, M. P., Struijs, P. A., Blankevoort, L., Welling, L., van Dijk, C. N., & Kerkhoffs, G. M. (2012). What is the evidence for rest, ice, compression, and elevation therapy in the treatment of ankle sprains in adults? *Journal of Athletic Training, 47*(4), 435–443. https://doi.org/10.4085/1062-6050-47.4.14

254. Block, J. E. (2010). Cold and compression in the management of musculoskeletal injuries and orthopedic operative procedures: A narrative review. *Open Access Journal of Sports Medicine, 1*, 105–113. https://doi.org/10.2147/oajsm.s11102

255. Reinl, G. (2014). *Iced! The illusionary treatment option*, 2nd ed. Gary Reinl.

256. Dubois, B., & Esculier, J. F. (2020). Soft-tissue injuries simply need PEACE and LOVE. *British Journal of Sports Medicine, 54*(2), 72–73. https://doi.org/10.1136/bjsports-2019-101253

257. Joyce, D., & Lewindon, D. (Eds.) (2015). *Sports injury prevention and rehabilitation: Integrating medicine and science for performance solutions*. Abingdon, UK: Routledge.

258. Fu, S. C., Rolf, C., Cheuk, Y. C., Lui, P. P., & Chan, K. M. (2010). Deciphering the pathogenesis of tendinopathy: A three-stages process. *Sports Medicine, Arthroscopy, Rehabilitation, Therapy & Technology, 2*, 30. https://doi.org/10.1186/1758-2555-2-30

259. Bickel, C. S., Cross, J. M., & Bamman, M. M. (2011). Exercise dosing to retain resistance training adaptations in young and older adults. *Medicine and Science in Sports and Exercise, 43*(7), 1177–1187. https://doi.org/10.1249/MSS.0b013e318207c15d

260. Beardsley, C. (2019, June 11). *Do you really need a deload?* Medium. https://medium.com/@SandCResearch/do-you-really-need-a-deload-64e7b4a4eb4f

261. Selye, H. (1950, June 17). Stress and the general adaptation syndrome. *British Medical Journal.* https://www.ncbi.nlm.nih.gov/pmc/articles/PMC2038162/pdf/brmedj03603-0003.pdf

262. Reaburn, P., & Jenkins, D. (Eds.) (1997). *Training for speed and endurance*. Unwin Hyman.

263. Issurin, V. (2008). Block periodization versus traditional training theory: A review. *The Journal of Sports Medicine and Physical Fitness, 48*(1), 65–75.

264. Prestes, J., Frollini, A. B., de Lima, C., Donatto, F. F., Foschini, D., de Cássia Marqueti, R., et al. (2009). Comparison between linear and daily undulating periodized resistance training to increase strength. *Journal of Strength and Conditioning Research, 23*(9), 2437–2442. https://doi.org/10.1519/JSC.0b013e3181c03548

265. Rhea, M. R., Ball, S. D., Phillips, W. T., & Burkett, L. N. (2002). A comparison of linear and daily undulating periodized programs with equated volume and intensity for strength. *Journal of Strength and Conditioning Research, 16*(2), 250–255.

266. Majeedkutty, N. A., Jabbar, M. A., Min, M. J., et al. (2018). Effect of linear and non-linear periodized resistance training on dynamic postural control and functional movement screen. *MOJ Yoga Physical Ther, 3*(1), 18–22. doi: 10.15406/mojypt.2018.03.00038

267. Bartolomei, S., Stout, J., Fukuda, D., Hoffman, J., & Merni, F. (2015). Block vs. weekly undulating periodized resistance training programs in women. *Journal of Strength and Conditioning Research, 29*(10), 2679–2687. doi: 10.1519/JSC.0000000000000948

268. Radaelli, R., Fleck, S. J., Leite, T., Leite, R. D., Pinto, R. S., Fernandes, L., & Simão, R. (2015). Dose-response of 1, 3, and 5 sets of resistance exercise on strength, local muscular endurance, and hypertrophy. *J Strength Cond Res., 29*(5), 1349–1358. doi: 10.1519/JSC.0000000000000758. PMID: 25546444

269. Schoenfeld, B. J., Contreras, B., Krieger, J., Grgic, J., Delcastillo, K., Belliard, R., & Alto, A. (2019). Resistance training volume enhances muscle hypertrophy but not strength in trained men. *Medicine and Science in Sports and Exercise, 51*(1), 94–103. https://doi.org/10.1249/MSS.0000000000001764

270. Carroll, K. M., Bazyler, C. D., Bernards, J. R., Taber, C. B, Stuart, C. A., DeWeese, B. H., et al. (2019). Skeletal muscle fiber adaptations following resistance training using repetition maximums or relative intensity. *Sports, 7*, 169. https://doi.org/10.3390/sports7070169

271. Dankel, S. J., Mattocks, K. T., Jessee, M. B. et al. (2017). Frequency: The overlooked resistance training variable for inducing muscle hypertrophy? *Sports Med, 47*, 799–805. https://doi.org/10.1007/s40279-016-0640-8

272. Schoenfeld, B. J., Ogborn, D., & Krieger, J. W. (2016). Effects of resistance training frequency on measures of muscle hypertrophy: A systematic review and meta-analysis. *Sports Medicine (Auckland, N.Z.), 46*(11), 1689–1697. https://doi.org/10.1007/s40279-016-0543-8

273. Nielsen, R. O., Buist, I., Sørensen, H., Lind, M., & Rasmussen, S. (2012). Training errors and running related injuries: A systematic review. *International Journal of Sports Physical Therapy, 7*(1), 58–75.

274. Lopes, C. R., Aoki, M. S., Crisp, A. H., de Mattos, R. S., Lins, M. A., da Mota, G. R., et al. (2017). The effect of different resistance training load schemes on strength and body composition in trained men. *Journal of Human Kinetics, 58*, 177–186. https://doi.org/10.1515/hukin-2017-0081

275. de Salles, B. F., Simão, R., Miranda, F., Novaes, J., Lemos, A., & Willardson, J. M. (2009). Rest interval between sets in strength training. *Sports Medicine (Auckland, N.Z.), 39*(9), 765–777. https://doi.org/10.2165/11315230-000000000-00000

276. Tomaras, E. K., & MacIntosh, B. R. (2011). Less is more: Standard warm-up causes fatigue and less warm-up permits greater cycling power output. *Journal of Applied Physiology, 111*(1), 228–235. https://doi.org/10.1152/japplphysiol.00253.2011

277. Rusin, J. (n.d.). *Ramp up your major lifts for performance and injury prevention.* https://drjohnrusin.com/ramp-up-performance-prevention/

278. Lorenz, D. (2011). Postactivation potentiation: An introduction. *International Journal of Sports Physical Therapy, 6*(3), 234–240.

279. Knapik, J. J., Orr, R., Pope, R., & Grier, T. (2016). Injuries and footwear (Part 2): Minimalist running shoes. *Journal of Special Operations Medicine, 16*(1), 89–96.

280. Escalante, G. (2016). Exercise modification strategies to prevent and train around shoulder pain. *Strength and Conditioning Journal, 39*. doi: 10.1519/SSC.0000000000000259

281. Ekstrom, R. A., Donatelli, R. A., & Soderberg, G. L. (2003). Surface electromyographic analysis of exercises for the trapezius and serratus anterior muscles. *The Journal of Orthopaedic and Sports Physical Therapy, 33*(5), 247–258. https://doi.org/10.2519/jospt.2003.33.5.247

282. Enoka, R. (2015). *Neuromechanics of human movement,* 5th ed. Champaign, IL: Human Kinetics.

283. Braith, R. W., Graves, J. E., Pollock, M. L., Leggett, S. L., Carpenter, D. M., & Colvin, A. B. (1989). Comparison of 2 vs 3 days/week of variable resistance training during 10- and 18-week programs. *International Journal of Sports Medicine, 10*(6), 450–454. https://doi.org/10.1055/s-2007-1024942

284. Yue, F. L., Karsten, B., Larumbe-Zabala, E., Seijo, M., & Naclerio, F. (2018). Comparison of 2 weekly-equalized volume resistance-training routines using different frequencies on body composition and performance in trained males. *Applied Physiology, Nutrition, and Metabolism, 43*(5), 475–481. https://doi.org/10.1139/apnm-2017-0575

285. Fleming, D., & Wickersham, S. (2012, July 10). *Piece by piece—starting with his head, ending with his body—Rams safety Adam Archuleta turned himself into a player with no limits.* ESPN Magazine. https://www.espn.com/espn/magazine/archives/news/story?page=magazine-20040913-article32

286. Keller, G., & Papasan, J. (2013). *The one thing: The surprisingly simple truth behind extraordinary results.* Bard Press.

287. Waitzkin, J. (2008). *The art of learning: An inner journey to optimal performance.* Free Press.

Index